NURSING
RESEARCH
SECRETS

NURSING RESEARCH SECRETS

Kathleen S. Oman, RN, PhD, CNS

Research Nurse Scientist
Division of Professional Resources
University of Colorado Hospital
Denver, Colorado

Mary E. Krugman, RN, PhD

Director, Division of Professional Resources
University of Colorado Hospital
Denver, Colorado

Regina M. Fink, RN, PhD, FAAN, AOCN

Research Nurse Scientist
Division of Professional Resources
University of Colorado Hospital
Denver, Colorado

Nursing Secrets Series Editor

Linda J. Scheetz, EdD, RN, CS, CEN

Assistant Professor, College of Nursing
Rutgers, The State University of New Jersey
Newark, New Jersey

HANLEY & BELFUS, INC.
An Imprint of Elsevier

HANLEY & BELFUS, INC.
An Imprint of Elsevier

The Curtis Center
Independence Square West
Philadelphia, Pennsylvania 19106

Note to the reader: Although the techniques, ideas, and information in this book have been carefully reviewed for correctness, the authors, editors, and publisher cannot accept any legal responsibility for any errors or omissions that may be made. Neither the publisher nor the editors make any guarantee, expressed or implied, with respect to the material contained herein.

Library of Congress Control Number: 2003102052

NURSING RESEARCH SECRETS   ISBN 1-56053-524-5

Printed in the United States

Last digit is the print number: 9   8   7   6   5   4   3   2   1

CONTENTS

CONTRIBUTORS

Katherine N. Bent, RN, PhD, CNS
Associate Chief, Nursing Service/Research, Denver VA Medical Center; Assistant Professor, University of Colorado Health Sciences Center, Denver, Colorado

Lisa Marie Bernardo, RN, MPH, PhD
Associate Professor, University of Pittsburgh School of Nursing, Pittsburgh, Pennsylvania

Mary A. Blegen, RN, PhD, FAAN
Professor, School of Nursing, University of Colorado Health Sciences Center; University of Colorado Hospital, Denver, Colorado.

Kathleen Coen Buckwater, RN, PhD
Associate Provost for Health Sciences, University of Iowa, Iowa City, Iowa

Rose Mary Carroll-Johnson, MN, RN
Editor, Oncology Nursing Forum, Valencia, California

Lauren Clark, RN, PhD
Associate Professor, School of Nursing, University of Colorado Health Sciences Center, Denver, Colorado

JoAnn G. Congdon, RN, PhD, CNS
Professor and Chair, Division of Health Outcomes, Populations, and Environments, School of Nursing, University of Colorado Health Sciences Center, Denver, Colorado

Katharine C. Cook, RN, PhD
Associate Professor, School of Nursing, College of Notre Dame of Maryland, Baltimore, Maryland

Dana R. Epstein, RN, PhD
Associate Chief Nurse for Research, Education and Research Service, Carl T. Hayden VA Medical Center, Phoenix, Arizona

Regina M. Fink, RN, PhD, FAAN, AOCN
Research Nurse Scientist, Division of Professional Resources, University of Colorado Hospital, Denver, Colorado

Mary Beth Flynn, RN, MS, CNS, CCRN
Clinical Nurse Specialist/Educator, University of Colorado Hospital; Joint Faculty Appointment, Senior Instructor, School of Nursing, University of Colorado Health Sciences Center, Denver, Colorado

Roxie L. Foster, RN, PhD, FAAN
Associate Professor, School of Nursing, University of Colorado Health Sciences Center; Chair of Pediatric Nursing, Clinical Director, Pain Service, The Children's Hospital of Denver, Denver, Colorado

Sandra G. Funk, PhD
Professor and Associate Dean for Research, School of Nursing, The University of North Carolina at Chapel Hill, Chapel Hill, North Carolina

Joanne Gladden, RN, PhD
Associate Professor, School of Nursing, College of Notre Dame of Maryland, Baltimore, Maryland

Colleen J. Goode, RN, PhD, FAAN
Vice President, Patient Services, and Chief Nursing Officer, University of Colorado Hospital, Denver, Colorado

Jan Hagman, RN, BSN, OCN
Nurse Manager, Division of Blood and Marrow Transplant, University of Colorado Hospital, Denver, Colorado

Katherine R. Jones, RN, PhD, FAAN
Professor, School of Nursing, University of Colorado Health Sciences Center, Denver, Colorado

Anne Marie Kotzer, RN, PhD
Director of Nursing Research, The Children's Hospital of Denver; Assistant Professor, School of Nursing, University of Colorado Health Sciences Center, Denver, Colorado

Mary E. Krugman, RN, PhD
Director, Divsion of Professional Resources, University of Colorado Hospital, Denver, Colorado

Barbara Krumbach, MS, RN, CNS, CCRN
Clinical Nurse Specialist/Educator, Division of Professional Resources, University of Colorado Hospital, Denver, Colorado

Joan K. Magilvy, RN, PhD, FAAN
Professor and Assistant Dean for Graduate Programs, School of Nursing, University of Colorado Health Sciences Center, Denver, Colorado

Patricia Moritz, PhD, FAAN
Professor and Dean, School of Nursing, University of Colorado Health Sciences Center; The Children's Hospital of Denver, Denver, Colorado

Kathleen S. Oman, RN, PhD, CNS
Research Nurse Scientist, Division of Professional Resources, University of Colorado Hospital, Denver, Colorado

Rosemary C. Polomano, RN, PhD, FAAN
Director, Outcomes Research, Department of Nursing, and Assistant Professor, Department of Anesthesiology, Penn State Milton S. Hershey Medical Center, Penn State College of Medicine, Hershey, Pennsylvania

Richard W. Redman, RN, PhD
Associate Dean, Academic Affairs, and Professor, School of Nursing, The University of North Carolina at Chapel Hill, Chapel Hill, North Carolina

David D. Shackelford, RN, BSN
Human Protections Coordinator and Research Subject Advocate, Children's Hospital of Pittsburgh, Pittsburgh, Pennsylvania

Souraya Sidani, RN, PhD
Associate Professor, Faculty of Nursing, University of Toronto, Toronto, Ontario, Canada

Martha H. Stoner, RN, PhD
Associate Professor Emeritus, School of Nursing, University of Colorado Health Sciences Center, Denver, Colorado

Cathy J. Thompson, RN, PhD
Assistant Professor, School of Nursing, University of Colorado Health Sciences Center, Denver, Colorado

Lisa K. Traditi, MLS, AHIP
Head, Education and Learning Resources Center, University of Colorado Health Sciences Center, Denver, Colorado

April Hazard Vallerand, RN, PhD
Assistant Professor, College of Nursing, Wayne State University, Detroit, Michigan

Carol P. Vojir, PhD
Associate Research Professor, School of Nursing, University of Colorado Health Sciences Center, Denver, Colorado

PREFACE

If we knew what we were doing it wouldn't be called research.
Mark Twain

Nurses are challenged to read, understand, and incorporate research findings into their clinical practice to provide current, effective, and evidence-based care. Evidence-based practice and research utilization are expectations in all areas of nursing. Conducting research, mostly an academic pursuit in the past, has found a significant place in clinical practice settings. Nurses are now asking research-focused questions, then designing and implementing studies to provide answers.

Our motivation for this addition to the Nursing Secrets Series® comes from our desire to support and mentor all nurses and nursing students in their journey into reading, using, and/or conducting nursing research. We are excited about nursing research and want to share this enthusiasm with our colleagues. Many excellent research books and resources are available, but practical wisdom and experience-based "secrets" are not always captured in textbooks. We have asked the experts to share their "secrets," and they have done so with the same passion and enthusiasm that they have for the research process.

These nursing experts (from both clinical and academic settings) have shared their experience and knowledge about a multitude of subjects. Although we have tried to be thorough, this book is not meant to be a comprehensive review of the topic. Rather it is intended to focus on commonly asked questions to stimulate further discussion and research. The authors have referenced many additional resources in their individual chapters.

We are grateful to our current and past University of Colorado Hospital Clinical Research Council Members for their ongoing efforts to keep research a strong and important focus in our clinical practice. We also acknowledge Colleen Goode, RN, PhD, FAAN, for her commitment and leadership in this process. We value our collaboration with the faculty at the University of Colorado School of Nursing for their research expertise and their contributions to this book. We thank Lisa Judd Jones for her assistance in the manuscript preparation, and special thanks are due to Linda Belfus and the staff at Hanley and Belfus for their editorial assistance, support, and willingness to believe in *Nursing Research Secrets*. It's no secret—we believe in nursing research.

Kathleen S. Oman, RN, PhD, CNS
Mary E. Krugman, RN, PhD
Regina M. Fink, RN, PhD, FAAN, AOCN

I. Getting Started

1. NURSING RESEARCH

Mary E. Krugman, RN, PhD

1. What is nursing research?

Research is any activity designed to investigate and find valid answers to a question that has been asked. There are many ways to investigate truths or learn more knowledge. For example, nurses seek knowledge daily in clinical practice, as they raise questions about patient care and use the nursing process of assessment, planning, implementation, and evaluation to answer clinical problems. Is this nursing research? How is the problem-solving approach different from nursing research? Burns and Grove[1] note that one of the distinguishing characteristics that sets nursing research apart from problem solving is the degree of systematic, diligent inquiry and investigation. Nursing research requires structured planning, organization, and persistence for uncovering knowledge. It is a more formal method of problem solving than the day-to-day strategies that nurses use to deliver patient care. The questions raised during clinical practice, however, provide a rich source of ideas for nursing research. The nursing profession has advanced over the past 25 years because of the astute clinical questions asked by nurses in all areas of professional practice.

2. Why is nursing research important?

Nurses hold a position of trust with the public and are regarded as advocates for patient well-being. Nursing care based on tradition rather than scientific evidence may not help the public. Care outcomes may be potentially compromised, resulting in the erosion of public confidence in the nursing profession In the 1880s Florence Nightingale established the prototype for nursing practice based on sound principles and evidence, but the nursing profession has struggled over the past century to overcome reliance on tradition, custom, and past experience. Nursing research is critical to developing knowledge based on tested reasoning, systematic findings, and evidence-based practice innovations. Quality outcomes associated with optimal patient health are not possible without a solid scientific basis for nursing interventions. Nursing continues to be viewed as an emerging profession because our body of knowledge is relatively modest compared with disciplines such as medicine and pharmacy. Research should be the foundation for nursing practice and document our significant contributions to patient care outcomes.

3. How did nursing research develop?

Polit and Hungler[2] note that "most people agree that research in nursing began with Florence Nightingale, who maintained detailed recorded observations about the

1

effects of nursing actions during the Crimean War" (p. 5). After a lengthy hiatus, nursing research surfaced again in the 1920s, focused on studying the demographic characteristics of nurses rather than building on the patient outcomes work first started by Nightingale. Research studying nurses as a population continued into the 1950s, with a shift to examining student nurses and the effects of educational programs. In 1952, nursing research gained ground with the publication of the first issue of *Nursing Research*, a journal specifically dedicated to reporting nursing research. The next milestone was Henderson and Simmons' survey of the status of nursing research since 1940.[2] It was not until the 1960s that clinical research began to be published, with studies of nursing care outcomes demonstrating the importance of establishing a scientific basis for nursing practice. Advances in nursing research continued into the 1970s and 1980s with the introduction of the research utilization movement (see Chapter 2). A significant achievement in the 1980s was the establishment of the National Center for Nursing Research, renamed the National Institute of Nursing Research in 1993. Hinshaw[3] outlines background on the development of this important advancement. Federal funding provided national recognition of the importance of nursing research to patient care outcomes. Further information about the history of nursing research can be found in many nursing research textbooks; a timeline of nursing research development is outlined in the *Encyclopedia of Nursing Research*.[4]

4. **What are the purposes and goals of nursing research?**
    - Discover the knowledge of the discipline
    - Uncover relationships
    - Describe phenomena
    - Explain and predict theories
    - Determine control over the elements of practice
    - Facilitate the development of clinical interventions to improve health outcomes and contribute to optimal care delivery

An early statement about nursing research, published by the American Nurses Association,[5] outlined the following purposes:
    - Develop knowledge about health and the promotion of health over the full life span
    - Learn more about the care of persons with health problems and disabilities
    - Gain knowledge of nursing actions to enhance individual ability to respond effectively to actual or potential health problems

Over the past 20 years, many commissions, councils, and organizations have further identified strategic plans and priorities for nursing research. Often the purposes and priorities for nursing research are driven by what types of nursing research are funded. For example, the National Institute for Nursing Research has identified five areas of major research focus:
    - Neurofunction and sensory conditions
    - Reproductive and infant health
    - Immune, infections and neoplastic disease
    - Cardiopulmonary and acute illness
    - Human development and health risk behaviors

Nursing research is essential for the development of scientific knowledge to promote evidence-based nursing care. Incorporating research into practice ensures a solid basis for nursing clinical actions.

5. What are the types of nursing research?

The two types of research are basic and applied. **Basic research** is conducted to establish facts or to test theories and thus to generate new knowledge. Basic research is also called fundamental research. Examples include nursing studies of adult perceptions to pain, the experiences of graduate nurses in their first position, the effects of chemotherapy on stomatitis, or attitudes of pregnant adolescents.

Applied research focuses on nursing interventions, procedures, processes, and methods of patient care. Nursing is an applied science that draws on many other disciplines for knowledge to apply to clinical practice. Examples include testing of different suctioning techniques for patients with endotracheal tubes, testing of different peripheral intravenous (IV) flush solutions, and application of anthropology concepts to nursing interventions for culturally diverse, terminally ill populations.

6. What is the difference between quality improvement and research?

This challenging question has stimulated much discussion among nurses and other health care disciplines. Quality improvement initiatives have grown in complexity and stature over the past 5–10 years, as regulatory agencies accrediting health care organizations mandate such activities. This question is important because of the process of institutional review board (IRB) approval. A performance improvement project does not have to be reviewed by an IRB to determine risks to human subjects. Federal regulations, however, require full scrutiny of an IRB of any research study. Research activities incorrectly classified as quality initiatives may not adequately protect patients, but if all quality projects were considered research, the burden on health care institutions and providers would be significant and probably result in fewer quality improvement projects.

Casarett, Karlawish, and Sugerman[6] outlined what they perceive as the distinction between the two activities. Quality projects are generally small-scale cycles of interventions designed to improve the process of care delivery and generally are not published. A major distinction is the level of assessment and intervention. For quality projects, patients usually are not randomized, as in a clinical trial. However, the line may be finely drawn, as when hospitals are required to benchmark outcomes of a particular procedures and place certain patients in one group for comparison with another. Another dilemma is the issue of publication, since disseminating findings of a quality project may be of benefit to other institutions.

Casarett et al.[6] suggest two criteria by which the two activities may be distinguished:
• The direct benefit to patients involved
• How the project imposes additional risks or burdens to the patient.

Chapter 19 reviews more information about informed consent, IRBs, and patient confidentiality. You should carefully review institutional requirements before undertaking any type of quality or research project.

7. If research was not taught in my nursing program, why should I learn it now?

Many nurses learned minimal information about research in their nursing programs. Often nurses feel uncomfortable about research, perceiving it as a complicated activity reserved for the few nurses with doctoral degrees. In the early decades of the profession, nursing curriculums lacked a solid foundation in research. Nursing had few prepared researchers—or even practicing nurses who understood the importance of using evidence as a basis for practice. Over the past 25 years, nursing graduates have become more knowledgeable about science and research. The profession is poised to make further gains, as a critical mass of the profession begins to grasp the importance of research to practice.

The fact that you learned little about research earlier in your career is not a problem. It is never too late to begin, regardless of your practice setting or basic nursing preparation. As a nurse, you have a higher level of responsibility to the public than simply doing your job. This professional responsibility includes life-long learning about the advances in both nursing and medicine and keeping up with recent changes in practice to deliver up-to-date care to your patients. Learning how to access computer search engines to find current articles, reading nursing and medical literature, asking questions, and sharpening your critical thinking skills to approach clinical problems with an attitude of inquiry are part of this lifelong learning and do not require a doctoral degree. The most important consideration is to begin thinking about research as an *essential* part of your practice, not as an option.

8. How does nursing research make a difference in patient care?

When you use evidence-based practice and are knowledgeable about current standards, you deliver safer and more efficient, effective care. Often nurses in practice do not realize the standards of care for a particular specialty are established through nursing research. Examples include the following:

- Nurse scientists are leaders in establishing clinical guidelines and national standards for such important care outcomes as pain and skin integrity.
- Best practices, based on research by nurses, have been developed for patients who are vulnerable to falls, or who suffer from chronic conditions such as Alzheimer's and diabetes.
- National projects such as the Thunder Project, sponsored by the American Association of Critical Care Nurses, and the Lunar Project, sponsored by the Emergency Nurses Association, have contributed to best practices in their specialties.

9. What is the difference between multidisciplinary and interdisciplinary research? Should nurses participate with other disciplines in research?

Fitzpatrick,[7] editor of *Applied Nursing Research*, observes that nurses should understand the distinction between multidisciplinary research and interdisciplinary collaboration and select the type of research best suited for the project. In **multidisciplinary research**, a multidisciplinary group, in which the nurse is a partner, formulates the research question from the perspective of many different disciplines, merging the viewpoints into one integrated project. In **interdisciplinary collaboration**, the nurse researcher maintains the nursing focus of the question but builds a team of experts to assist in either understanding the question more fully or helping to analyze the results.

Fitzpatrick notes that nurse researchers should build interdisciplinary initiatives because care delivery is complex, multifaceted, and based on team interaction. Cronenwett[8] also argues that the basis of the science of nursing must be interdisciplinary—if nurses are to continue to develop as leaders in the areas of evidence-based practice and research. She notes that when nurses hold back from collaborating with teams, they lose an opportunity for interesting other disciplines in their work and gaining new knowledge from collaboration. Chapter 9 gives more information about incorporating other disciplines into research.

10. Where do I begin, if I know nothing about nursing research?
One of the easiest ways is to talk with other nurses about their experiences in research. Nurses who engage in evidence-based practice, research utilization, or conduct research can share with you how they got started and what steps they took to gain greater comfort and confidence. Participation in journal clubs and quality improvement activities is an excellent way to gain beginner skills, especially by working with others who may have more experience. Chapter 4 gives more information about journal clubs and along with Chapter 5, focuses on further developing skills and knowledge in research. Look for workshops, courses, or classes on nursing research. The local School or College of Nursing will offer courses in which you may be able to enroll under special student status. Some teaching health sciences center hospitals have continuing education programs that offer nursing research courses. Often local research conferences or symposiums provide another avenue to become updated on nursing or other discipline research and a forum for interacting with nurse researchers. Grand rounds are often focused on research; make a point of attending them. Textbook and on-line resources can provide a knowledge base. Computer listservs associated with specialty organizations may permit you to connect and communicate with others in your field who are also trying to learn more about research. The key to beginning the exploration is to ask questions, be open to new ideas, and not be afraid to say that you do not know and would like to learn more.

11. Do I have to hold a doctoral degree to become involved in nursing research?
Absolutely not. Your background, level of expertise, and knowledge drive the depth to which you are involved in nursing research. All nurses, regardless of educational background, can learn about research, read about research, and incorporate research findings into practice. These are essential competencies that any nurse should hold for professional practice. Regardless of level of education, nurses can learn how to search the literature for evidence to verify practice in policies and procedures. This is one easy way to start participating in research activities without holding any special degree and provides a sense of accomplishment by documenting your institutional practices with evidence. If you obtained a baccalaureate degree, your curriculum was developed using the guidelines of the American Association of Colleges of Nursing and includes research- and evidence-based concepts as essential elements. Because each academic program has a different way of implementing these concepts, some nurses may start their careers with a practice-based research foundation, whereas others have a more theoretical orientation to research. Often baccalaureate-prepared nurses serve as data collectors in clinical projects and may take an active role in a quality or research project under the guidance of a nurse with a master's or doctoral degree. Nurses holding master's degrees may conduct research and serve as coordinators of research and/or data collectors for nursing or other discipline-related research. Nurses who are doctorally prepared have expertise in research design, the complexity of the research process, statistical analysis, and skill in analyzing findings. Whether you hold a basic or advanced degree or never have had a research course does not matter. There is a place for everyone in the research enterprise. The only boundaries are those within yourself.

REFERENCES

1. Burns N, Grove SK (eds): The Practice of Nursing Research: Conduct, Critique, and Utilization, 4th ed. Philadelphia, W.B. Sanders, 2001.
2. Polit DF, Hungler BP (eds): Nursing Research: Principles and Methods, 5th ed. Philadelphia, J.B. Lippincott, 2001.
3. Hinshaw AS, Feetham SL, Shaver JLF (eds): Handbook of Clinical Nursing Research. Thousand Oaks, CA, Sage Publications, 1999.
4. Fitzpatrick JJ (ed): Encyclopedia of Nursing Research. New York, Springer Publishing Company, 1998.
5. American Nurses' Association Commission on Nursing Research: Generating a scientific basis for nursing practice: Research priorities for the 1980's. Nurs Res 29:219, 1980.
6. Casarett D, Karlawish JH, Sugerman J: Determining when quality improvement initiatives should be considered research: Proposed criteria and potential implications. JAMA 283:2275–2280, 2000.
7. Fitzpatrick JJ: Multidisciplinary and interdisciplinary research: What it is and what it is not. Appl Nurs Res 15(2):59, 2002.
8. Cronenwett L: Research, practice and policy: Issues in evidence based care [keynote address]. Midwest Nursing Research Society, March 3, 2001, Chicago.

2. EVIDENCE-BASED PRACTICE

Colleen J. Goode, RN, PhD, FAAN

1. Define evidence-based practice.

Evidence-based practice is conceptually defined as the use of current best evidence in making decisions. The term evidence-based practice is usually used in reference to health care decisions. However, the term is also used in making decisions about management, educational programs, or any practice discipline. The term *current best evidence* implies that interventions have been tested and that evidence supports which interventions produce the best outcomes.

2. What definitions of evidence-based practice are found in the current literature?

- Sackett[1] defined evidence-based practice as the conscientious, explicit, and judicious use of current best evidence in making decisions about the care of individual patients. The practice of evidence-based medicine involves integrating individual clinical expertise with the best external clinical evidence available from systematic research.
- In 1992, the Evidence-Based Medicine Working Group,[2] primarily composed of Canadians, defined evidence-based medicine as deemphasizing intuition, unsystematic clinical experience, and pathophysiologic rationale as sufficient grounds for clinical decision making. The emphasis instead is placed on examination of evidence from clinical research.
- Stetler and colleagues[3] developed a definition for evidence-based nursing patterned after the Evidence-Based Medicine Working Group definition. Evidence-based nursing de-emphasizes ritual, isolated and unsystematic clinical experience, and ungrounded opinions and traditions as a basis for nursing practice, stressing instead research findings, appropriate quality improvement data, other operational and evaluation data, the consensus of recognized experts, and affirmed experiences.
- Mulhall[4] suggests that evidence-based nursing practice incorporates evidence from research, clinical expertise, and patient preferences into decisions about health care.
- Goode and Piedalue[5] developed a definition for multidisciplinary evidence-based practice based on the synthesis of knowledge from research; retrospective or concurrent chart review; quality improvement and risk data; international, national, and local standards; infection control data; pathophysiology; cost effectiveness analysis; benchmarking data; patient preferences; and clinical expertise.
- Titler and colleagues[6] published a refined Iowa Model of Evidence-Based Practice and defined evidence-based practice as the conscientious and judicious use of current best evidence to guide health care decisions.

3. What type of research is used for making evidence-based decisions?

The medical profession usually requires the use of prospective, randomized, controlled trials for making evidence-based decisions. They are considered the gold standard or the strongest evidence that can be used as a basis for practice decisions. In the nursing profession, there is support for using robust experimental studies, observational studies, descriptive studies, and correlational studies to determine evidence-based practice. Limiting the research base to prospective, randomized, controlled trials limits evidence-based nursing practice. When the effectiveness of a medication is tested, a randomized, controlled trial is appropriate to determine whether the drug is safe and effective. For determining the best evidence related to care models for patients with Alzheimer's disease, experimental and nonexperimental research may be the best evidence available. It is important to critique the research rigorously to determine whether it is scientifically sound and whether it has been replicated and to ensure that it will cause no harm.

4. What is the difference between evidence-based practice and research utilization?

The research utilization (RU) movement began in the early 1970s in the United States; this term originally was used by nurses. Much of the literature focused on the process for transforming research into practice. Research-based plans of care and protocols were developed and used as the basis for nursing practice. Before the RU movement began, nursing practice was usually based on tradition, trial and error, or intuition.

The evidence-based practice movement began in England in the early 1990s. This movement focused on the use of randomized, controlled clinical trials integrated with the clinical expertise of the physician for making medical decisions. Stelter and colleagues[7] differentiate between RU and evidence-based practice by identifying how RU provides the preparatory steps for research-related actions that, when implemented and sustained, result in evidence-based practice.

5. What are the WICHE and the CURN RU Projects?

The first federally funded RU project, sponsored by the Western Interstate Commission for Higher Education (WICHE), defined the process for RU and taught nurses how to base practice on research. A nurse clinician, paired with a nurse educator from a school of nursing, defined a clinical problem, gathered research related to the problem, and developed research-based interventions to address the problem. An evidence-based plan of care for grieving spouses, whose loved one was in a coronary care unit and had a high probability of dying, was among the published outcomes from the WICHE project.[8] This landmark publication gives an excellent example of how research-based nursing practice can improve outcomes.

Another federally funded study that had a profound impact on nursing practice was the Conduct and Utilization of Research (CURN) project. The CURN project gathered and synthesized available research to establish ten research-based nursing protocols. The project used a team approach whereby a group of nurses critiqued the research, developed the protocol, and implemented the protocol on their acute care unit. The protocols developed during the CURN project have greatly influenced nursing practice. For example, nurses now understand the importance of a closed urinary drainage system in preventing urinary tract infections and the critical nature of preoperative teaching in reducing postoperative complications.

6. Why has the RU movement been replaced by the evidence-based practice movement?

The RU movement was extremely valuable in facilitating the nursing profession's understanding of the importance of a scientific basis for practice. However, the movement provoked some criticisms:

- The term *research utilization* was a nursing term, neither used nor understood by other disciplines.
- The importance of patient preferences was not addressed. Patients are demanding a stronger voice in decisions about their health care.
- The cultural, religious, or other beliefs and values of the person override even the best research-based protocol. If the patient does not want the intervention because of personal beliefs, it is not done. This issue was not addressed in the research utilization movement.
- The RU movement did not evaluate other sources of evidence in making health care decisions.
- The importance of integrating the clinical judgment that practitioners acquire through professional education and clinical experience was not incorporated.

7. What started the evidence-based practice movement?

The evidence-based practice movement began in England in the early 1990s. The National Health Service of the United Kingdom dictated that the decisions about the provision and delivery of clinical services would be based on evidence related to clinical effectiveness and cost. Because resources were limited, there was a push to eliminate interventions that did not demonstrate improved outcomes. The desire was to provide clinically effective care with available resources.

8. What is the Cochrane Collaboration?

In 1972, a book about health services effectiveness and efficiency was published by Cochrane, a British epidemiologist.[9] The health care profession was clearly not ready for Cochrane's ideas about the need to determine whether medical interventions were effective and whether the profession was efficiently delivering care. In 1993, with a new emphasis in England on evidence-based practice, the Cochrane Collaboration was founded. This group was composed of representatives from nine countries who focused on teaching and practicing through an evidence-based approach. Today the Collaboration has centers around the world dedicated to teaching and practicing evidence-based medicine. The Cochrane library houses the Database of Systematic Reviews and the Database of Abstracts of Reviews of Effectiveness. This synthesis of randomized controlled trials has had a major impact on medical practice.

9. What are the AHCPR guidelines? Discuss their influence on evidence-based practice.

The work of Cochrane and colleagues jump-started evidence-based practice in England and Canada and has had great impact in the United States. However, the Agency for Healthcare Policy and Research (AHCPR), now called the Agency for Healthcare Research and Quality (AHRQ), also had a major influence on evidence-based practice in the United States. Established in 1989 to enhance the quality and appropriateness of health care services, AHRQ developed guideline panels and clinical practice guidelines to assist providers in making evidence-based decisions. These guidelines were developed by a panel of experts who rigorously critiqued the research and rated the strength of the recommendation based on the scientific evidence. The consensus of the panel experts was also considered as evidence but given a lower rating compared with a meta-analysis. Nurses not only have served on many panels but also have been chairs or cochairs of panels. For example, the expert panel on Pressure Ulcer Prediction and Prevention was chaired by Nancy Bergstrom, an expert nurse scientist in this field.

10. What are the components of an evidence-based multidisciplinary practice model?

The University of Colorado Hospital model illustrates an evidence-based clinical practice model. Exploration of the evidence begins in the center or core of the model. Clinicians should use research as the basis for clinical decision-making whenever an adequate research base is available to guide practice. The nine sources of evidence attached to the research core can supplement evidence obtained from research or, when research is not available, provide the best available evidence (see questions 11–20 for detailed descriptions). They are as follows:

- Pathophysiology
- Cost-effectiveness analysis
- Benchmarking data
- Clinical expertise
- Infection control data
- International, national, and local standards
- Quality improvement and risk data
- Retrospective or concurrent chart review
- Patient preferences

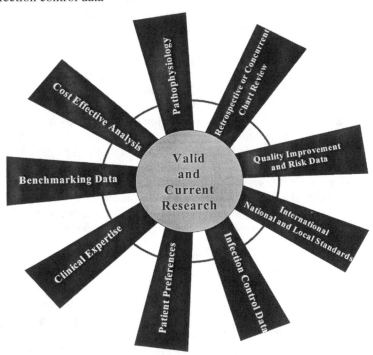

Evidence-based multidisciplinary practice model used at the University of Colorado Hospital. © University of Colorado Hospital.

11. How is research evaluated?

Evaluating clinical studies to determine their validity involves critically appraising both their merits and limitations. All types of research should be evaluated for their contribution to the evidence. Basic research skills and knowledge of statistics are required to evaluate and interpret a study. The reviewer must look for the most current research so that the latest evidence is included in the review. Haller, Reynolds, and Horsley's[10] criteria include studies that are scientifically sound, replicated, and cause no harm to patients. Changes in practice should not be based on one study with a small sample.

12. How does pathophysiology guide clinical decisions?

Pathophysiology, the science of the function of cells, tissues, organs, and how these functions are altered by disease, is a frequent source of evidence used by all clinicians for making clinical decisions. For example, pathophysiologic evidence guides decision making of a nurse practitioner if abnormal cells are identified on a Pap smear.

13. Explain the role of cost-effectiveness analysis.

Cost effectiveness alone does not imply that an intervention should be adopted. Adoption depends on whether the benefit is sufficiently large relative to the risks and costs. A cost-benefit analysis related to the use of ultrasound for detection of bladder distention in neurology patients addresses the reduction in frequent catheterizations and provides the evidence needed to change practice and purchase needed equipment. Evidence from cost-effectiveness analysis is becoming more important in the struggle to contain health care costs.

14. What are benchmarking data?

Some institutions have better quality and cost outcomes than others for certain types of patient populations and clinical therapies. It is beneficial to gather evidence related to "best practice" and to determine what is different in the institution where the outcomes are better. This benchmarking process provides a way to gather evidence to improve clinical decision making. Hospitals that belong to the University HealthSystem Consortium share clinical data and costs. For example, data indicate that patients admitted to hospital X's neonatal intensive care unit with extreme prematurity have shorter lengths of stay, lower costs, and fewer complications than patients at other like facilities. Such data are adjusted for severity and regional variations in costs. By studying the evidence from the "best practice" hospital, one can determine what changes need to be made to improve outcomes.

15. How important is clinical expertise?

Clinical judgment based on reflection and knowledge of the patient is an important source of evidence. Clinicians move from a status of novice to expert as they acquire proficiency and clinical judgment through experience and education. Clinical expertise must be integrated with the best available clinical evidence.

16. How are infection control data used for clinical guidelines?

Infection control surveillance provides evidence related to the incidence of infections and the causative organisms so that appropriate interventions can be instituted.

For example, infection control practitioners provide data related to the incidence of ventilator-acquired pneumonia and determine whether rates are in line with national norms. When a new evidence-based protocol for changing ventilator circuits is instituted, continued monitoring of ventilator-acquired pneumonia rates provides data for outcomes related to the new protocol.

17. Explain the role of international, national, and local standards.

Evidence may also be provided by international and national standards of care such as those developed by the Oncology Nursing Society, Centers for Disease Control, or the American Association of Critical Care Nurses. For example, the Centers for Disease Control provides standards related to care of patients with infectious disease. These standards provide evidence to guide practice and help to ensure quality of care.

18. How are quality improvement and risk data used to guide clinical practice?

Data related to the incidence of skin breakdown, medication errors, surgical complications, mortality, other adverse occurrences, and sentinel events provide evidence to support implementation of a new protocol. For example, quality data about an increased incidence of patient falls can be used to support implementation of a process improvement initiative and development of a new prevention protocol. An adverse outcome related to conscious sedation can provide evidence that the current protocol is not working or that additional training of staff is needed in a specific department.

19. Why is retrospective or concurrent chart review important?

The patient's medical record provides a wealth of evidence, such as patient allergies or changes in vital signs. The record provides a rich history that can tell us how the patient responded to a specific medication, procedure, or treatment in the past. The history can also provide evidence related to the patient's family and alert clinicians to look for specific familial problems. Evidence related to response to current interventions and diagnostic testing may also influence decision-making.

20. Discuss the role of patient preferences.

The patient's religious and cultural preferences and other patient information, such as living wills and advance directives, are an essential source of evidence. Clinicians must respect the preferences of the patient and family, providing ample opportunity for patient input into decision making. If the patient prefers not to receive a specific intervention or treatment, it should not be done.

21. How have clinicians used the University of Colorado Hospital's (UCH) evidence-based practice model to improve prevention of pressure ulcers?

In 1999, UCH's institutional quality improvement team and evidence-based practice council reviewed current skin practices based on an increase in skin breakdown in a patient care unit. The Skin Champions of Change, a research group at UCH, explored the evidence related to prevention of pressure ulcers. This team of direct care providers, led by a clinical nurse specialist and research nurse scientist, used scientific methods to determine baseline pressure ulcer occurrence at the hospital. In addition, a baseline random survey of nurses was done to determine their knowledge of risk factors associated with pressure ulcers and their beliefs about skin care. Documentation patterns were also collected.[11]

The evidence-based Braden Skin Risk score was added to inpatient nurse documentation flow sheets, and staff received inserviced training and competency testing on its use. Evidence related to skin and wound assessment was presented in the staff education and training sessions. The education provided by Champion nurses included case exemplars, revision of documentation forms, development of an evidence-based skin care algorithm and treatment goals.

Pressure ulcer prevalence decreased from 9% to 4% after these interventions. Results from a random registered nurse sample (n = 115 before intervention and n = 95 after intervention) revealed that nurses' knowledge increased from 58% to 77%. These evidence-based interventions positively impacted skin care outcomes.

22. How has evidence-based practice influenced respiratory care at UCH?

The practice of routinely changing ventilator circuits at specified frequencies began in the 1960s when reports demonstrated that respiratory care equipment was associated with increases in nonsocomial pnuemonia. It was assumed that changing ventilator circuits frequently would decrease ventilator acquired pneumonia. Studies in the literature indicated that this assumption may not be true. The UCH evidence-based practice model examined the evidence related to this issue. Evaluation of research, infection control data, and CDC standards indicated a need to change practice. Evidence supported change of circuits only when they were soiled and of suction catheters every 48 hours rather than daily. Policy changes were made, and staff received inservice training. Data collected previous to the change and 6 months after the change showed a decrease in the incidence of ventilator-acquired pneumonia.

23. Discuss the effect of evidence-based practice on the treatment of acute cystitis in women at UCH.

An evidence-based project was undertaken to generate an evidence-based practice guideline for the treatment of uncomplicated acute cystitis in a female population, to determine the extent to which the guideline would be used by providers, and to measure the cost and quality of outcomes. Evidence from research, chart review, infection control, and cost analysis was used to establish the guideline. The implementation of an outpatient practice guideline resulted in a significant change in antibiotic prescribing and a trend toward a change in ordering cultures and clinic visits. There was also a significant decrease in treatment costs.

24. Should patients and families ask for evidence so they can participate in making decisions about their care?

It is important for clinicians to communicate to patients and their family evidence-based information so that patients can make informed decisions about the plan of care. For example, providers can inform patients, during preoperative and postoperative teaching, about the research evidence indicating that early ambulation is one of the most important interventions for prevention of postoperative pneumonia and deep vein thrombosis. Obviously, clinicians must present information in a form that can be easily understood by the patient. Recipients of care are becoming more informed about health and illness and asking thoughtful questions. The growth and wider availability of the Internet will greatly increase access to health information. Accurate evidence-based information has the potential to enhance the quality and appropriateness of health care.

25. Are process and outcome measures important in evidence-based practice?

The outcomes from evidence-based clinical care are determined not only by the strength of the evidence but also by the quality of the management of the interventions and the delivery of the interventions. When an evidence-based clinical practice change is implemented, it is important to evaluate the process for carrying out the intervention and the outcome. If the clinicians do not carry out the intervention as intended, the expected outcome may not occur. For example, an evidence-based pain management protocol may not be effective because providers do not assess pain appropriately, barriers may make it difficult to carry out the intervention, or resistance from providers or system issues may make it difficult to implement the pain management intervention. The expected outcomes should include as many dependent variables from the research studies as clinically reasonable. Outcome criteria become the evaluation tool for objective monitoring after implementation of an evidence-based practice change.

26. What does the future hold for evidence-based practice?

Schools of nursing are including evidence-based practice throughout the baccalaureate, masters, and doctoral curriculum. A new doctoral program started at one university makes evidence-based practice the focus of study. More nurses than before are highly motivated to become evidence-based practitioners. In addition, many health care organizations are working to establish a culture in which evidence-based practice is an expectation. Professional nurses are increasingly aware of the need to base decisions on the best available evidence. The future holds great promise for the growth of evidence-based nursing practice.

REFERENCES

1. Sackett DL, Rosenberg WM, Gray JAM, Haynes RB: Evidence-based medicine: What it is and what it isn't. Br Med J 312:71–72, 1996.
2. Evidence-Based Working Group: A new approach to teaching the practice of medicine. JAMA 268:2420–2425, 1997.
3. Stetler CB, Brunell M, Giuliano KK, et al: Evidence-based practice and the role of nursing leadership. J Nurs Admin 28:45–53, 1944.
4. Mulhall A: Nursing, research and the evidence. Evidence-Based Nurs 1:4–6, 1998.
5. Goode CJ, Piedalue F: Evidence-based clinical practice. J Nurs Admin 29:15–21, 1999.
6. Titler MG, Kleiber C, Steelman VJ, et al: The Iowa model of evidence-based practice to promote quality care. Crit Care Nurs Clin North Am 13:497–509, 2001.
7. Stetler CB: Updating the Stetler model of research utilization to facilitate evidence-based practice. Nurs Outlook 49:272–279, 2001.
8. Dracup KA, Breu CS: Using nursing research findings to meet the needs of grieving spouses. Nurs Res 27(4):212–216, 1978.
9. Cochrane AL: Effectiveness and Efficiency: Random Reflections on Health Services. Nuffield Provincial Hospitals Trust, 1972.
10. Haller KB, Reynolds MA, Horsley JA: Developing research-based innovation protocols: Process criteria and issues. Res Nurs Health 2:45–51, 1979.
11. Flynn MB, Fink R: Committing to evidence-based skin care practice. Crit Care Nurs Clin North Am 13:558–568, 2001.

3. OVERCOMING THE RESEARCH-PRACTICE GAP

Cathy J. Thompson, RN, PhD

1. What is a research-practice gap?

A research-practice gap refers to the disparity between the *availability* of new knowledge to improve nursing practice and its actual *use* by practicing nurses. The term was coined in the 1970s to reflect the awareness that nursing research findings were not routinely used in practice, despite their publication and dissemination. The awareness of this gap forced nurse researchers, nurse educators, and nurse administrators to examine the reasons behind its existence. This new awareness has led to translate nursing research findings in a way that makes sense in the clinical setting; and to disseminate research findings in popular nursing journals. Many nursing journals have added monthly features to highlight nursing research findings relevant to their readers' practice settings.

2. How have barriers to conducting and participating in clinical research been assessed?

Funk, Champagne, Wiese, and Tornquist[1] developed and tested the BARRIERS to Research Utilization Scale, which consists of a 29-item, Likert-type scale with additional qualitative questions to elicit perceptions of barriers and facilitators of research utilization from staff nurses, administrators, and educators. Thompson[2] devised the Research Factor Questionnaire to ascertain factors that affect research use, including personal and professional characteristics, organizational perceptions of research culture, interpersonal communications, and influences of mass media on research utilization. Both instruments are based on Rogers' Diffusion of Innovations[3] theoretical constructs and have demonstrated reliability and validity. In a multisite study, Thompson, Fink, Bonnes, et al.[4] reported that time to implement research and lack of authority to change practice were the greatest barriers identified by nurses. These findings supported the results of other researchers.[1,5,6]

3. What types of barriers have been identified?

Barriers can be real or imagined and are typically labeled as personal, professional, or organizational in nature.
- **Personal barriers** include a deficiency of research knowledge; lack of material or financial resources; limited individual motivation; a negative research attitude; and lack of perceived power to change practice.
- **Professional barriers** include job requirements that may not acknowledge the use and/or conduct of research; absence of support from nursing and/or health care colleagues; poor dissemination or communication of research findings; and lack of time.
- **Organizational barriers** include inadequate administrative support for nursing research; lack of incentives and/or resources to pursue or conduct research; and organizations that discourage staff from questioning their clinical practice.

4. How do I know if research findings are good enough for implementation into practice?

No magic formula tells you when research findings are definitely ready for implementation. However, two general criteria can help you assess whether a particular research finding is ready for use in nursing practice.

- Change in practice should not be based on the results of *one* study, even if the sample size is large. There is always a possibility that the results of any one study may be due to chance, regardless of how well designed the study.
- The more often a study is replicated with the same or similar conclusions, the more confidence one has in the reliability and validity of the results and their usefulness to practice.

5. What specific questions should nurses ask to assess the clinical readiness of research findings?

Haller and colleagues[7] developed the following set of questions:

- Does the research have a base of more than one study?
- Have the studies established scientific merit? In other words, were the study results statistically and/or clinically significant? Did the study follow accepted research guidelines and use reliable and valid tools? Were the design and conduct of the study scientifically rigorous? Were appropriate data analytic techniques used? Were conclusions were congruent with the data?
- If the findings are implemented, are the patient benefits greater than the risks?
- Are the research findings relevant to your practice setting?
- Is it feasible to implement the research findings in your institution?
- Do you have the appropriate resources for their implementation? (Examples include human, financial, organizational, and material resources.)
- Do you have a plan for evaluation of these findings in your patient population?

If the answer to these questions is yes, the findings are ready for implementation. Ongoing evaluation of the new practice change relative to patient outcomes is important. Evaluation of the practice change may lead to the reconsideration of the use of this research in your particular setting—the research may not impact your patient population as expected. Be sure to report your results so that others may learn from your experience.

6. What research models are available to facilitate research utilization?

Many research utilization models have been devised to assist clinicians in implementing research-based practice. Some of these models use an algorithm-type approach. For example, the Iowa Model of Evidence-Based Practice to Promote Quality Care incorporates the steps of the research process infused with decision points and multiple feedback mechanisms that take into account unit/institutional priorities, societal, and environmental changes affecting health care, and the consideration of all forms of evidence, in addition to research-based studies.[8] Another model is the Multidisciplinary Evidence Based Practice Model developed by staff at the University of Colorado Hospital[9] (See Chapter 2).

7. How does organizational culture affect the conduct of research in a clinical setting?

Organizational culture is extremely important in setting the tone for research utilization. Nurses who feel supported by administrators (including nurse managers) are more apt to question the status quo and feel empowered to make changes in practice to benefit the patient.

Funk et al.[1] reported that the perceptions of barriers varied among clinicians, administrators, and academicians. Clinicians felt that the greatest barriers to research utilization were related to administrative and organizational influences. Administrators cited the setting and individual nurse characteristics as the most significant barriers. Research utilization has been significantly correlated with organizational climate or culture in other studies as well.[5,10]

8. **How can nurse administrators influence research utilization?**
   - Establishing expectations that all nurses will practice using research- and evidence-based practice, as reinforced by the institution's nursing philosophy and nursing job descriptions.
   - Charging standing committees with ensuring that policies and procedures, standards of care, and organizational processes are based on sound research and evidence.
   - Providing resources that promote nursing research and assist staff in conducting and evaluating studies, such as employment of a nurse researcher/scientist, unit- or service-based clinical nurse specialist (CNS), Nursing Research Committees or Councils, subscriptions to nursing research journals, and internet access.
   - Instituting incentives and providing time for nurses who would like to participate in research conferences, research studies, journal clubs, research courses, or graduate degree programs.

9. **What do you need to know about your institution and administration before you can facilitate research-based clinical practice?**

Try to ascertain whether your institution is supportive of change and nursing research. Some questions that may help you gauge this support include:
   - Does the institution have a written philosophy of nursing that includes the significance of research to practice?
   - Does the philosophy speak to the provision of quality patient care and refer to evidence-based practice outcomes?
   - Does the nursing philosophy state that care will be state-of-the-art?
   - Is the overall institutional atmosphere collaborative and inclusive or autocratic and exclusive?
   - Is shared governance/shared leadership the leadership style at your institution? Examine your organizational structure.
   - Are nurses in prime administrative positions that can influence policy and procedure?
   - What type of educational preparation do the nurses in administrative and research positions have?
   - Is there a nurse researcher or nurse scientist position in the structure?
   - Are nurse educators or advanced practice nurses (e.g., CNS; nurse practitioner [NP]) part of the organizational structure and involved in the research mission?
   - Are the committees and councils multidisciplinary or dominated by one discipline?

- Is there evidence that current literature and research form the basis of committee/council decisions?
- Do nurses chair some of the committees or councils? Is there a nursing/clinical research committee or council?
- Are there visible efforts to get nurses involved in institutional governance?
- Is there visible and tangible support for evaluating current practice and changing practice if warranted?

10. How can a clinical research committee or council help and support the research process?

The purpose of a clinical research committee/council (CRC) is to promote, evaluate, and initiate clinical research in the institution; it is a wonderful resource for nurses and other health care professionals. The CRC can focus on generating research that is clinically relevant and cost-effective and promotes positive patient outcomes.

The CRC members are the cheerleaders for clinical research in the institution. They can guide and mentor staff through the research critique and proposal processes. They may be involved in disseminating research results, promoting research activities in the institution, and/or recruiting nurses and others for research projects. The CRC may function as a review board for graduate student nursing proposals for research to be conducted in the institution. Council members may act as facilitators of unit or service-based journal clubs and research workshops.

CRC members may develop material resources, such as research self-learning modules to assist health care providers to learn or review research basics, or produce an institutional research manual to guide potential researchers through the policies and procedures of proposing and conducting a research study. The CRC members may be responsible for maintaining research bulletin boards or disseminating research findings and promoting research activities through institutional newsletters. Some CRCs also administer intramural research funds to assist with the expenses for the conduct of research studies, attendance at research conferences, or production of research posters or presentations.

If your institution provides this valuable resource, take advantage of it! Attend meetings to see how your talents may be used or how you can learn more through interacting with colleagues on research topics. If your institution does not have this type of resource, you can play a key role in initiating a CRC.

11. How do I get a clinical research committee or council started?

The first step is to ensure buy-in from the people in charge. You may want to check with your unit manager or educator, CNS, or chair of the Institutional Review Board. These people should be able to give you an idea of whether a CRC would be accepted. At some point an institutional administrator will probably have to approve the formation of the committee, especially if it is to be a standing committee and if meetings will be held during work time.

The second step (or it may be first, depending on your viewpoint), assess interest from colleagues, both nurses and other health care providers, by answering the following questions.

- Do you have enough people with research interest to make this group successful? Who will be involved? How many participants are enough? How many are too many?

- Who/where are your resources? Do you have any colleagues with research expertise to help lead the committee/council? Are health care researchers already on staff? Is a nurse researcher or nurse scientist on staff or available for consultation? Is there a school of nursing nearby?

Invite nurse researchers and nursing faculty to lend expertise and advice for forming and facilitating this committee. Once you've received a positive response from administration and your colleagues, it is time to form your council and establish formal outcomes.

12. Who should participate as members of the CRC?

The CRC may include all health care providers interested in research and represent service lines or individual units. Participants may include advanced practice nurses (e.g., CNS, NP), staff nurses, nurse educators, nurse managers, nursing faculty, nurse researchers, pharmacists, respiratory therapists, social workers, physicians, and chaplains. Collaboration among all health care providers is crucial to developing a practice environment that supports research.

13. How do you determine the logistics of council meetings?

Once the group is formed you can decide on the logistics of the meetings—how often to meet, where, what time/day, rotation of time/day, and other organizational considerations. Choose someone to chair the committee. Many CRCs share the responsibilities of chairing between a staff nurse and a nurse researcher. The CRC usually meets on a regular basis with a formal agenda. Meetings should be publicized and open to all interested staff.

At your first meeting develop a mission statement—what is the purpose of your CRC? Use your purpose to guide activities. Take it slowly. Get the group established and then slowly initiate and promote your activities. In addition, be sure to document the outcomes of your activities.

14. How can I learn more about the research process?

Keep up with the literature; read current research studies in your clinical area. Go to the library and pick up a clinically based research journal, such as *Applied Nursing Research*, and read about studies in your area. Participate in a journal club; if none is available, start one on your unit or patient care area (see Chapter 6). Volunteer to assist with an ongoing research project. Talk to advanced practice nurses in your institution about research and why it is important. Take a research class at a local college. As with any skill, it takes practice to understand the research process and its implications for practice.

15. How do I get my colleagues involved in a research project?

Get your colleagues involved in research by sparking their interest. What are the clinically important questions? Brainstorm to decide which questions are important to study on your unit or patient care area. Clinical questions come from bedside practice, research literature, and professional organizations. Once a question has been identified, select a few people to do a search of the literature to find out whether the area has been adequately studied already. Assign the articles for a research journal club meeting and have the group critique the articles. Summarize the studies and discuss the research findings. Is the nursing practice currently used research-based or not? Is there is enough research on your topic? If not, you may want to get a group together to design and conduct a study.

Nurses have to believe that research is valued in your unit and institution and that research-based practice is the expectation of professional nursing practice. Some institutions mandate research involvement through their philosophical statements, which are usually integrated into the nursing job descriptions. In other institutions, research involvement is part of clinical merit programs, such as clinical ladder models.

16. What kinds of research opportunities are available for the nurse clinician?

Nurses may participate formally in research or on the research team in the following roles:

- Principal or co-investigator
- Study coordinator or project director
- Research assistant
- Data collector

Clinicians may participate informally by providing routine nursing care, such as collecting physiologic data or documenting outcomes, for patients enrolled in approved studies conducted by health care colleagues. Whenever you care for a patient using a protocol, clinical guideline, or clinical pathway, you participate in research. Additionally, assessing new products for utility and cost is a research activity. Product review committees assess new products for cost-effectiveness, efficacy, and effectiveness. Research findings are used to support the decision to purchase the product.[11]

17. What research has identified the characteristics of nurses who participate in research activities and those who do not?

The research-practice gap phenomenon generated many studies associated with research utilization. Individual nurse characteristics play a significant role in the incorporation of research into practice. Predictors of the nurse's use of research in practice include a positive research attitude, awareness of organizational supports for research, and past exposure to research via research courses.[6] Nurses who participate in research activities are more apt to use research in practice than those who do not participate in research activities.[6,12]

18. Who can I go to for research help? Who are my resources?

Granger and Chulay[11] remind us that even experienced researchers seek help for their research projects. Their book, *Research Strategies for Clinicians*, is an excellent resource for nurses interested in research. They suggest finding a person to act as your research mentor—someone with research experience who is willing to work with you on an ongoing basis.

- If your institution employs a nurse researcher or nurse scientist, he or she should be helpful in pointing you in the right direction. The nurse researcher has a broad overview of the types of studies conducted in the facility and can inform you of the resources available to hone your research knowledge. The nurse researcher can help develop your research plan and make sure that your study meets the requirements of ethical and meritorious research. She or he can help you analyze data and give tips about presenting research findings.
- Seek out a clinical nurse specialist (CNS). CNSs are trained in research methods, and facilitation and conduct of research are considered a major role of the

CNS.[13] The CNS can help to identify the clinically important questions for your patient population and assist in the design, implementation, and presentation of your study. What areas are you concerned about regarding patient care or nursing systems? Your nurse educator may also be of assistance.

- Nurse faculty who are researchers are good sources of research information and opportunities. Remember physicians and allied health colleagues. Many studies benefit from the expertise of different disciplines in designing and conducting clinically relevant studies. Patients are the ultimate beneficiaries of collaborative research.
- Friends and colleagues in neighboring institutions can also serve as research resources or provide opportunities to collaborate in multisite studies. Lindquist, Treat-Jacobson, and Watanuki[9] noted that multisite research is valuable to promote change in nursing practice. Certain clinical questions are more effectively studied by using several institutions.

19. How can I get more involved in conducting research?
- Whenever you collect data (e.g., vital signs, blood samples, lab values) on a patient enrolled in a study, you are participating in research. The role of data collector is vital to the success of the study. The researchers conducting the study depend on *accurate* collection of samples and recording of data. These data are the basis for the study findings and recommendations. If they are inaccurate, the researchers may be led to false conclusions.
- Identify resources on your nursing unit, in the institution, and in the community, as noted in the preceding question. Are any studies currently being implemented in your area of expertise? If so, talk to the investigators—let them know of your desire to learn more about research and increase your involvement. Ask them to keep you in mind for future studies.
- Take a research class at the nursing school. Talk to the faculty teaching the course. They should be able to identify fellow faculty who need research assistants for their research projects, which is an excellent way to get first hand research experience.

20. Do I need funding for doing unit-based research?
The answer to this question depends on the scale and scope of your study. You can design studies that do not require funding. Questions related to funding include the following:
- Is the study plan already designed?
- Should special equipment be purchased or special training provided for data collectors/or investigators?
- Do you need to design and duplicate data collection forms, or can you use existing forms?
- How will the study coordinator and/or data collectors be paid?
- Is research part of the job expectations or do you have to come in on your days off?
- Do you need help entering the data or analyzing the data?

Many unit-based studies are replications of studies of interest: the research plan and study instruments may be already designed. In some instances, the unit/institution will help you conduct the study by paying for your time and offering limited in-kind services (services provided at no charge) for unit-based research. In-kind services can include copying, secretarial support, or the services of a statistician. Time to conduct the study may be the most challenging consideration and involve payroll expense. The conduct of research may be considered an expectation of your role (e.g., CNS) or of your clinical level (e.g., clinician IV) and may be negotiated with your nurse manager. Some nurses conduct research on their own time. Some studies may require outside funding (see Chapter 8 for more details on funding research).

21. Will anyone else be interested in the results of your unit-based study?

Of course! The study that you conduct, whether a replication study or an original study, will assist others who serve a similar patient population in deciding whether to use nursing research findings in practice. Your study may change practice in your setting and promote positive outcomes for patients in your institution and beyond.

22. After conducting a research study, do I have an obligation to report and disseminate insignificant findings?

Yes. Research is not completed until it is disseminated. Research needs to be replicated to increase confidence that the results will improve nursing practice and promote positive patient outcomes. You will be instrumental in helping to close the research-practice gap.

23. How do I get my colleagues excited about using research in practice?

Nurses get excited about research when they see that what they do makes a difference in patient care. Nurses who feel empowered generally have more positive attitudes toward their work and work environment. When nurses identify the "what ifs?" of practice and then participate in studying such questions, a sense of ownership and pride evolves. If the study produces tangible and positive results, nurses feel validated (the question that they identified *was* important), and they are encouraged to examine their practice further. Basing practice on the most current and valid research and accepted evidence enhances a nurse's identity as a professional.

24. What organizational strategies can I implement to promote research utilization?

- Make organizational support of nursing research *visible*. Administrative leaders play important roles in promoting research-based practice.
- Provide Internet access for nurses to read and evaluate research available online. Get a subscription to the nearest medical library for full-text access to articles.
- Start a unit- or service-based journal club (see Chapter 6). Provide time for interested nurses to participate. Negotiate patient coverage so that as many staff members as possible can participate.
- Write the expectation of research- and evidence-based practice into the nursing philosophy and job descriptions. Administration is obligated to provide opportunities for the staff to fulfill this expectation.

25. How are research findings incorporated into institutional policy and procedures?

Several studies have shown that nurses tend to follow institutional policy.[2,15,16] Nurse administrators, therefore, have an influential role in promoting research-based practice. A commitment from administration that all policies and procedures should be evidence-based directs the policy and procedure (P&P) committee to ensure that this is the case. As P&Ps are reviewed and the research literature is critiqued, changes may be made to the policy. The references are cited in the policy and identified as a citation at the end of the policy.

26. What if new research findings contradict the current policy?

After you have critiqued the studies for scientific merit, bring the findings to the awareness of the chairperson of the P&P committee. Offer to revise the policy and procedure in question, citing research-based references. Again, if there is not enough evidence to support a change, more research is needed before changes to practice are made in your patient care area.

27. How do I resolve a situation in which nurses want to implement a research-based intervention and a particular physician is against it?

There are two keys to this dilemma: put the patient at the center of the debate (remove the "turf" issue from the equation), and make the physician your ally in this cause. Physicians respond to a research-based, data-driven process:

- Summarize the research and evidence supporting your claims.
- Have the studies available for the physician's perusal.
- Identify how the patient will benefit from the change in procedure.

If the physician is still unsure:

- Suggest a pilot or trial period for the new intervention. Invite the physician to be a member of the research team.
- Document and track how the patients respond to the research-based intervention. How you evaluate outcomes will vary with the purpose of your intervention. For example, is there a decrease in complication rates? Do wounds heal faster? Are patients and/or families more satisfied with their care?
- Share your results.

28. How can I reinforce and encourage staff support of research-based practice?

The key is to help staff members realize that they make a difference in patient care. Change is difficult; recognize that it takes time.

Provide incentives for nurses to participate in the research process. Reward clinicians who are instrumental in disseminating to their colleagues research-based information pertinent to your patient population.

- A bookstore gift certificate and paid-time-off to attend a research conference are examples of tangible rewards. An acknowledgement in a newsletter, a poster, or bulletin board postings describing the individual research activities provides personal benefits.
- Start a "Research Mentors" bulletin board and highlight one person a month. Put this board in a prominent place, where family members can read too!
- Post thank-you letters from patients and families that can be linked with changes in practice. Celebrate these accomplishments!
- Showcase the research projects being conducted on your unit or patient care area. Make this recognition as public as possible. This is good public relations for nursing and your unit to your health care colleagues in other units and disciplines, to family members, and to the community.

- Institute a research newsletter that covers either unit-based or house-wide research news. Highlight unit and personnel research activities.
- Track and post patient outcomes related to research- and evidence-based practice changes to encourage and motivate staff.
- Highlight nursing research activities during Nurses' Week celebrations.

Create formal research teams.

- Divide staff interested in specific problems into teams to research clinical problems, design, and conduct research studies.
- Team members could present the results of the study locally, regionally, and nationally. An article submitted for publication should be the final product.

Provide resources to encourage and motivate staff to continually assess their practice.

- Subscribe to several nursing journals that highlight clinically relevant research. Keep these accessible to the staff in the break room or nursing lounge.
- Have several research texts on hand. Invest in a subscription to your medical library to provide access to research articles online.
- Develop a "Research Bulletin Board." Include a section to post a research article pertinent to the care of your patient population. Change the article once a month. Include information about research studies being implemented in the unit or facility. Be creative in the bulletin board design to peak the interest of the staff.
- Require clinicians who attend clinical and research conferences with unit funds to present a summary of the experience, new findings, etc., to the other staff members after they return.

REFERENCES

1. Funk S, Champagne M, Wiese R, Tornquist E: Barriers to using research findings in practice: The clinician's perspective. Appl Nurs Res 4: 90–95, 1991.
2. Thompson CJ: Extent and factors influencing research utilization among critical care nurses. Houston, Texas Woman's University, 1997 (unpublished doctoral dissertation; university microfilms no. 9818572).
3. Rogers EM: Diffusion of Innovations, 3rd ed. New York, The Free Press, 1983.
4. Thompson CJ, Fink R, Bonnes D, et al: The effect of organizational strategies on the promotion of research utilization: A multi-site report. Presentation at the Thirteenth Annual Rocky Mountain Regional Interdisciplinary Research Symposium: Evidence Based Practice: Climbing to New Heights, Denver, CO, 2002.
5. Pettingill MM, Gillies DA, Clark CC: Factors encouraging and discouraging the use of nursing research findings. Image 26(2):143–147, 1994.
6. Rizzuto C, Bostrom J, Suter WN, Chenitz WC: Predictors of nurses' involvement in research activities. West J Nurs Res16(2):193–204, 1994.
7. Haller KB, Reynolds MA, Horsley JA: Developing research-based innovation protocols: Process, criteria, and issues. Res Nurs Health 2(2):45–51, 1979.
8. Titler MG, Kleiber C, Steelman VJ, et al: The Iowa Model of Evidence-Based Practice to Promote Quality Care. Crit Care Nurs Clin North Am 13:497–509, 2001.
9. Goode CJ, Piedalue F: Evidence-based clinical practice. J Nurs Admin 29(6):15–21, 1999.
10. Champion VL, Leach A: Variables related to research utilization in nursing: An empirical investigation. J Adv Nurs 14:705–710, 1989.
11. Granger BB, Chulay M: Research Strategies for Clinicians. Stamford, CT, Appleton & Lange, 1999.
12. Bostrom J, Suter WN: Research utilization: Making the link to practice. J Nurs Staff Devel 9(1):28–34, 1993.
13. Hamric AB, Spross JA, Hanson CM: Advanced Practice Nursing: An Integrative Approach, 2nd ed. Philadelphia, W.B. Saunders, 2001.
14. Lindquist R, Treat-Jacobson, D, Watanuki S: A case for multi-site studies in critical care. Heart Lung 29:269–277, 2000.
15. Brett JLL: Use of nursing practice research findings. Nurs Res 36(6):344–349, 1987.
16. Coyle LA, Sokop AG: Innovation adoption behavior among nurses. Nurs Res 39(3):176–180, 1990.

4. SEARCHING THE LITERATURE

Lisa K. Traditi, MLS, AHIP

1. What is a literature search?

A literature search is a systematic and thorough search of all types of published literature to identify as many items as possible that are relevant to a particular topic. A well-done search of the literature includes a review of primary and secondary sources, gray literature (see question 21), and ongoing research.

2. Why do a literature search?

- To provide a conceptual framework for your research or clinical question
- To validate and direct your research or clinical decision-making
- To answer a question
- To solve a problem

3. How do I put my research question into a searchable format?

Before you start asking your question in a database, ask yourself a few questions about what you need to know. Think about the specific information that you hope to get from your literature search. For instance, do you need to know about every kind of intervention for improving all types of diabetes care, or do you need to compare the effectiveness of interventions targeted at health care professionals and aimed at improving outcomes for adult patients with insulin-dependent diabetes? The following two questions can help you put your question into a searchable format.

1. What is the research question or clinical problem that I want to solve?
   Be as specific as possible. Evidence-based practice proponents advise using the four **PICO** elements to build your question:
   - **P**atient or problem: an adult with type I diabetes
   - **I**ntervention (e.g., cause, prognostic factor, treatment, etc.): educational outreach visits by a nurse
   - **C**omparison intervention (if necessary): compared with no educational intervention
   - **O**utcome(s): improved patient outcomes
2. What are my searching goals?
   Prepare before starting your database search by doing the following:
   - Break down the search topic. Continuing with the example above, identify the search topics one by one: type I diabetes, patient education, patient outcomes, morbidity, mortality, therapy, adult.
   - Select the major concepts: type I diabetes, patient education, and outcomes.
   - Start your search with the major concepts only. In most databases, especially those that use a controlled vocabulary (see question 13), you will have better luck if you search each term individually. Once you have searched each term, you can combine search sets with Boolean logic operators (and, or) (see question 4).

- Consider synonyms and variations of the words. Think of other ways to search your major concepts:
  - (a) Should you search for patient education or diabetic patients with education as a subheading or teaching materials or all of the above?
  - (b) Should you explode (see question 15) the heading of diabetes mellitus or search using the more specific term for type I diabetes?
  - (c) If you are searching in a database that does not use a controlled vocabulary, consider using the terms type 1 or insulin-dependent diabetes as well as type I diabetes in your search.

4. What is Boolean logic? Which Boolean logic operators will you need to use?

Named after the nineteenth-century mathematician George Boole, Boolean logic is a form of algebra in which all values are reduced to either *true* or *false*. In database searching, Boolean logic is a way to combine search terms in a logical way, using the words *and*, *or*, and *not*. Machines cannot think, but phrasing your question in Boolean logic helps the computer "understand" the relationship between the concepts that you are trying to retrieve.

After creating sets of citations that include the key elements of your search, you may wish to combine two or more of these sets. Sets can be combined in the following ways:

1. **And**
   - All terms must appear in each reference.
   - Using *and* narrows the retrieval of citations.

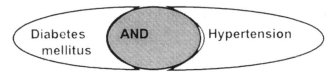

2. **Or**
   - Either of the selected terms may appear in each citation (used to include similar terms or concepts).
   - Using *or* increases the number of citations.

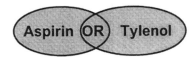

3. **Not**
   - The term will not appear in the reference (used to eliminate terms that may be included in some of the citations but are not relevant to the topic. *Use with caution*).
   - Using *not* decreases the number of citations.

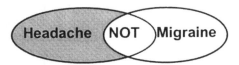

5. How will I limit my search?

Most databases that use a controlled vocabulary provide specific methods for limiting citations to years of publication, age groups, or other parameters

- **Years of publication**. Think about the time period that is important to your question. Remember that some adverse reactions and side effects may have been reported in earlier studies.
- **Age group(s)**. Use the appropriate age group limits for the database. The Cumulative Index to Nursing and Allied Health (CINAHL) age groups are listed below. Other database age groups may vary, but most databases that use a controlled vocabulary also use some sort of age group categorization as part of the limit options available to you. In CINAHL, for example, the only way to successfully limit your search to the elderly is by using the age groups limit "Aged" and "Aged, 80 and over" in the database's limit function.

AGE LIMIT	AGE COVERAGE
Pregnancy	
Fetus	From conception to birth
Newborn infant	Birth to 1 month
Infant	1–23 months
Preschool child	2–5 years
Child	6–12 years
Adolescent	13–18 years
Adult	19–44 years
Middle aged	45–64 years
Aged	65–79 years
Aged, 80 & over	80+ years

- **Language**. A limit to English restricts retrieval to articles written in the English language. Foreign language articles with English abstracts are also eliminated by a limit to English.
- **Human or animal**. A limit to human restricts retrieval to articles primarily about human subjects, retaining articles about both human and animal subjects. If you limit by age group you do not need to use this limit.
- **Publication type**. Using the publication type limit restricts your retrieval to specific types of publications.

Useful CINAHL Publication Types

Research (indicates a research study using data collection, methodology, discussion of results)

Clinical innovations

Clinical trial

Consumer patient teaching materials

Critical path

Nursing interventions

Practice guidelines

Systematic review

Useful Medline Publication Types

Review: restricts retrieval to articles that are reviews of a subject. For National Library of Medicine (NLM) databases this includes all review types: review literature; review of reported cases; review, academic; review, multicase; review, tutorial; and meta-analysis.

Abstract: restricts retrieval to publications with abstracts. The only abstracts included in Medline are those provided by the publisher. NLM Indexers do not write additional abstracts for articles indexed in Medline.

Clinical trial: restricts retrieval to all types and phases of clinical trials. This is a quick way to limit your results to evidence-based practice.

Patient education handout: a new publication type for MEDLINE.

- **Journal subsets**. In Medline you can limit your search by any of a number of journal subsets, including *nursing journals*. The CINAHL database contains 25 subsets of broad journal categories such as *allied health journals* or *core nursing journals*. You can restrict your retrieval to any of these subsets by a limit to journal subset.

6. **Which database is best for answering my question?**

Think about whether your question will more likely be answered by nursing literature, medical literature, or the literature of some other health field. Get to know the database you are using. Does the database use a controlled vocabulary? How do you limit your search? Which areas of health care does the database cover? How many years does the database cover? The descriptions of several databases follow, although this list is by no means complete.

- **Cumulative Index to Nursing and Allied Health (CINAHL)** provides authoritative coverage of the literature related to nursing and allied health, including the disciplines of cardiopulmonary technology, emergency services, health education, medical records, occupational therapy, physical therapy, physician assistant, radiologic technology, social service/health care, and surgical technology. Selected journals in the areas of consumer health, biomedicine, and health sciences librarianship are also indexed. In total, more than 500 journals are regularly indexed, and online abstracts are available for more than 150 of these titles. CINAHL also provides access to health care books, nursing dissertations, selected conference proceedings, standards of professional practice, educational software, and audiovisual materials in nursing.

- **Health and Psychosocial Instruments (HAPI)** provides a centralized resource for identifying a variety of measurement instruments in the health fields and psychosocial sciences that are of interest to practitioners, educators, administrators, and evaluators. Actual measurement tools are not available in the HAPI database, but HAPI records provide references to the primary sources for questionnaires, interview schedules, checklists, index measures, coding schemes/manuals, rating scales, projective techniques, vignettes/scenarios, and tests.

- **HealthSTAR** contains citations to the published literature of health services, technology, administration, and research and focuses on both clinical and nonclinical aspects of health care delivery. The following topics are included:

evaluation of patient outcomes; effectiveness of procedures programs, products, services and processes; administration and planning of health facilities, services and manpower; health insurance, health policy, health service research, health economics and financial management; laws and regulations, personnel administration, quality assurance, licensure and accreditation. The database contains citations and abstracts to journal articles, monographs, technical reports, meeting abstracts and papers, book chapters, government documents, and newspaper articles from 1975 to the present.

- **MEDLINE** or **PubMed**, produced by the National Library of Medicine since 1966, is widely recognized as the premier source for bibliographic and abstract coverage of biomedical literature. Abstracts are included for about 67% of the records. MEDLINE includes information from Index Medicus, Index to Dental Literature, and International Nursing Index as well as other sources of coverage in the areas of allied health, biologic and physical sciences, humanities, and information science as they relate to medicine and health care, communication disorders, population biology, and reproductive biology. Also available via PubMed at <http://www.ncbi.nlm.nih.gov/PubMed>. PubMed includes HealthSTAR, PreMEDLINE, and other related databases.

- **PsycINFO** covers the professional and academic literature of psychology and related disciplines, including medicine, psychiatry, nursing, sociology, education, pharmacology, physiology, linguistics, and other areas. Coverage is worldwide and includes references and abstracts to journals and dissertations in more than 30 languages and to book chapters and books in the English language.

- **EMBASE** (Excerpta Medica Database) from Elsevier Science is a major biomedical and pharmaceutical database well known for its international scope and timely, in-depth indexing. EMBASE now contains more than 9 million records from 1974 to the present from over 4,000 journals published in 70 countries; approximately 450,000 records are added annually. Over 80% of recent records contain full author abstracts. EMBASE features coverage of drug research, pharmacology, pharmaceutics, pharmacy, side effects and interactions, and toxicology; human medicine (clinical and experimental); basic biomedical sciences; biotechnology, biomedical engineering and instrumentation; health policy and management; pharmacoeconomics; public, occupational and environmental health, and pollution; substance dependence and abuse; psychiatry; forensic medicine; and alternatives to animal testing.

- **Micromedex** pioneered the concept of peer-reviewed clinical information systems by establishing and supporting a full-time internal editorial staff of over 50 pharmacists, toxicologists, physicians, and nurses. Micromedex includes monographs and other resources on drug dosing, pharmacokinetics, drug interactions, complementary and alternative medicine, acute and chronic disease states, toxicology, patient education, and a large set of diagnostic pearls and tools.

7. What is the difference between Ovid MEDLINE and PubMed?

The MEDLINE portion of the two databases is the same; the search interface differs. Ovid MEDLINE allows you to start with a search that uses the controlled vocabulary and to choose the Medical Subject Heading (MeSH) that you desire. PubMed automatically maps the search terms that you enter to the MeSH and combines those terms with the words that you entered as Textword searches. You usually get a larger list in PubMed than in Ovid MEDLINE.

The scope of the two databases is also different. Ovid MEDLINE includes only MEDLINE, whereas PubMed includes citations from MEDLINE, PreMEDLINE, and other related databases. PreMEDLINE is a database of the current citations in the process of being indexed. Ovid also provides access to a combined MEDLINE/PRE-MEDLINE database, which may be available to you.

The Ovid MEDLINE search interface is more accommodating if you are combining two or more subjects; it is also easier to limit your search in Ovid. In addition, with Ovid you can search databases from producers other than the National Library of Medicine, such as CINAHL, an important nursing resource, using the same search software.

PubMed, on the other hand, includes convenient features, such as the "see-related articles" feature that allows you to use one "best" article to link to others like it.

Both Ovid MEDLINE and PubMed include the ability to limit your retrieval to clinically significant studies. Both link to some full-text articles but not necessarily in the same journals. If your goal is to search your topic thoroughly, consider using both Ovid MEDLINE and PubMed, as well as other subject-appropriate databases.

8. Do I need to do my search in more than one database?

In many cases, yes. CINAHL, MEDLINE, and other databases do not index exactly the same journal articles, and no database covers the entire world of health-related literature.

9. If the results from my search are too large or too small, what can I do?

Narrow the search	Broaden the search
• Restrict to focus, using the major topics of your question.	• Do not restrict to focus.
• Refine the search; think of more specific terms.	• Look at search results. Evaluate what you have so far, and look at subject headings for clues to further refine your search.
• Add a subject heading (have you left out an important concept?).	
• Apply subheadings. Using the subheading of drug therapy nets better results than using drug therapy as a subject heading—i.e., diabetes mellitus/drug therapy rather than diabetes mellitus and drug therapy.	• Remove subheadings.
	• Remove limits.
	• Delete any unnecessary subject headings.
	• Explode subject headings.
• Apply limits. Consider appropriate year, age, and language limits to narrow your results.	

10. Am I answering the basic research question?

Always keep in mind your original question. It's easy to get sidetracked by interesting but irrelevant findings. Review the titles and abstracts in your search results. Does it look like you are getting article citations that will lead to your answer?

11. Which criteria should I use to evaluate my findings?

Some specific ways to evaluate information resources—books, journal articles, or web pages—are to filter for relevance and scientific validity, look for currency and relevancy of the source, and assess expertise or authority. The *Users Guides to the Medical Literature* is an excellent resource for evaluating specific types of articles. A complete list of the articles in this series and the databases in which they are compiled is referenced in the bibliography of this chapter.

12. Why do I need to know about CINAHL subject headings, MeSH, or other controlled vocabularies?

Databases that use a controlled vocabulary allow much greater precision. With a controlled vocabulary you do not need to search for synonyms, think about plurals or derivations of your word, or try to search every possible spelling. Databases that use Textword only searching allow greater freedom to use slang terms or new phrases. For example, the CINAHL database is indexed by subject specialists who read each article completely, then assign terms to describe (as specifically as possible) the content of the article. The terms come from a "controlled vocabulary"—a standardized list of vocabulary and definitions called subject headings.

The idea behind a controlled vocabulary is that all articles about the same concept are assigned the same standardized subject heading, regardless of the exact words or synonyms the that author uses. For example, one author may use the phrase *whooping cough*, another may use the word *pertussis*, but both articles are indexed under whooping cough, the CINAHL term for the disease. The most effective way to search CINAHL is to use the controlled vocabulary terms whenever possible. The CINAHL subject headings list is designed in a "tree structure," with broader headings followed by narrower headings.

Controlled Vocabulary Tree Structure Comparison: Diabetes Mellitus

CINAHL	MEDLINE
Diabetes mellitus	Diabetes mellitus
Diabetes mellitus, insulin-dependent	Diabetes, gestational
Diabetes mellitus, non-insulin-dependent	Fetal macrosomia
Diabetic angiopathies	Diabetes mellitus, experimental
Diabetic foot	Diabetes mellitus, insulin-dependent
Diabetic retinopathy	Wolfram syndrome
Diabetic coma	Diabetes mellitus, lipoatrophic
Hyperglycemic hyperosmolar nonketotic coma	Diabetes mellitus, non-insulin-dependent
Diabetic ketoacidosis	Diabetic angiopathies
Diabetic nephropathies	Diabetic foot
Diabetic neuropathies	Diabetic retinopathy
Diabetic foot	Diabetic coma
Pregnancy in diabetes	Hyperglycemic hyperosmolar nonketotic coma
Diabetes mellitus, gestational	Diabetic ketoacidosis
Fetal macrosomia	Diabetic nephropathies
	Diabetic neuropathies
	Diabetic foot
	Obesity in diabetes
	Prediabetic state
	Pregnancy in diabetics
	Fetal macrosomia

13. Why can't I just search with text words or the words that I use regularly?

You can search any database using text words, but you get only what you enter. For example, if you want to search for non–insulin-dependent diabetes, do you enter "type II diabetes," "type 2 diabetes," "type two diabetes," or "non–insulin-dependent diabetes"? You have to know exactly how the author spelled the words. With a controlled vocabulary, you choose the designated term, and all of the articles with spelling variations will be retrieved.

14. When I search in CINAHL or MEDLINE, I often get a list of subject headings with the options to choose the Explode box or the Focus box. When should I choose one or the other?

The **explode** option is available only in databases with a thesaurus or controlled vocabulary. Since articles are indexed to the most specific term possible, it is not always possible to retrieve everything on a topic by choosing a broad index term. The explode option ensures that you retrieve all articles on a broad topic area. To explode a search term means to search an index term and all of its narrower terms. Index terms are arranged in a hierarchy, with broader concepts near the top of the hierarchy and more specific terms near the bottom. The explode process searches the indicated term as well as every other term under it in the hierarchy. For example, in the CINAHL tree in question 12, if you choose to explode the main term of *Diabetes mellitus*, you will get any article indexed to all of the more specific terms indented under diabetes mellitus. You may prefer to explode only one of the narrower terms, such as diabetic angiopathies, which would net you all the articles indexed under that term as well as all articles indexed under diabetic foot or diabetic retinopathy.

The **focus** option ensures that the subject heading is the main concept in the articles retrieved. This option narrows your search by excluding articles in which the subject heading is only a minor point.

Both Explode and Focus options may be selected at the same time because they have different functions.

15. How do I find articles about clinical evidence?

Many databases now offer "expert searches" that use proven, evidence-based search strategies. In PubMed, use the Clinical Queries button on the left-hand navigation bar to see a good example. Your local library may have developed expert searches for your use.

16. Which databases have been built especially for this purpose?

- **EBN Online** is the electronic full text of the current issue of *Evidence-Based Nursing*, including figures and tables, and extra "web-only" material. *Evidence-Based Nursing* is a quarterly journal designed to alert practicing nurses to important and clinically relevant advances in treatment, diagnosis, etiology, and prognosis. Published by the BMJ Publishing Group and the Royal College of Nursing, *Evidence-Based Nursing* selects and examines every aspect of the best international nursing research. Available at <http://ebn.bmjjournals.com/>.
- The **Joanna Briggs Institute** (JBI) is an international research collaboration for evidence-based nursing and midwifery based at the Royal Adelaide Hospital and Adelaide University. Established in 1996 in recognition of the

need for a collaborative approach to the evaluation of research and its integration into nursing practice, the JBI collaboration identifies areas for which nurses most urgently require summarized evidence on which to base their practice, to carry out systematic reviews of international research, and to conduct trials in areas where good evidence is not available. Available at <http://www.joannabriggs.edu.au/>.

- **Cochrane Database of Systematic Reviews** includes the full text of completed and in-process systematic reviews conducted by the Cochrane Collaboration. The Cochrane Collaboration, an international network of individuals and institutions committed to preparing, maintaining, and disseminating systematic reviews of health care, has produced this database since 1991. Participants in the review process use explicit and rigorous methods to identify, critically appraise, and synthesize relevant studies from the published medical literature. Available at <http://www.cochranelibrary.com/cochrane/default.HTM>.

- **Best Evidence** is a small but growing database of full-text articles from two journals, the *ACP Journal Club*, a publication of the American College of Physicians, and *Evidence-Based Medicine* from 1991 through 1999. The two journals merged in 2000. The editors screen the top clinical journals to identify studies that are both methodologically sound and clinically relevant, then write enhanced abstracts and provide commentaries on the value of the articles for clinical practice. Available via OVID as the ACP Journal Club database and at <http://www.acponline.org/catalog/electronic/best_evidence.htm>.

- **PEDro**, an initiative of the Centre for Evidence-Based Physiotherapy (CEBP) at the School of Physiotherapy of the University of Sydney, is a database of physiotherapy evidence with abstracts of randomized controlled trials and systematic reviews in physical therapy. Available at <http://ptwww.cchs.usyd.edu.au/pedro/>.

- **Bandolier** is a print and Internet journal, using evidence-based practice techniques to provide advice about particular treatments or diseases for health care professionals and consumers. The content is tertiary publishing, distilling the information from secondary reviews of primary trials and making it comprehensible. Bandolier is created under the direction of Henry McQuay, Professor of Pain Relief, Churchill Hospital, University of Oxford. Andrew Moore, MD, edits Bandolier, which is produced from the journal *Pain Research*. Moore and McQuay are members of the Centre for Evidence-based Medicine. Available at <http://www.jr2.ox.ac.uk/bandolier/>.

- **EMBASE**, the Excerpta Medica database, is a biomedical and pharmacologic database that gives access to the most up-to-date information about medical and drug-related subjects. The primary focus of EMBASE is drug research and pharmacology. The EMBASE journal collection is international, with over 4,000 biomedical journals from 70 countries. Updated weekly, EMBASE is available online via the major database vendors: DataStar, DIALOG, DIMDI, LEXIS/NEXIS, Ovid Online, and STN. It is also possible to access EMBASE on the Internet through ScienceDirect at <http://www.sciencedirect.com/>.

17. How do I find full-text articles on line?

First, check with your local health sciences library, which may subscribe to electronic journals on your behalf. Some journals offer free access for some or all of their issues; PubMed attempts to link to most of these. Online journals offer many advantages, such as the convenience of accessing articles from the desktop. However, not every journal is available online.

18. Will I get all of the information I need from database searching?

The answer depends on your original reason for doing a database search. You may find sufficient journal citations that, once you have read the full article, will provide the answers that you seek. You may need to refer to a textbook, website, human expert, or other resource for your answer. Health-related databases are wonderful tools, but they are not the only resource that you should consider when asking your research question.

You may have noticed that for many systematic reviews, the authors report that they did a "hand search" of the literature. Hand searching, which is often necessary to do the most complete literature search possible, involves reviewing bibliographies of articles, books, and conferences in your topic area.

19. When should I use a general web search tool and when should I use a subject-specific database?

When you need to search the World Wide Web, a bewildering array of search services is at your command. General web search tools claim to search the entire web, and many of them, such as Google, are becoming increasingly sophisticated at finding resources in the health sciences. A general web search tool rarely searches all available websites all of the time. Rather, most general web search tools search a snapshot of the entire web. This is one reason that you get different search results with different web search tools. Subject-specific databases have done some of the work for you, allowing you to search a smaller group of preselected websites appropriate for your field. Again, for the most thorough results, search your topic in 2–4 web-based search tools and compare your findings to determine whether you are getting what you need.

20. What is "gray literature"? How do I find it?

Gray literature, or fugitive publications, may include conference proceedings, theses, dissertations, technical reports, market research reports, technical specifications and standards, and other documents not published commercially. Gray literature by its nature can be difficult to find. Often the best place to start is with researchers in your field of interest. Health sciences libraries can assist you with your search for gray literature.

21. What is the purpose of programs such as ProCite, Reference Manager, and Endnote?

ProCite, Reference Manager, and Endnote are bibliographic database software programs produced by ISI ResearchSoft at <http://www.isiresearchsoft.com/>. They allow you to create your own local database of article, book, and website citations, which you can sort by subject and author. These programs also work with word-processing programs to help create footnotes and bibliographies in a desired format.

22. How can I order photocopies of references that I find?

Most online full-text journal producers offer a fee-based service through which you can order articles. You may find it less expensive to go in person to your local health sciences library. Contact your closest health sciences library or public library for assistance (see question 26).

23. How do I report on the literature search process in my grant or articles?

Review the grant proposal requirements or journal for which you are writing. The literature review section of the articles that you have read offers clues about how to report the process that you used to find your articles.

24. How can I stay up to date on my research topic?

Learn about the databases, websites, and other resources that offer the best net coverage of your topic. Then review the help files, or ask an expert if these resources have an automated update system to which you can subscribe. For instance, OVID has a feature called AutoSDI/AutoAlert (SDI), which is used to retrieve the newest documents meeting your search criteria whenever a database is updated. SDIs are intended to help users stay up-to-date on a specific topic and learn of new documents by favorite authors. The user establishes a search strategy once, then automatically receives periodic e-mail messages containing all new documents retrieved by the strategy with each new database update. The user does not have to re-key the search, limit it to the latest update, or even know when the database has been updated.

25. Why should I use a library or librarian if everything is online?

As many have already discovered, not everything is online. At this stage in the evolution from print to online information, online access may be best described as a valuable adjunct to, but not a replacement for, print information. Librarians spend years learning and staying updated in the field of library science. Use their expertise to help you save time in the research process, to help you find difficult concepts in the literature, and to reassure you that you have found the right answer to your information question.

26. Where can I go to get help with my literature search?

Ask your friendly neighborhood health sciences librarian. He or she is trained to help health care professionals get and use information. Contact the National Network of Libraries of Medicine to discover the health sciences library closest to you—http://nnlm.gov/ or 1-800-338-7657. If you do not have a health sciences librarian nearby, ask for help from your local public library. Also, discover the colleagues around you who have strong searching skills and cultivate their friendship. Take advantage of classes offered at professional conferences to learn about new resources or to add to your existing skill set.

BIBLIOGRAPHY

1. Denison Memorial Library. Available at <http://denison.uchsc.edu>.
2. Glasziou P, Guyatt GH, Dans AL, et al: Applying the results of trials and systematic reviews to individual patients [editorial]. ACP J Club 129:A15–A16, 1998. Comments: ACP J Club 129(3):A17, 1998.
3. Gordon Guyatt, Rennie Drummond (eds): Users' Guides to the Medical Literature: A Manual of Evidence-Based Clinical Practice. Chicago, AMA Press, 2002.
4. Haynes RB, McKibbon KA, Walker CJ, et al: Computer searching of the medical literature. An evaluation of MEDLINE searching systems. Ann Intern Med 103:812–816, 1985.

5. Haynes RB, Wilczynski N, McKibbon KA, et al: Developing optimal search strategies for detecting clinically sound studies in MEDLINE. J Am Med Inform Assoc 1:447–458, 1994.
6. Hunt DL, McKibbon KA: Locating and appraising systematic reviews. Ann Intern Med 126:532–538, 1997. Comments: Ann Intern Med 128:322–323, 1998; 128:323, 1998.
7. Kirpalani H, Schmidt B, McKibbon KA, et al: Searching MEDLINE for randomized clinical trials involving care of the newborn. Pediatrics 83:543–546, 1989.
8. McKibbon KA: Using 'best evidence' in clinical practice [editorial]. ACP J Club 128:A15, 1998.
9. McKibbon KA, Walker-Dilks CF, Wilczynski NL, Haynes RB: Beyond ACP Journal Club: How to harness MEDLINE for review articles [editorial]. ACP J Club 124:A12–A13, 1996.
10. McKibbon KA, Walker-Dilks CJ: Beyond ACP Journal Club: How to harness MEDLINE for diagnostic problems [editorial]. ACP J Club 121(Suppl 2):A10–A12, 1994.
11. McKibbon KA, Walker-Dilks CJ: Beyond ACP Journal Club: How to harness MEDLINE for therapy problems [editorial]. ACP J Clu. 121(Suppl 1):A10–A12, 1994. [Published drratum appears in ACP J Club 121:A11), 1994.]
12. McKibbon KA, Walker-Dilks CJ: Beyond ACP Journal Club: How to harness MEDLINE to solve clinical problems [editorial]. ACP J Club 120(Suppl 2):A10–A12, 1994.
13. McKibbon KA, Walker-Dilks C, Haynes RB, Wilczynski N: Beyond ACP Journal Club: How to harness MEDLINE for prognosis problems [editorial]. ACP J Club 123:A12–14, 1995.
14. Sackett D, Straus S, Richardson WS, et al: Evidence-Based Medicine: How to Practice and Teach EBM, 2nd ed. London, Churchill Livingstone, 2000.
15. Walker-Dilks CJ, McKibbon KA, Haynes RB: Beyond ACP Journal Club: How to harness MEDLINE for etiology problems [editorial]. ACP J Club 121:A10–A11, 1994.

5. READING, UNDERSTANDING, AND CRITIQUING RESEARCH REPORTS

Kathleen S. Oman, RN, PhD

1. What is meant by critique?

Critique is associated with critical thinking and appraisal, not merely criticism. Critique is directed at the product of the research, not the author. An intellectual critique of research involves a careful assessment of all aspects of a study to judge the merits, limitations, meaning, relevance, and significance, based on previous research experience and knowledge about the topic.[1]

2. Why should we critique research reports?

Critique is essential to strengthen scientific investigation and utilization of research findings in practice. All studies have strengths and limitations. Ryan-Wenger[2] has stated that before we use research to change our clinical practice, we must evaluate it for credibility, integrity, and potential for replication. Through critical appraisal a research report can be evaluated for its strengths and limitations, feedback can be provided to the researcher, and determinations can be made about the applicability of research findings to clinical practice. A researcher or consumer of research must critique a study to interpret the findings in light of the following:
- Can I believe the results?
- Is the work applicable to my clinical setting?
- Can I build on or replicate this research?
- Do these findings lead to increased understanding of the topic?
- Are the findings consistent with previous studies?
- Are the findings ready to implement in practice?

3. What process or method can be used to critique a study?

Numerous examples of critique forms are published in the literature. Because nurses and other health care professionals have different scopes of understanding and knowledge of the research process in general, as well as varied experiences in critiquing research and evaluating its scientific merit and clinical relevance, a consistent approach provides a structured format that helps improve critiquing skills. In addition to using a standardized format, it is essential to read and practice critiquing. The more experience that one has in critiquing research reports, the more proficient one becomes. A journal club is an excellent format to learn to critique articles. Being part of a group engaged in reading and critiquing research helps us learn from each other and can actually be fun (see Chapter 6).

4. Give examples of a critique form.

There are many examples of critique forms in the literature. The Research Report Critiquing Form, developed by Colleen Goode,[3] is an example of a critique form used at University of Colorado Hospital (Appendix A). Rasmussen et al.[4] have developed a brief critique form for both quantitative and qualitative studies. In reviewing more than one research report, it is helpful to use the Research Report Summary Form (Appendix B) to compile data from the literature review.

The critique process has been divided into nine sections: purpose and/or problem statement, literature review, hypotheses and/or research questions, research methodology/design, variables, data collection and measurement, data analysis/results, clinical implications, and limitations. Before critically reviewing a report it is wise to read through it once to obtain a general idea of what the researcher is attempting to achieve.

5. How are the purpose and/or problem statement, literature review, framework, and hypotheses evaluated?

The purpose of the study, problem, or research question should be clearly stated in a research report. The choice of research design depends on the research question. Review of the literature should be stated in an organized fashion with recent and relevant information. The theoretical or conceptual framework can be derived from nursing or other health-related disciplines. The conceptual framework serves as an organizing structure to guide and direct all aspects of the research process. An hypothesis translates the problem statement into a precise, unambiguous prediction of expected outcomes.[5] Hypotheses are subject to testing through various methods in the research design.

Questions to Consider for Critique

THE RESEARCH PROBLEM	REVIEW OF LITERATURE	THEORETICAL/CONCEPTUAL FRAMEWORK	HYPOTHESIS
Is the problem clearly and concisely stated?	Is the literature review logically and clearly organized?	Does the report attempt to link the problem to a theoretical or conceptual framework?	Are the hypotheses clear, testable, and specific?
Is the problem adequately narrowed into a researchable problem?	Does the review provide a critique of the relevant studies?	Is the theoretical framework easily tied to the problem or does it seem forced?	Does each hypothesis express a predicted relationship between two or more variables?
Does the problem statement give precise information about the variables to be studied?	Does the review include recent literature?	If a conceptual framework is used, are the concepts adequately defined? Are the relationships among these concepts clearly identified?	Do the hypotheses logically flow from the theoretical or conceptual framework?
Can the research problem be answered with empirical evidence?	Is the cited research pertinent to the research problem?		Do the hypotheses indicate the general population of interest?
Is the problem significant to nursing or other clinical services?	Are important relevant references omitted?		Are the independent and dependent variables operationally defined?

(Table continued on next page.)

Questions to Consider for Critique (cont.)

THE RESEARCH PROBLEM	REVIEW OF LITERATURE	THEORETICAL/CONCEP-TUAL FRAMEWORK	HYPOTHESIS
Is the relationship of the identified problem to previous research clear?	Does the review conclude with a brief synopsis of the literature and its implications for the problem under investigation?		Are extraneous or intervening variables identified?

6. How is the research process evaluated?

A review of the research process should include an evaluation of the research design, population sample, data collection instruments, and procedure. The research design provides operational definitions for all variables and should be appropriate for the research problem. Data collection methods should be clearly described with attention to checks on validity and reliability. The research procedure describes how the project was carried out. Statements about consent and protection of the subjects' rights should be included.

More Questions to Consider for Critique

RESEARCH DESIGN	SUBJECTS/ SAMPLING	DATA COLLECTION METHODS	RESEARCH PROCEDURE
Is the research design adequately described?	Is the population identified and described?	Are data collection methods appropriate for the study?	Has the study been reviewed and approved by an investigational review board?
Is the design appropriate for the research problem (experimental, quasi-experimental, or nonexperimental)?	Is the sampling method described and appropriate?	Are the data collection methods clearly identified and described?	Are the procedures used to execute the design clearly described to permit replication?
Does the research design control for threats to internal and external validity of the study?	Is the sample size adequate? Is it representative of the population?	Are the reliability and validity of the measurement instruments acceptable?	Are procedures for ensuring constancy of conditions described?
What procedures are used to control for individual differences? Are these procedures the most effective ones possible?	Are the sample criteria for inclusion and exclusion into the study identified?		Are procedures for preventing contamination between treatment groups discussed?
	Is there any sampling bias in the chosen method?		Is the setting of the study appropriate for the research question?
	Does the report indicate the response rate?		Was informed consent obtained from subjects?
			Were the rights of the subject protected?

7. How should data analysis methods and results be evaluated?

- The statistical analyses performed should be appropriate for answering the research question. The type of analysis needs to be appropriate for the level of measurement for each variable.
- Reliability and/or validity of instruments used with this sample need to be reported.
- The results section should be clear and logically organized and need to answer the research question.
- The tables and figures should be clear and understandable.

8. How are the clinical implications and limitations of the study evaluated?

The discussion is a compilation of what was found as well as what conclusions can be drawn from the findings. Caution should be used in evaluating the discussion, for it is easy to overgeneralize the findings. In the discussion, the need for replication studies prior to initiating the findings into practice should be considered. The following questions should be considered in evaluating the conclusions and clinical implications section of the research report.

Conclusions

- Are the conclusions clearly stated and in a meaningful fashion?
- Are the conclusions based on the data obtained?
- Does the investigator distinguish between actual findings and interpretations?
- Are the findings discussed in relation to previous research and to the theoretical/conceptual framework?
- Are the limitations of the results identified?
- Is there evidence of bias in the interpretations?
- Does the interpretation distinguish between clinical and statistical significance?

Clinical implications, limitations, and recommendations for future research

- Are the implications of the findings for clinical practice described?
- Are the implications discussed in terms of retention, modification or rejection of a theoretical or conceptual framework?
- Is consideration given to the study's limitations in discussing its implications?
- Are recommendations for future research identified?
- Are there recommendations on how the study's methods could be improved?
- Is the study reproducible?

9. What other aspects of the research report should be critiqued?

This section addresses some overall quality aspects of the report, including the title, abstract or summary, reference list, and writing style.

- Is the title clear? Does it include the important variables and the population being studied?
- Does the abstract restate the problem? Does it briefly describe the methodology and the results?
- Are the references complete and in a consistent style? Are they recent, do they include classic citations if available?
- What is the overall writing style like? Is the report clearly written? Is it logically organized? Is correct grammar used? Are words spelled correctly?

In evaluating research reports, not all elements of the critique process or identified questions apply to each study, and judgments are always subjective. However, using a checklist or having a systematic way of evaluating research reports helps nurses to judge more accurately the applicability of the findings to their practice.

10. What criteria are used for critiquing qualitative research?

The evaluative criteria for qualitative studies differ from those presented thus far. Qualitative studies seek to gain a greater understanding of phenomena and life experiences. This goal is accomplished through interviews, observation, and art. Thus, the evaluation of qualitative studies focuses on whether the findings truly reflect the phenomena or experience, as the reader knows it. The following criteria[6-10] are used for evaluating qualitative studies:

1. **Auditability (or confirmability)**. Can the reader follow the decision trail of the researcher from data collection through conclusions? This criterion fits with the concept of reliability in the quantitative method. Key questions to consider include:

- Did the authors provide a description of the strategies used to collect and analyze the data?
- Were the characteristics of the informants/participants described and was the process used to choose them included?
- Were the social, physical, and interpersonal contexts associated with data collection described?
- Did more than one researcher perform the theoretical coding?

2. **Credibility**. Is the experience recognizable? Is there support for its truthfulness? This criterion is similar to the concept of internal validity. Questions to consider include:

- Were the personal or intellectual biases of the researchers identified and their impact on the research process explored?
- Were multiple methods of data collection (triangulation) used to look for patterns of convergence?
- Did the researchers validate their findings with the research subjects?
- Were contradictory instances searched out and analyzed?

3. **Fit (or transferability)**. Are the findings generalizable to other settings? This criterion is comparable to external validity. Questions to ponder include:

- Did the researchers validate the representativeness of the data?
- Are the data described in enough detail to allow the reader to judge the appropriateness of applying the findings to other settings?
- Did the sample include the full range of possible cases or settings?

Applying these criteria to qualitative research is an important step in evaluating rigor and quality. They may not apply to every qualitative design.

APPENDIX A

University of Colorado Hospital
Research Report Critiquing Form

AUTHOR:

TITLE:

JOURNAL:

YEAR: VOLUME: ISSUE: PAGES:

Purpose and/or Problem Statement:
Clearly stated? Relates to title of paper? Precise information about variables studied?
Researchable and significant problem?

Literature Review (Conceptual or Theoretical Framework):
Do the authors relate literature to a framework? Is the literature relevant to the study?
Logically and clearly organized? Include recent literature? Were primary sources used? Are
important findings related to the problem(s) reported?

Hypotheses and/or Research Questions:
Is there a clear and specific question(s) or hypothesis(es)? Logically flow from con-
ceptual/theoretical framework? If hypotheses tested, are they operationally defined with pre-
dicted relationships between variables? Are the study variables identified in the research
question/hypothesis?

Research Methodology/Design:
a. Setting for the research: Context clear? Related to research problem?

b. Subjects, sample size, and selection: If population, is it identified and described? Is
    sample size adequate and representative of population? Is sampling bias evident? Was the
    assignment of patients to treatment/intervention randomized? Are the number of subjects
    adequate (30+) for quantitative study?

c. Research design: Appropriate for research problem? Adequately described?

Variables (Nursing interventions, patient characteristics, or patient behaviors):
Are key variables clearly and precisely defined? Are there any undefined variables? Are they
identified by type?
a. Independent: Causes the effect that is being studied. Found in experimental, quasi-experi-
    mental, and correlational studies.

b. Dependent: Measured effect or outcome thought to result from or depend on the indepen-
    dent variable. Found in experimental quasi-experimental and correlational studies.

(Cont'd.)

APPENDIX A (Continued)

Variables *(cont'd.)*:
c. Intervening or Study Variable: Characteristics or qualities that are to be measured, identified, or described. Found in exploratory and descriptive studies.

Data Collection and Measurement:
a. Methods of data collection: Clearly described? Appropriate to study?

b. Instruments used:
Reliability (consistency): Does the author report reliability of the instrument?
Validity (accuracy): Does the author report validity of the instrument?
Are reliability and validity acceptable?

c. Study Procedure: Constancy of procedure conditions? Contamination prevented? Subject rights protected?

d. Statistical tests used: Level of significance? Appropriate tests for answering questions?

Data Analysis/Results:
Logically organized and presented? Analysis appropriate for level of measurement? Information answers research question? Tables and figures clear and relevant? How large/precise was the treatment effect?

Clinical Implications:
Are conclusions stated in meaningful fashion? Does the investigator distinguish between actual findings and interpretation? Are implications discussed in relation to previous research and theoretical/conceptual framework? Can the results be applied to my patient care? Were all clinically important outcomes considered? Are the likely treatment benefits worth the potential cost/adverse effects?

Limitations:
Are limitations of results identified? Is there evidence of bias in interpretation? Implications for practice described? Recommendations for improvement/future research based on limitations? Potential biases reported? Limitators such as sample size noted?

Prepared by: _____

This form was developed by Colleen Goode, PhD, RN, FAAN, based on Gehlbach, Stephen H. Interpreting the Medical Literature, 3rd ed. New York: McGraw-Hill, Inc., 1993.

APPENDIX B
Research Report Summary Form

Author **Title**			
Purpose **Research Design** Setting Sample Variables Independent Dependent Measurement **Results/Clinical Implications** **Limitations**			

Evidence of a research base from summarized reports
Is there replication? Scientific merit? Risk to patient? Client applicability? Cost? Benefits?

1992 Horn Video Productions - Ida Grove, Iowa 51445

REFERENCES

1. Burns N, Grove S: Critical analysis of nursing studies. In The Practice of Nursing Research: Conduct, Critique, and Utilization, 3rd ed. Philadelphia, W.B. Saunders, 1997, pp 647–665.
2. Ryan-Wenger N: Guidelines for critique of a research report. Heart Lung 21:394–401, 1992.
3. Goode CJ, Butcher LA, Cipperly JA, et al: Research Utilization: A Study Guide, 2nd ed. Ida Grove, IA, Horn Video Productions, 1992.
4. Rasmussen L, O'Conner M, Shinkle S, Thomas MK: The basic research review checklist. J Contin Educ Nurs 231:13–17, 2000.
5. Polit D, Hungler B: Nursing Research: Principles and Methods, 6th ed. Philadelphia, J.B. Lippincott, 1999.
6. Sandelowski M: Rigor or rigor mortis: The problem of rigor in qualitative research revisited. Adv Nurs Sci 16:1–8, 1993.
7. Burns N: Standards for qualitative research. Nurs Sci Q 2:44–52, 1989.
8. Beck C: Qualitative research: The evaluation of its credibility, fittingness, and auditability. West J Nurs Res 15:263–266, 1993.
9. Mays N, Pope C. Assessing the quality in qualitative research. Br Med J 320:50–53, 2000.
10. Byrne M: Evaluating the findings of qualitative research. AORN J 73:703–706, 2001.

BIBLIOGRAPHY

1. Gehlbach S: Interpreting the Medical Literature, 3rd ed. New York, McGraw-Hill, 1993.
2. Greenhalgh T: How to Read a Paper: The Basics of Evidence Based Medicine. London, BMJ Publishing Group, 1997.
3. Haughey B: Evaluating quantitative research designs: Part 1. Crit Care Nurse 14:100–102, 1994.
4. Haughey B: Evaluating quantitative research designs: Part 2. Crit Care Nurse 14:69–72, 1994.
5. Liehr P, Houston S: Critiquing and using nursing research: Guidelines for the critical care nurse. Am J Crit Care 2:407–412, 1993.
6. Munro B: Statistical Methods for Health Care Research, 3rd ed. Philadelphia, Lippincott-Raven, 1997.
7. Pett M: Non-parametric Statistics for Health Care Research: Statistics for Small Samples and Unusual Distributions. Thousand Oaks, CA, Sage Publications, 1997.
8. Sandelowski M: The problem of rigor in qualitative research. Adv Nurs Sci 8:27–37, 1986.
9. Shekelle P, Andersson G, Bombardier C, et al: A brief introduction to the critical reading of the clinical literature. Spine 19(Suppl 18S):2028S–2031S, 1994.
10. Strubert H: Evaluating the qualitative research report. In Lobiondo-Wood G, Haber J (eds): Nursing Research: Methods, Critical Appraisal and Utilization, 3rd ed. St. Louis, Mosby, 1994, pp 481–499.
11. Topham D, DeSilva P: Evaluating congruency between steps in the research process. A critique guide for use in clinical nursing practice. CNS 2:97–102, 1988.
12. Tornquist EM, Funk SG, Champagne MT, Weise RA: Advice on reading research: Overcoming the barriers. In Clinical Methods. Philadelphia, W.B. Saunders, 1993, pp 177–183.

6. JOURNAL CLUBS

Jan Hagman, RN, BSN, OCN, and Mary E. Krugman, RN, PhD

1. What is a journal club?

A journal club is much like a popular book club. A select group of people meet to discuss a written piece of work. In lieu of a piece of literature, a journal club reviews a research article. Although book clubs usually are composed of a group of friends, journal clubs usually consist of a group of professionals with a discipline in common. Journal club participants may be all nurses or all respiratory therapists, but ideally they are a multidisciplinary group. This approach allows for a broader overview of the research critiqued. Members of the journal club are better able to keep abreast of issues or trends that may affect the care that they give to patients.

2. Why start a journal club?

Health care professionals strive to provide excellent care that is up to date and cost-effective. Using evidence in practice contributes to improved patient outcomes. Evidence-based practice is defined as the "use of the best clinical evidence from systematic research in making patient care decisions".[1] Journal clubs assist greatly in this goal. By reviewing current research in a particular patient care issue, we can find evidence to support what we do or evidence that prompts us to examine our current practice more closely.[2] By including multiple disciplines in journal clubs, we can explore different viewpoints and gain greater knowledge about a topic. Group discussions should include whether the article is valid, what methods the authors used, and whether the conclusions can be supported. In holding such discussions with our peers we increase collegiality and develop as professionals.

3. What are the goals of journal clubs?

Nolf[3] notes that journal clubs are most often formed for practicality, socialization, promotion of scholarship and professional growth, and development of enhanced knowledge. Journal club interactions improve critical thinking skills and have been reported to serve as a powerful tool for education among all disciplines. The tradition of holding journal clubs originated over 100 years ago in the medical profession.[4,5]

4. How are the meetings set up?

Journal clubs should meet the needs of the participants. It is helpful to survey the staff members who are interested in attending a journal club to determine the best time and place. Often journal clubs are held in a staff conference room. The room should be large enough to hold all participants and to allow open discussion in a quiet, private space without constant interruptions. If the journal clubs are held at lunchtime, members can brown-bag their lunch while an article is reviewed. Journal clubs can also be held away from the hospital or clinic. This approach allows a more relaxed atmosphere and is helpful in team building. It is best to hold the journal club on a designated day and time, such as the first Thursday of every month at noon.

The article to be reviewed at the meeting should be distributed at least 2 weeks before the meeting to allow participants time to read and review it. Articles are chosen usually by the person who will lead the journal club session. They should be on a topic of interest to all participants.

5. How do you publicize journal clubs?

Journal club meeting times should be posted in a visible, frequently viewed area. A copy of the article should be available in a designated spot, such as a bulletin board, for participants to pick up at their convenience. Articles may also be placed in employee mailboxes. An additional way to publicize meetings is via e-mail. This method is helpful for multidisciplinary journal club meetings. It also can be used to remind people that the meeting is approaching. See Appendix A for an example of a journal club notice.

6. What are the roles of the participants in a journal club?

Membership in a journal club is usually voluntary. However, in many institutions it is strongly encouraged. Members should show commitment to the journal club by attending and being prepared to discuss the article. Each member should read the research article and complete a critiquing form in advance of the meeting. Members should arrive at the meeting prepared to discuss the article and provide input. Member preparation facilitates a more focused and concise discussion. Participants may expand on the topics that affect or change practice at future meetings. Members alternate acting as the leader of a session.

7. Discuss the role of the leader.

The role of the session leader is to focus the team on the article using information analyzed by the critiquing tool. The leader chooses the article to be presented, based on the club's disciplinary background and relevance to practice. The leader is responsible for distributing the articles and critiquing tool to the journal club members at least 2 weeks before the meeting to ensure adequate time for article review and preparation. The leader moderates the discussion during the meeting, keeping the flow of conversation on track and helping each participant contribute his or her ideas.

8. What is a facilitator?

Although it is not required, it is helpful to have a facilitator at your meetings. A facilitator is a person with a background in research. It is helpful if the facilitator has participated in research and/or has published research articles. During the meeting, the facilitator acts as a mentor, resource, and guide for the leader and the team. The table below summarizes the roles and functions of the various participants in journal clubs.

Journal Club Roles and Functions

ROLE	FUNCTION
Members	• Attends meetings regularly • Prior to the meeting, reads the assigned research article and completes a critiquing form • Alternately acts as the leader of a session

(*Table continued on next page.*)

Journal Club Roles and Functions (cont.)

ROLE	FUNCTION
Leader	• Chooses the article to be presented, based on the club's disciplinary background and relevance to their practice • Distributes the articles and critiquing tool to the journal club members at least two weeks prior to the meeting • Focuses team on the article using information analyzed by the critiquing tool. • Moderates the discussion during the meeting, keeping the flow of conversation on track and helping each participant contribute his/her ideas
Facilitator	• Has background in research and may have experience in publishing research articles. • Acts as mentor, resource, and a guide for the leader and the team

9. How are the articles selected for discussion and review?

It is best to identify a group of journals that are most likely to relate to the clinical work of the practice area. Both clinical and research journals may be included, depending on the goals of the group. The table of contents or individual journal article abstracts may be posted for staff information. As the leader rotates, he or she is responsible for reviewing the table of contents of identified journals since the last meeting. Articles are selected that most directly apply to the area of practice and/or are judged to be most relevant.

10. Where are the critiquing tools obtained?

Reviewing and critiquing research articles are integral parts of the research process. Numerous examples of critique forms have been published in the literature (see Chapter 5). Using a consistent approach for critiquing an article provides a structured format that helps improve critiquing skills. Repeated use of a critique form assists journal club members in judging all aspects of an article, including its merits and limitations, relevance, and significance. Journal club members gain increased skills by using a structured critique form. However, all questions on a critique form may not pertain to each research article.

11. What are the benefits of joining a journal club?

Joining a journal club may increase professional confidence and self-esteem, through the knowledge that your practice is based on scientific findings. Journal clubs allow another avenue to learn current patient care methods. Journal club members are more confident in the justification and explanation of standards and procedures based on research results. Members learn critical appraisal skills for assessing the validity and applicability of research results for the incorporation of findings into patient care. Journal clubs can promote team building among peers. As members rotate into the role of the leader, they can improve their communication and leadership skills. Ultimately patients benefit from nurses' and other health care professionals' participation in journal clubs. Journal clubs can also stimulate ideas for the conduct of research.[6,7]

12. Can continuing education (contact hour) credits be awarded for journal club meetings?

In most institutions the journal club leader may submit an application for continuing education contact hours as determined by the length of the meeting. This strategy provides an incentive to participate in a journal club for disciplines requiring continuing education credits.

13. What resources are available to assist in developing a journal club?

Resources for starting a journal club can be found in a variety of places. You may begin by finding out whether your hospital has a research committee. Is someone assisting other areas in setting up a journal club? Are other professionals already participating in journal clubs? Can you attend as an observer? Is your facility associated with a school of nursing, medical school, or school of pharmacy? Finally, look into professional organizations that may be promoting journal clubs, such as the American Association of Critical Care Nurses and the Oncology Nursing Society.[3,4]

APPENDIX A: Announcement of Journal Club Meeting

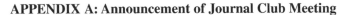

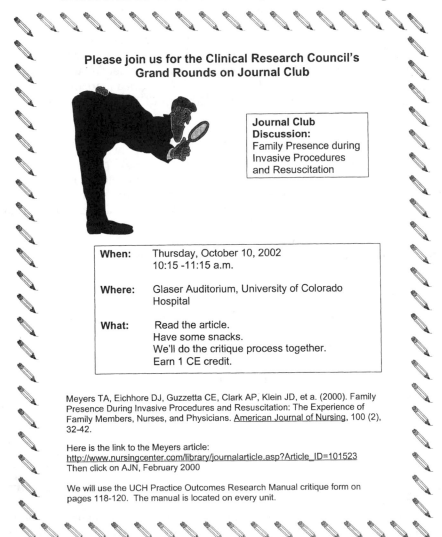

Please join us for the Clinical Research Council's Grand Rounds on Journal Club

Journal Club Discussion: Family Presence during Invasive Procedures and Resuscitation

When: Thursday, October 10, 2002
            10:15 -11:15 a.m.

Where: Glaser Auditorium, University of Colorado Hospital

What: Read the article.
            Have some snacks.
            We'll do the critique process together.
            Earn 1 CE credit.

Meyers TA, Eichhore DJ, Guzzetta CE, Clark AP, Klein JD, et a. (2000). Family Presence During Invasive Procedures and Resuscitation: The Experience of Family Members, Nurses, and Physicians. American Journal of Nursing, 100 (2), 32-42.

Here is the link to the Meyers article:
http://www.nursingcenter.com/library/journalarticle.asp?Article_ID=101523
Then click on AJN, February 2000

We will use the UCH Practice Outcomes Research Manual critique form on pages 118-120. The manual is located on every unit.

REFERENCES

1. Goode CJ: What constitutes the "evidence" in evidence-based practice? Appl Nurs Res 13(4):222–225, 2000.
2. Tibbles L, Sanford R: The research journal club: A mechanism for research utilization. Clin Nurse Spec 8:23–26, 1994.
3. Nolf B: Journal club: A tool for continuing education. J Contin Educ Nurs 26:238–239, 1995.
4. Speers AT: An introduction to nursing research through an OR nursing journal club. AORN J 69(6):1232–1236, 1999.
5. Linzer M: The journal club and medical education over one hundred years of unrecorded history. Postgrad Med J 740(63):475–478, 1987.
6. Shearer J: The nursing research journal club: An ongoing program to promote nursing research in a community hospital. J Nurs Staff Devel 11:104–105, 1995.
7. Johnson JM, Reineck C, Daigle-Bjerke A, et al: Understanding research articles: A pilot study of critical readings of research publications. J Nurs Staff Devel 11:95–99, 1995.

7. DEVELOPING THE RESEARCH QUESTION

Roxie L. Foster, RN, PhD, FAAN

1. What is a research question?

In many ways a research question is like any other question; it identifies what we want to know. A research question, however, must be more thoughtfully constructed than many other questions. It forms "an explicit query about a problem or issue that can be challenged, examined, analyzed, and will yield useful new information"[1] (p. 2).

2. Why does the research question require so much thought?

Ambiguous questions lead to vague answers. A clear and concise research question focuses the inquiry to produce meaningful results. Attention to the research question is well worth the effort because a well-constructed question directs the study's design, data collection methods, and analysis. Once you identify precisely what you want to know, the rest of the research process falls logically into place.

3. How do I develop the research question?

There are four steps in developing the research question. Through these steps, a general topic area is increasingly focused until the research can be precisely represented and clearly understood from one or more questions or hypotheses.

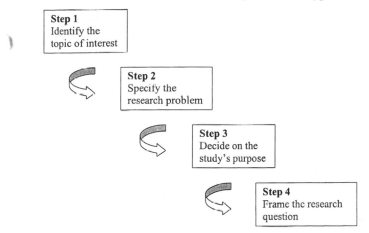

Steps in developing the research question.

4. How do I find a research topic?

A number of sources for research topics are listed in the table below. Keep in mind, however, that this list is designed to spark ideas, not to be exhaustive. Once you begin to think in terms of researchable ideas, you will find them everywhere.

You will become aware of potential research topics in your professional encounters with clients and colleagues, as you read professional and lay literature, as you learn about agendas for health reform, as you listen to the news during your daily commute, and every time you ponder, "I wonder what would happen if. . .?"

Sources of Research Topics

SOURCE	EXAMPLE
Clinical experience	A nurse colleague relates his dissatisfaction with pain management for 10-year-old Virginia, who had a laparoscopic appendectomy yesterday. Despite aggressive administration of opioid analgesics, Virginia continues to report pain of 4 on a 0–5 scale. He confides, "I really think anxiety is a lot of her problem. She's lying still and rigid and seems afraid to try to move. If I could just get her to relax and think about something else I think she'd feel a lot better. As it is, I've spent half the shift with this one child." You discuss mutual experiences and frustrations and agree that there must be a better way.
Nursing literature	An article you discussed at journal club questions the routine use of dexamethasone in preventing or decreasing postextubation stridor.[5] You know dexamethasone is routinely used prior to extubation in your PICU/NICU settings and realize that the evidence may not support this practice.
Societal concerns	With increasing health care costs, the limited science base to support clinical practice impedes the ability to "rationalize care and emphasize what is effective in producing desirable patient outcomes"[4] (p. 13). You wonder how this might apply to outcomes in your practice.
Previous research	A study just completed on your unit found that children's satisfaction with postoperative pain management was unrelated to the severity of postoperative pain.[3] You wonder if better family education about pain management would change these results.
Theory	Caring theory is consistent with your personal philosophy of care and you wonder about the relationships between caring behaviors and patient outcomes in your practice.[4]
Feedback from patients and families	The wife of a patient with dementia confides that the caregiving role has become overwhelming. She has few family members to help her and no longer has any close friends. There is no one who seems to understand what she is going through. You wonder if a computer-assisted support group would help to sustain in-home care for patients with dementia.
Special interest groups	In a monthly newsletter, you notice the list of research priorities for a gerontological nursing society to which you belong. You realize that two of these priorities reflect issues in your clinical practice.

Informed by Talbot [4] and Polit & Hungler[2]

5. How do I choose one topic from all of the choices?

Making the options concrete and explicit can help with your decision. Consider these suggestions:

- Make a list of all the topics that interest you.
- Highlight the topics about which you are most passionate and/or the ones that represent the most troublesome concerns or issues for your practice. Brink and Wood[1] advised, "If it keeps nagging at you, you probably have an interest that will sustain you throughout the research" (p 3). Do a cursory review of the

literature to see how much information is available about the topic. (See Chapter 4 for help in searching the literature.)
- Discuss your interests with colleagues. Articulating your thoughts can help to clarify the areas of greatest interest or concern.
- Identify windows of opportunity. Sometimes the topic is right because the time is right, and delay may cost you vital support. Backing by administration, peers, and funding agencies waxes and wanes with social/political agendas. It is wise to strike while the iron is hot.

6. What if the topic has been studied before?

Previous research does not limit further study; instead it helps to focus additional inquiry. Rarely is any phenomenon so well studied that additional research cannot further illuminate its properties and actions. When little is known about a phenomenon, the purpose of research is to explore and describe. As knowledge accumulates, research can be designed to evaluate associations with other variables, predict outcomes, and identify causes and effects.

7. How do the research topic and research problem differ?

The research topic is much broader than the research problem. Research problems focus on a particular way of looking at the topic or situation. Even when a research topic seems quite focused, there are almost always a number of ways to approach it. The following problems are among several that could be derived from the clinical vignette presented in question 4:
- It is difficult to distinguish between pain and anxiety.
- Analgesics alone may be inadequate to provide effective pain relief.
- Nurses do not feel competent in using relaxation strategies with children.
- Inadequate pain relief increases the level of acuity.

8. How do I identify the right research problem?

If there were a *right* problem, it would indicate that other problems are *wrong*. Such is not the case. There are simply different ways of framing the issue. Your task is to identify the problem that aligns most closely with your interests and resources at a given time. To do so, first elucidate all of the problems that you can think of in relation to the given topic. Review the bulleted suggestions in question 5 for choosing a research topic to help narrow the problem list. Ask yourself which of the problems poses the greatest threat to patient care. *The stronger your argument for the significance of the problem, the stronger the significance of conducting research to reduce or resolve it.*

9. Once I identify a clinical problem, how do I know if it is appropriate for research?

Appropriateness can be evaluated in terms of researchability and feasibility. A problem is researchable when:
- The answer is not a known or accepted fact or something you can look up
- Existing evidence is inadequate to guide clinical judgments
- An answer is discoverable through systematic inquiry
- Resolving the problem will make a substantial difference in the cost, process, or outcomes of patient care

Feasibility of researching the problem involves consideration of your expertise and resources. Among those resources are administrative support; availability of necessary consultants, including a human subjects review panel; time to plan and conduct the project; adequate fiscal and physical resources, cooperation and/or collaboration of peers; access to the population of interest; and an unquenchable spirit of inquiry. (See Chapter 8 for further discussion of feasibility.)

10. What is the relationship between the problem and the research purpose?
   The research purpose is a declarative statement that tells how you intend to study the problem. Problems can be addressed in a number of ways, depending on your interests and resources. For example, for the problem, "It is difficult to distinguish between pain and anxiety," the following are among many possible purpose statements. Each of these purpose statements approaches the problem differently and will result in a different research design.
   • To describe a patient's lived experiences of pain and anxiety after surgery.
   • To examine the relationship between patients' postoperative pain and anxiety.
   • To compare ratings of patients' postoperative anxiety between nurses who used a standardized assessment instrument and those who did not.

11. What should I consider when constructing the purpose statement?
   The first rule of thumb for writing purpose statements is to make them simple and concise. Avoid combining several purposes in one statement. Instead, write separate statements or create a stem followed by an itemized list. For example, the purposes of this study are to describe (a) patients' lived experiences of anxiety and (b) nurses' lived experiences in assessing anxiety.
   The second rule of thumb is to choose verbs that precisely indicate what you will do. These verbs link directly to the study design. For example, a descriptive design is appropriate when the purpose is to *explore* or *describe*. A correlational design is indicated when the purpose is to *examine the relationship*. An experimental design is used when the purpose is to *compare* two or more groups.

12. When should I include research aims in the proposal?
   Research aims or objectives are itemized statements that convey what you plan to do in the course of the research. When used, they typically follow the purpose statement. Aims are usually broader in scope than questions or hypotheses. They can be helpful when the purpose, questions, and hypotheses fail to communicate the whole picture. For example, you may want to include an aim about the interpretation or dissemination of the results.

13. How does the purpose statement help me frame the research question?
   Once the purpose of the research is clear, the research question simply restates the purpose in question form. When the purpose and research question are this closely related, some researchers omit the purpose statement and state only the research question to avoid redundancy.[2] When it is possible to achieve more specificity about the purpose, however, you can do so by writing clear, simple questions.

14. What are the guidelines for writing research questions?
   To write the research question, you must think ahead to the study's design and methods. The research question should reflect not only what you will study but how you will study it.

- Construct questions that forecast the design and methods (see table below).
- Avoid the stems "do," "does," and "is" that imply the question can be answered by yes or no.
- Avoid the use of "should" or "could," which ask for opinions.
- Construct clear, simple questions.
- Avoid complex questions, such as "How do patients rate their postoperative pain and anxiety?" Instead, separate questions about pain and anxiety by writing one question for each of the key variables: "How do patients rate their postoperative pain?" "How do patients rate their postoperative anxiety?"
- Do not worry about redundant wording between questions. It is appropriate to sacrifice unique wording for the sake of clarity.

Relationship Among the Research Purpose, Question, Design, and Methods

PURPOSE	QUESTIONS STEMS	DESIGN	DATA COLLECTION METHODS	DATA ANALYSIS METHODS
To describe/ To explore/ To understand a phenomenon	What? When? Where? How?	Descriptive	Qualitative (e.g., interviews, focus groups, participant observation, card sorts, field notes, diary) Quantitative (e.g., surveys, questionnaires, record review)	Qualitative Descriptive statistics (e.g., mean, mode, median, standard deviation)
To examine/ To predict the relationship between 2 or more variables, sets, or groups	What is the relationship? Which best predicts?	Correlational	Quantitative (e.g., surveys, questionnaires, record review)	Correlation Regression
To examine/ To compare differences between 2 or more variables, groups, or sets	Why? What is the effect? What is the difference?	Experimental	Quantitative (e.g., surveys, questionnaires, record review)	Tests for group differences (e.g., t-test, ANOVA)

ANOVA = analysis of variance.

15. What is a research hypothesis?

An hypothesis is a statement that predicts the relationship between measurable variables and, thus, predicts the outcome of a specific aspect of inquiry involving quantitative methods. Ideally, researchers use theoretical and/or empirical evidence to support the prediction. Hypotheses can be constructed with less evidence, using the researcher's logic or clinical experience,[2] but poorly substantiated predictions are not as useful in guiding analysis and interpretation of results.

16. When should I use an hypothesis instead of a question?

It is not necessarily an either/or question. Because an hypothesis "translates the research question into a prediction of expected outcomes"[2] (p. 104) it is narrower in scope than the research question and, thus, may not be redundant with the question. Viewing the research question and hypothesis as tools to communicate the focus of your research helps to eliminate their mystique and places you, the researcher, in charge.

17. How is an hypothesis written?

Research hypotheses can be stated in either nondirectional or directional language. Nondirectional hypotheses predict the existence of a relationship, whereas directional hypotheses predict the nature of that relationship. For example:

- Nondirectional: Patients' postoperative anxiety is related to the intensity of their pain.
- Directional: Patients who experience greater pain have greater anxiety.

Another type of hypothesis is the null or statistical hypothesis. The null hypothesis has been described as "a ritualized exercise in devil's advocacy" in which "one assumes as a basis for argument that there is no systematic difference between the experimental and control scores"[3] (p. 9) The null hypothesis is denoted as H_0.

- H_0: Anxiety ratings will be the same for patients who received training in relaxation and those who did not.

Null hypotheses are used less often than research hypotheses, perhaps because null hypotheses can seem convoluted and difficult to interpret. One way to think about the null hypothesis is to compare it to the legal assumption of innocence. "The variables are assumed to be 'innocent' of any relationship until they can be shown to be 'guilty' through statistical procedures"[2] (p. 109).

18. How do I know when it is time to stop refining the question or hypothesis?

It is time to go on to other aspects of the research proposal when you have achieved as much clarity and specificity as you can at the time. In actuality, you will probably find yourself revisiting the purpose, questions, and hypotheses more than once as you formulate the design and methods. Working through details of design, methods, and procedures often yields insights that direct further refinement.

REFERENCES

1. Brink PJ, Wood MJ: Basic Steps in Planning Nursing Research. From Question to Proposal. Boston, Jones & Bartlett, 2001.
2. Polit DF, Hungler BP: Essentials of Nursing Research. Methods, Appraisal, and Utilization, 5th ed. Philadelphia, Lippincott, 2001.
3. Abelson RP: Statistics as Principled Argument. Hillsdale, NJ, Lawrence Earlbaum, 1995.
4. Talbot LA: Principles and Practice of Nursing Research. St. Louis, Mosby, 1995.

BIBLIOGRAPHY

1. Foster RL, Varni JW: Measuring the quality of children's postoperative pain management: Initial validation of the child/parent total quality pain management (TQPM) instruments. J Pain Symptom Manage 23:201–210, 2002.
2. Jacox A, Suppe F, Campbell J, Stashinko E: Diversity in philosophical approaches. In Hinshaw AS, Feetham SL, Shaver JL (eds): Handbook of Clinical Nursing Research. Thousand Oaks, CA, Sage, 1999, pp 3–17.
3. Jansaithong J: The use of dexamethasone in the prevention of postextubation stridor in pediatric patients in PICU/NICU settings: An analytical review. J Soc Pediatr Nurs 5:182–191, 2001.
4. Watson J: Assessing and Measuring Caring in Nursing and Health Science. New York, Springer, 2002.

II. Planning the Study

8. FEASIBILITY AND FUNDING

Patricia Moritz, PhD, FAAN

1. What does feasibility mean for a research study?

Think of feasibility as the background work that must be done *before* a study can be implemented. It is the scholarly equivalent of the "due diligence" that a corporate official must undertake before committing a company's resources to a new venture or investment. Once a research question is identified, the first question an that investigator must ask is whether the study is feasible—is it doable?

- Are the necessary elements (research team, access to clinical sites and subjects, and financial and material resources) available or obtainable?
- Are the required data available and accessible?
- Can the project be carried out effectively?

A proposed study may fail if feasibility is not examined thoroughly. Perhaps most importantly, funding organizations expect you to identify and resolve feasibility issues before you even submit an application for financial support.

2. When should feasibility be considered?

You should study a project's feasibility as early as possible—and always before a study is initiated. In any professional activity, unexamined assumptions and unanticipated details will derail a project. Thus you must consider thoroughly the feasibility issues for each aspect and phase of a proposed study, and you need to revisit these issues routinely and be alert for the emergence of new issues after the study is underway. Successfully completing the feasibility inquiry is often a required component of proposals for approval or funding of research, but there is no "cookbook" for this process.

3. What factors are considered in examining the feasibility of a study?

- The location where the study will be conducted and how access to that location will be assured
- Whether human or animal subjects will be involved
- Whether subjects will be available and whether it is reasonable to assume that they will be interested in the study
- Whether the study will have a therapy, intervention, or clinical program that will be the experimental treatment in the study
- What resources are needed to conduct the study and whether they can be obtained if they are not already available

Only the investigator and research team can plan a strategy for each of these parameters. For a team that is new to an area of research, the feasibility review—sometimes called a feasibility study—may take longer than it will for a team that has been working for some time in that particular research area.

4. Why is study location an important aspect of study feasibility?

A study's location usually has two elements, reflecting the typical research scenario in which data are collected at one place and analyzed at another.

- One is the location (e.g., offices, laboratories) where the investigators will be housed while they are carrying out the study.
- The other is the actual location or site where the study is conducted (i.e., where data are collected and/or observations are made).

A major feasibility issue related to the location is whether it has the physical features and other resources to provide both security and proper management of the study's data—especially for any confidential information that is generated by the study.

The study location may be one particular clinical setting (e.g., hospitals, home care agencies, rehabilitation facilities) or a combination of clinical facilities. Before beginning a study, multiple levels of approvals are usually obtained and a number of safeguards are established to gain access to clinical settings. No one can simply approach subjects and get clinical data from patient records, even if the investigator works in the setting as a nurse. A crucial part of the feasibility assessment for any clinical setting is to determine what is required to conduct a clinical study there: how access is obtained, who gives access, what assurances and protections must be put in place by the investigator, and what the site's human subject protection requirements are.

At a minimum the investigator should have the research question, design, and plans for study implementation completed and ready to give to people contacted in the clinical setting. In reality, obtaining such access takes time and is at the discretion of those who are responsible for patient safety and security and those who review research proposals for possible implementation at that site. Investigators should be mindful that such review may take some time—perhaps a lot of time—because sites must focus first on clinical responsibilities and secondarily on other issues such as research proposals.

5. What are the feasibility issues concerning human and animal subjects?

Including either people or animals in research requires that you proactively put certain protections in place. These protections are required by the federal government, by organizations where the research is conducted, or by sponsors through outside funding. To determine the feasibility of such a study, you *must* determine what these requirements are.

The major emphasis for nurses is on people as subjects, because only a limited number of nurse investigators focus on animal models in their research. Specific information about protecting the welfare of research animals can be obtained at the website of the National Institutes of Health at <www.nih.gov>. If you cannot meet the welfare requirements for research animals, the study is not feasible. The same is true for human subjects.

Most institutions at which research is conducted have, or are affiliated with, an institutional review board (IRB), which is responsible for reviewing all research that includes human subjects and for assuring that the necessary protections are in place in each study. *IRBs should review all research proposals with human subjects*, even if the investigator believes that no harm will come to the people in the study or that it is exempt from full review. Protections are stringent because of the need to protect human subjects from any harm. Additional, special protections exist for certain human subjects, such as pregnant women, children, and prisoners. These protections are covered in Chapter 11.

6. It has been said that all ethnic populations need to be included in a study. How can this goal be feasible?

For a study in which the data are to be obtained from people, the more representative the sample of the population or group that has the health problem or is the focus of the intervention under study, the better and more useful the study will be. A major goal of research design is to ensure that the findings of the completed study can be generalized and replicated as broadly as possible. Otherwise, generalizability would be limited only to those included in the study. Thus, researchers should make every possible effort to include in their study sample all of those who have the clinical condition being studied—including representation from a wide variety of ethnic groups. A convenience sample of all college students, for example, would limit the generalizability of a study's results if the problem under study occurs in adults of all ages. To be useful, the same study would have to be repeated with a more representative sample.

There is an unfortunate history in the United States of using research subjects who were convenient to the investigator or more easily controlled. The control issue occurred in the past when there was worry over the impact of one gender's physiologic processes on study results. An extreme example was the use of male subjects in studies of women's health problems, because of concern that menstrual cycles and related symptoms may be confounding issues. Convenience samples are used when the investigator knows the limitations of such an approach and is interested primarily in knowing, for example, whether an intervention has any effect at all. Convenience samples are usually used when an area of research is new and exploratory. Under such circumstances, this more limited approach is acceptable.

A grant application to a funding agency that proposes to use a convenience sample would be expected to show the results of a feasibility study that had examined the availability of people who had the health problem or who already demonstrated a potential need for the intervention under study. The approach in this type of feasibility study is to examine the profile of those identified with the health problem in the research literature and then to determine the profile of these groups, including ethnic groups, in the geographic area where the study is to be conducted. For a small-scale initial study, limiting to a single geographic area may be acceptable if most but not all involved groups are represented. For larger-scale studies, it may be necessary to work with colleagues in other geographic areas to increase and balance the sample so that all involved groups are included.

Some federal funding agencies require—sometimes as a prerequisite for any funding—representation of the ethnic and racial groups that have the problem under study. Thus, by the time an investigator has reached the point of such funding, he or she should have clearly demonstrated, through feasibility and pilot studies, sufficient experience to know how to reach all groups for inclusion.

7. What are the feasibility considerations for a study in which a therapy or intervention will be studied?

- The independent variables must be clearly defined and specified.
- The intervention must be available for use in the study.

• The intervention must be controllable by the investigator.
• For comparison purposes, there must be one or more control groups that does not receive the treatment.

If the study is to use a therapy such as a drug or device that the investigator did not design or does not own, access to the product must be negotiated, and related agreements must be signed and in place before you apply for funding assistance. If the design of the study requires a placebo for a control group, the investigator must determine how to obtain a sham. For an intervention study in which the strategy requires development of an interpersonal relationship as part of the intervention, such as counseling or public health home visiting, a placebo control group may be required for a quality design. If the experimental group is to receive a drug treatment or a one-time intervention, some type of a sham treatment group may be needed as a control group; otherwise, it would be obvious to the control group that they did not have the intervention. Good design also requires that the clinician carrying out the intervention be blinded as to which is the actual treatment group. Use of placebos is controversial and is at times unethical. You should seek expert consultation in designing a study that includes a placebo.

8. Is it feasible to use a placebo control group in my intervention study?

The major feasibility question for any therapy or intervention study is whether a placebo can safely be used without compromising the health or well-being of any of the subjects. Another important question is whether a reasonable placebo can be produced and used. A placebo, or sham therapy or procedure, can be carried out in a study only if it is ethical to do so, given the design of a study. One can never deny a required therapy, when the efficacy is known, to a group of subjects simply because it makes for a stronger research design. However, if a study's purpose is to examine an interpersonal intervention, such as a relaxation technique, carried out by a nurse, it makes sense to have a placebo group that receives an interaction event but not a relaxation technique per se. Such a placebo control may be a friendly visitor on a schedule similar to that of the actual experimental intervention group. Any investigator considering a placebo control group is advised to seek early advice from experts and their institutional review board about the ethical and appropriate use of placebos as part of the feasibility considerations.

9. What should be considered if I simply want to get data from a clinical agency?

Even though most of us deal with patient data in our clinical settings every day, such data are not always legally or ethically available for study purposes. Recent changes in federal law have increased the security requirements for access to patient records and to clinical data linked to individual patients. There are distinct requirements for maintaining considerable distance between those who are not directly caring for a patient and the patient's clinical records or a site's automated records. Some circumstances may require permission from all patients whose data will be used before their records can be accessed. This new law, called the Health Insurance Portability and Accountability Act (HIPAA), and its full impact will be felt through this decade.

Investigators who are designing a study that requires only access to clinical data should contact the clinical agencies targeted for the study and determine their requirements for data access. The investigators can then determine how feasible it will be to gain access to the data. Before submitting an application to fund a proposal in which clinical site data access is one part of the larger data set, you must still examine the requirements for access to determine whether costs are associated with obtaining the data. Examining this aspect of feasibility in a timely manner assists in developing an adequate budget in a funding proposal.

10. Once I have looked at all aspects of feasibility, what do I do with the information?

The information is useful for completing the final version of your research proposal and for developing any grant application to a funding source. As an investigator proceeds through the various steps of a feasibility review, there is an obvious gain in helpful information, along with the confidence that there are fewer obstacles in the way of the implementation. The investigator usually also finds that completing each of the answers to the feasibility questions generates new insights—and can generate even more questions that need to be asked. Despite one's natural eagerness to get on with what appears to be a promising project, no one wants to be in the position of encountering one or more show-stopping problems after planning a study, obtaining funding, and arriving at the launch-point of implementation—especially if those problems might have been discovered or anticipated with a little more work up front.

The quality and thoroughness of your feasibility efforts are indispensable elements in establishing a career in research and in developing a history of successful funding for the work that you love. They are also your major tool for ensuring that Murphy's law and its correlates have only a minor impact on the research projects that you design.

11. What does research funding mean?

Funding refers to the provision of resources to support the actual conduct of the research—such as financial support for the investigator and research team; necessary resources, such as copies of measures or pharmaceuticals to be used; and compensation to the employer for the time required by staff to conduct the research. The funding of research can be *intramural* (from the investigator's place of employment, such as a hospital research committee) or *extramural* (from a source external to the investigator's place of employment, such as a federal or state agency, or foundation, or clinical society).

Some intramural research support funds only the time needed by the investigators to conduct the study and funds few or none of the additional resources. Extramural research funding is almost always preceded by a scientific or technical review of the research proposal for scientific merit. Such reviews are done by panels of experts—usually peers of the investigators—who are experts in the content and the methods used in the studies that they review. Reviewers also consider and make recommendations about the goodness of fit of the proposals with the program objectives of the funding agencies. In addition, the reviewers are asked to determine the reasonableness of the scientific return for the overall cost of the research. In other words, they are asked, because resources are limited, what will be the scientific return for the expenditure of these limited funds?

Although scientific merit is an important aspect of the review, funders also ask reviewers to consider appropriateness of the human protections (or animal welfare) specified in the application. The reviewers determine human subject safety based on the information in the application and not on second-guesses or assumptions about what the investigator intended.

12. How do I identify organizations that fund research in my area of interest?

Organizations that fund research are looking for the best possible scientific proposals focused on cutting-edge health problems and health care issues that are congruent with their mission. Such organizations fund research that meets the parameters defined in public notices about their funding programs. Funding sources for nursing research are numerous and varied. The best first steps for an investigator who is new to seeking research funding is to consult with colleagues who have already achieved such funding and to search the websites of organizations known to provide support for research in specific areas.

Some organizations support new investigators who are seeking their first grant support; others are more clearly focused on supporting experienced investigators; and still others support both. Clinical and nursing honor societies have research programs, usually with limited funds. These sources of funding, such as Sigma Theta Tau, Oncology Nursing Society and Foundation, the American Nurses Foundation, the American Association of Critical Care Nurses, the Emergency Nurses Association, and the Association of Perioperative Registered Nurses, provide varying levels and types of research funding. Such funding may be limited at times to members and at other times to registered nurses with certain credentials. It is important to search the website of organizations to which an investigator belongs and those of others that fit with the clinical focus of the study. The level of funding from such groups can be as small as a few hundred dollars or as large as $10,000; they often require a goodness of fit between the principal investigator and the focus of the study.

Sample of Potential Funding Sources

ORGANIZATION NAME	WEB ADDRESS
American Association of Critical Care Nurses	http://www.aacn.org
American Association of Neuroscience Nurses	http://www.aann.org
American Nephrology Nurses' Association	http://www.annanurse.org
American Nurses Foundation	http://www.nursingworld.org/anf
American Organization of Nurse Executives	http://www.aone.org
American Psychiatric Nurses Association	http://www.apna.org
Association of Perioperative Registered Nurses	http://www.aorn.org
Emergency Nurses Association	http://www.ena.org
National Nursing Staff Development Organization	http://www.nnsdo.org
Oncology Nursing Society and Foundation	http://www.ons.org
Sigma Theta Tau	http://www.nursingsociety.org

13. How do organizations that fund research operate?

Generally, organizations that fund research make it well known that they do so. It is much easier today than in the past to gain access to such information. A library or web search on the topical focus of the research that an investigator wishes to carry out may bring up such organizations. A more targeted approach for nurses is to search the websites of clinical, honor society, and general nursing organizations, such as the American Nurses Association site, Nursingworld, which has links to the American Nurses Foundation and other nursing organizations. Sigma Theta Tau provides new investigator support and has joint grant programs in which they partner with other organizations. The size and complexity of the grant vary. Many nursing specialty organizations also have research programs of various sizes that usually are targeted to their mission.

Funding organizations usually have some process that determines whether the proposed research fits with their stated mission. Such missions are published and usually incorporated into the various calls for grant applications and proposals. Investigators ignore such information at their own peril and at the cost of wasted effort, because they may devote much work to develop a superb proposal that is outside of the scope of the funder's mission.

Funding organizations almost always want annual and final progress reports and hold investigators accountable for conducting the research as planned and within the approved time plan and budget. Funders have been known to stop funding when the work is not going as expected or seems to be done inadequately.

14. Explain peer review.

Organizations that fund research usually select experts to conduct a scientific review of grant applications and provide feedback about the application's merit. This process, called peer review, is highly valued in the scientific community because a group of experts has given impartial feedback. Some new investigators seek peer review for some indication of the quality of their work.

15. Because I am doing a nursing research study, do I have to limit myself to organizations that fund nursing research?

Not necessarily. Nursing research represents studies that are pertinent to the knowledge base for nursing practice, health care delivery, and the myriad questions that nurses ask. Nursing research is conducted by investigators with a number of different scientific and clinical backgrounds; not all of them are nurses or prepared in nursing science. The importance of the research is that it will expand the boundaries of our knowledge in nursing.

The various organizations that fund nursing research understand what it is about and appreciate the complexities involved in carrying it out. Such funding organizations usually focus on the content of the research and the goodness of fit with their funding programs. Federal funding is available from the National Institute of Nursing Research (NINR) at the National Institutes of Health (NIH) as well as other sources that have missions compatible with nursing research. Among these are the Agency for Healthcare Research and Quality (AHRQ), the Centers for Disease Control and Prevention (CDC), and the other institutes of the NIH, such as the National Institute of Mental Health and National Institute of Aging. All of the national institutes can be found through the NIH website at www.nih.gov. NINR can be reached directly at www.nih.gov/ninr. AHRQ is found at www.ahrq.gov and the CDC at <www.cdc.gov>.

16. If my study is small, what funders may be interested in it?

Small in research usually means small in complexity, which suggests that few dollars are needed to complete the study. At times, the best source of such funding is intramural (from the investigator's employer or the site where the study will be carried out). For other funders to be interested, a first test of the study is whether it is directly related to building scientific knowledge or is more of a clinical imperative for a particular site. This distinction is important, because small studies may not be the next step in building an area of scientific knowledge, which is a requirement of almost all funding sources.

If the first test is met, several funding sources are available for small studies, including the American Nurses Foundation, Sigma Theta Tau, and the clinical specialty organizations that fund research. Private or local foundations sometimes fund small-scale research that fits with their mission and that is limited to a geographic area.

17. Why should I bother with getting funding if I can afford to fund the research myself?

One aspect of the application process that should be important professionally to investigators and research teams is peer review of the proposal. Such review is considered by some to be a gold-standard endorsement that the research is of high quality, scientifically meritorious, and worthy of being carried out. It also provides some idea of how others, who are knowledgeable in your area of research, view the proposal. In addition, some editors expect to see a footnote to research articles about the source(s) of funding. It is better to know the judged quality of the scientific merit of a study before you carry it out than later, when you cannot get the results published because of questions about its design, methodology, or other issues.

18. Can I send the same application to more than one funding source at the same time?

Maybe. An investigator must be careful not to lose credibility with a funding organization. Some sources of extramural funding make it clear in their literature that the organization does not expect an applicant to submit the same application to multiple institutions. It is important to follow such requirements. At times, it is necessary to submit to more than one funding source because the size, complexity, and scale of the study (and thus its cost) are beyond the resources of one funding organization. Under such circumstances, it is important to communicate with each of the potential funding agencies to determine their interest in the planned study and their potential willingness to work with multiple funders. The investigator should make clear in each of the research applications the full scope of the study, the funding agencies to which other applications have been submitted, and what part(s) would specifically be funded by each organization. By doing so, you ensure that everyone involved in the review and potential funding of the application knows what is occurring from the beginning.

When an investigator has a research proposal under review by a funding organization and it is not clear that that funder will be able to support the study, it is generally considered acceptable to submit the proposal to another funding organization. However, if the first organization is able to fund the application, the second submission should be withdrawn. It is never appropriate, nor permissible under federal rules, to have more than one funding source for exactly the same work (referred to as double-dipping).

19. Once I am funded, what requirements will I have to meet?

When investigators receive word that their study is being funded, they should begin to plan for the initiation of the study. Once the actual funds have been received and processed, new staff and other resources required to carry out the study can be obtained. It is the investigator's responsibility to conduct the study with integrity, in an ethical manner, within the required parameters of human subject protections, and within the financial limitations of the resources provided by the funder. The investigator should remember that the funder will not provide additional years of funding if the previous year's work has not been carried out as planned.

At some point (about two-thirds or three-fourths through the first grant year), the funding organization will require an annual report if the funding is for several years or a final report when the study is completed under a single-year award. This report is crucial to any additional funding, because it informs the funder about the quality of the work performed by the investigator and the research team as well as progress toward meeting the study's full requirements.

20. If the study is not completed, will the funds have to be paid back?

The answer depends on the circumstances and the policies of the funding agency. Investigators may get sick or die. Under such circumstances, the study clearly cannot be completed. But the situation is different when an investigator decides to change focus before a study is completed or simply does not manage time and other resources well and runs out of money before the study is finished. In such cases, the funding organization may require that all or part of the funds be returned. However, there are safeguards because, in most cases, the research awards are made to the employing institution of the investigator and not directly to the person conducting the study. In such situations, the institution has considerable authority over the investigator and the extramural funds, although the conduct and integrity of the study rests with the investigator and research team. If an investigator decides not to complete a study, the institutional authorities—with the permission of the funding organization—usually can transfer responsibility for the study to another investigator.

21. Is the research expertise of the investigator considered when funding decisions are made?

Without question, the research preparation and expertise of the investigator—or the lead investigator if a team is involved—are considered in the review of a research grant application. A scoring system of some sort usually is used by funding agencies, and several common areas of scientific quality measurement are considered in determining a score. Among these are the research question itself and whether it is on the cutting edge from a scientific perspective, design integrity and study feasibility, quality and expertise of the research team, resources available for the conduct of the study within the investigator's setting, and degree of innovativeness of the research. The expertise and research experience of the investigator can influence positively and directly the enthusiasm of a group of reviewers for a well-designed study. Similarly, a lack of experience can be a hindrance.

22. If I am just beginning my career in research, what type of funding is available?

Most funding agencies assume that preparation for a career in research begins with the completion of a doctoral program in an area of research. Nurses have doctorates not only in nursing research but also in related areas, such as social and behavioral sciences, epidemiology, physiology, and health services research. Several sources also provide small-scale funding to nurses who lack such preparation to carry out discrete clinical studies.

The National Institutes of Health provides funding for those who are in doctoral programs as well as postdoctoral research fellowships. These fellowship awards provide annual stipends but do not directly support the actual studies being conducted. Other sources of funding are needed. The National Institute for Nursing Research (NINR) is the best initial contact for a nurse with research training or a nurse enrolled in a doctoral program who is in the early stages of considering or implementing a research career. You can find information about research funding, the Institute's areas of research, and staff contacts for research areas at <www.nih.gov/ninr>.

After a new investigator has experience in research and in publishing the results, multiple types of research career development awards, commonly called K Awards, are available from NIH. Several require a research mentor who can provide guidance as needed and advice when sought. These awards can also be found through the NINR website. At this stage of his or her career, the investigator is beginning to build a small team of colleagues, such as statisticians, research assistants, and consultants, who also participate in the research.

Once the new investigator is ready for more complex research, the size of the study team increases with added investigators and other team members. At this stage the traditional NIH research grant, called the R01, is sought. This mechanism is versatile; some awards are small, whereas others are quite large, depending on the complexity of the study and the readiness of the research team and principal investigator.

23. This process seems quite complex—is it worth it?

Without question! Everyone who has had major research accomplishments and awards started at the beginning stages. It may seem difficult at first, but with time and experience it becomes second nature. It is also important to have your research reviewed and judged by peer colleagues; peer review leads to a better understanding of the quality of your own work in comparison to others and helps you to become known in the field of your research. Even Harold Varmus, former Director of the National Institutes of Health and Nobel Laureate, funded all of the research that lead to the Nobel Prize through NIH grants. Give it a try—colleagues are available to assist you.

BIBLIOGRAPHY

1. Reif-Lehrer L: Grant Application Writer's Handbook. Boston, Jones & Bartlett, 1995.
2. Ries JB, Leukefeld CG: Applying for Research Funding: Getting Started and Getting Funded. Thousand Oaks, CA, Sage Publications, 1995.

9. PUTTING TOGETHER THE RESEARCH TEAM

Kathleen Coen Buckwalter, RN, PhD

1. Do I really need a team to carry out my nursing research?

The answer depends largely on the size and complexity of the research project under investigation. Many people believe that the era of the investigator who works alone is past because the type of research questions now addressed by nurses require multiple skills and areas of expertise and access to diverse settings and populations. Nursing research can benefit from a variety of theoretical and methodologic perspectives as well as from collaboration with colleagues to share the workload.

2. What are the major advantages of a research team?

A primary advantage of a research team is the opportunity to blend team members with various types of expertise. Other key advantages include mentorship of novice researchers by senior investigators, facilitation of entry into data collection settings and obtaining IRB approval at research sites, access to subjects and subject recruitment to increase sample size, and enhanced resources that can result from pooled finances, equipment, or consultants. Collaboration means the sharing of talent, expertise, and workload.[1]

3. What are the most common models of research collaboration?

The most common form of collaboration is the **investigator-staff model**. This approach generally uses staff assistants for data collection and management. For example, a research project may require interviews with family caregivers of persons with dementia in a region of the country with a large Hispanic population. In this case, to overcome potential cultural barriers and to promote reliable and valid data collection, a research assistant may be hired who is Hispanic and speaks fluent Spanish. Often staff may transcribe or code data as well.

In the **investigator-team model** of collaboration a group of investigators forms a team to undertake research of mutual interest. Often this approach combines the expertise of researchers from several different disciplines (e.g., nursing, medicine, social work) or investigators with different areas of methodologic expertise (an expert in phenomenologic research and another in factor analytic statistical techniques).

A third model is essentially a combination of the first two: a team of investigators with staff assistants.[2]

4. What other schemes are used to classify forms of research collaboration?

Stone[3] defines the following forms of collaborative research: (1) intranursing, (2) interdisciplinary, (3) intrainstitutional, and (4) interinstitutional. Intranursing collaborative research brings together nurses with different areas of expertise to examine a research question, whereas an interdisciplinary collaborative research group includes researchers from various disciplines other than nursing. Research conducted by individuals within the same institution, such as one university hospital, is called intrainstitutional. A project that involves collaborators from different institutions, such as a multicenter clinical trial, is designated as interinstitutional research.

5. Is there a difference between an interdisciplinary and a multidisciplinary research team?

Although the terms *interdisciplinary* and *multidisciplinary* are often used interchangeably, subtle differences do exist. As adapted from Walker et al.,[4] multidisciplinary research teams handle different aspects of the research process independently and from their own disciplinary perspectives. Various aspects of the research problem may be subdivided and treated in parallel, with each team member responsible only for his or her own area. An interdisciplinary research team, on the other hand, suggests that team members from different disciplines approach the research process in a more coordinated manner, sharing mutual goals, resources, and responsibility for conduct of the research.

6. What characteristics are particularly important for members of an interdisciplinary research team?

Successful interdisciplinary research teams require that members are able to put aside traditional disciplinary concerns and engage in creative dialogue with other team members. The term *interpersonal competence* describes the ability of team members to appreciate the skills and uniqueness of others; the term *mutuality* describes team members who acknowledge and appreciate different ways of doing things and who value differences among the professions.[4] Willingness to negotiate and compromise to reach group consensus are important characteristics.[3]

7. What are the chief characteristics I should look for when inviting or hiring research team members to collaborate?

Effective research team members are able to do the following[3]:
• Accept new ideas and perspectives
• Be open and tolerant of review and critique
• Negotiate and compromise
• Function independently and interdependently
• Be conscientious in completing their assignments
• Be ethical, and able to trust and share their ideas with others

Research team members also need to be accountable and accept responsibility for their designated contributions to the research effort. Ideally, team members should care about the research goals, be able to have fun together and take pride in creating a team identity.

8. What characterizes an unsuccessful research team?

In contrast to the attributes listed above, unsuccessful research teams are characterized by inadequate knowledge and experience; poor leadership; poorly defined, ambiguous roles and responsibilities; conflicting goals; lack of openness; and poor listening and communication skills. Relational factors such as personality clashes and "power-plays" or "one-upsmanship" among team members also spell disaster.

9. Who should be on the research team?

The answer varies according to the nature of the research. The principal investigator (PI) should carefully analyze his or her own strengths and limitations as related to the goals of the research project and then seek to fill any voids with qualified team members who share a mutual commitment to the research objectives. For example, if the design of the project is complex and calls for data entry and statistical analyses beyond the investigator's level of comfort or available time and resources, it makes sense to bring on board a statistician as a team member or consultant. Likewise, if one aspect of the research project involves outcomes related to medication side effects in oral health care, it may be wise to include a pharmacist and/or dentist as members of the research team. To the extent possible, the research team leader should seek out colleagues with similar research philosophies and work habits.

10. Describe the optimal size and disciplinary composition of the research team.

There are none. Team size and composition are driven by the nature of the research as well as fiscal resources. Some projects may require only research assistant(s) who help the PI with discrete functions such as literature review or data collection activities. Others require interdisciplinary collaboration from a variety of clinical and methodologic specialists. Still other projects, especially those conducted in academic health centers, seek to involve students or pre- and postdoctoral fellows to provide them with course credit and/or experience as a member of a research team. Finally, to increase sample size or permit access to subjects and diversity among research participants, many projects need multisite data collection; in such cases, the research team by necessity is larger and embraces coinvestigators and collaborators from a variety of settings. Most multisite investigations require some form of external support to fund investigators at diverse locations as well as the means to meet and communicate with other team members regularly.

11. Describe other special considerations in the composition of a research utilization team.

If the purpose of the project is research utilization (RU), defined as a process of using research findings as a basis for practice,[5] rather than the conduct of research, staff nurses are essential members of the team. Staff nurses question current practice, identify practice areas that may benefit from examining research findings, ask critical questions such as "What does this mean for my practice?," serve as informal leaders, and champion the needed research-based practice changes among their peers. Staff nurses can also participate in the critique and synthesis of studies.[6] Additionally, RU teams should include advanced practice nurses (APNs) who operationalize RU activities by leading others in critiquing studies, synthesizing findings, determining what the findings mean for current practice, and implementing and evaluating changes in practice. Finally, nurse executives and managers are important members of the RU team because they set the tone and expectations regarding research and practices, allocate resources, and ensure an organization commitment to evidence-based practice. Some practice agencies are fortunate enough to be able to hire a nurse scientist who can provide consultation and direction for the staff related to RU activities.[7]

12. What if no one in my home institution has the particular expertise that I need to carry out the research project?

In this case, the nurse researcher may first investigate the interests of faculty members from nearby academic settings. Development of research consortia can be an effective method of sharing expertise and resources. For example, practitioners at three Veterans Administration (VA) hospitals in Iowa identified acute confusion as an escalating clinical problem. They developed a consortium with nurse scientists and statistical consultants at the University of Iowa College of Nursing to study collaboratively the incidence and prevalence of acute confusion (delirium) in patients and residents.

Once the problem and its risk factors were described, a multisite clinical trial was initiated to intervene in this pervasive problem, which is associated with high morbidity and mortality rates. Advantages of the consortium included the methodologic expertise of the nurse scientists in designing a rigorous study using reliable and valid measures and assistance with data collection and analysis. The consortium approach also enabled an increased sample size in diverse settings—in this case, two long-term care VA hospitals and one acute-care VA facility.

If no potential collaborators are available in the immediate proximity, the researcher may identify potential consultants by turning to meetings or directories of regional research societies, such as the Midwest Nursing Research Society or the Eastern Nursing Research Society, contacting experts who frequently publish their research in journals of specialty organizations such as the Oncology Nursing Society or Critical Care Nurses. Another potential source is the research directories of national organizations such as Sigma Theta Tau and the American Academy of Nursing, many of which have research interest sections.

13. Describe some of the unique challenges facing research teams.

When multiple people are collecting, coding, and entering data, concerns about integrity of the intervention and the consistency and accuracy of the data are paramount. Conflict and frustration can also emerge if some team members try to impose their own ideas or research ideologies on other members of the team. Finally, a major issue confronting most research teams has to do with authorship and publication/presentation issues. All team members must receive credit and recognition for their contributions to the research effort, and it is strongly suggested that authorship issues be agreed upon, in writing, soon after the research team is constituted. This approach helps to avoid misunderstandings and conflicts that can impede the collaborative research process.

14. What authorship guidelines are available for the research team?

The nursing literature identifies various patterns for assigning publication credit; no one method is "best." Among the strategies cited[1]:
- Authors listed according to extent of contribution
- Topic originator as first author with others listed according to extent of contribution
- Authors listed in alphabetical order with equal credit to all team members designated by a footnote
- Participants who need publication credit the most (i.e., academics facing promotion and tenure decisions) listed first with all other authors listed alphabetically.

Many nurse researchers prefer the approach outlined in the Publication Manual of the American Psychological Association (APA)[8] which states, "Authorship is reserved for persons who make a primary contribution to and hold primary responsibility for the data, concepts, and interpretation of results for a published work. Authorship encompasses not only those who do the actual writing but also those who have made substantial scientific contributions to a study." The APA recommends that the name of the principal contributor should be first in authorship, with other authors listed in terms of descending contribution. For additional discussion on authorship see Chapter 25.

15. What other guidelines for group research have been developed?

Based on her survey of 176 researchers, Thiele[1] developed the following guidelines for group research which she recommends each potential member of the group receive when considering participating in a collaborative research effort:
- Designation of principal investigator (PI)/group leader
- Responsibilities of the PI
- Responsibilities of team members
- Process for deciding authorship for articles or other written materials resulting from the study; where to submit abstracts for presentations/posters; presenter(s); recognition of efforts and contributions of members; acknowledgment of members' contributions to group efforts on written documents; and extension of the research and/or spin off projects
- Assignment of tasks
- Tentative time schedule of research
- Access to data by group members and nongroup members

16. What are the major responsibilities of the PI or research group leader?
- Ensuring effective communication among all team members
- Facilitating decision making
- Determining assignment of responsibilities
- Grant preparation, including budget
- Overall integrity of the data collection and analyses effort
- Preparation of all reports to funding agencies

Even when a statistical consultant is part of the research team, the PI must have sufficient knowledge of the research design and data to work effectively with the statistician, make sense of the findings, and interpret the data. The team leader is responsible for coordinating and managing all aspects of the research effort but may delegate such tasks as convening meetings and conference calls to a project director, if funding is available for such a position.[3]

17. What are the key responsibilities of research team members?
- To know their respective assignments in the research project (task clarity)
- To complete them in a timely and accurate manner
- To participate actively in team meetings
- To ask questions of the other members of the team when anything is unclear or unacceptable

18. What factors contribute to effective team meetings?

Convenient time and location for the research meetings are important for good attendance of all team members. Most groups prefer a set time and place, but in some circumstances both may vary to accommodate the changing schedules of team members, to rotate the location to make meetings more convenient for interinstitutional studies, or to observe new data collection sites. Other essential aspects include open communication so that all research team members have an opportunity to speak, an agenda to guide the work of the team, and accurate record keeping, including dissemination of minutes that reflect issues discussed and decisions made by members of the research team. A designated "secretary" who takes ongoing notes is an effective strategy. After the PI has reviewed the meeting minutes, they can be disseminated via e-mail attachment to all participants.

19. What special challenges must be overcome for effective multisite team meetings?

Although face-to-face communication between members of the research team is always desirable, it is not always possible. Especially for multisite studies, the majority of team meetings may be conducted via videophone or speaker phone. It is therefore critical to have all telecommunications equipment in good working order and to attend to such seemingly minor details as team members who reside in different time zones, so that all researchers expect the call at the same time. For one multisite study involving nurse researchers from the University of Iowa in Iowa City, the University of Minnesota in Minneapolis, and the Mayo Clinic in Rochester, Minnesota, the PI rotated the quarterly face-to-face meetings so that every three months team members traveled to Iowa City, Minneapolis, or Rochester and once a year met half-way in a neutral location. This approach takes planning and cooperation as well as budgetary considerations for travel, meals, and lodging, but it also sends team members an important message: all team members and data collection sites are important to the ultimate success of the research effort. Furthermore, the PI can better understand and trouble-shoot problems with personnel or research procedures at any given site.

20. What strategies help to maintain consistency of the research across sites?

The PI is responsible for the overall integrity of the research process. The data collection procedures and delivery of the intervention must be consistent at all research sites—a particular challenge when coinvestigators are located many miles away. Methods to deal with this potential problem include detailed written protocols/procedures and centralized training. If it is not possible for all investigators to come to a central site for training, alternatives such as videotaping "model" interviews with informants and showing the tapes to interviewers at distant sites until they become familiar with the interview protocol are acceptable. The off-site interviewers are then videotaped and their interview style critiqued by members of the research team and refined as necessary until their styles are determined to be equivalent to the style of the PI.[2] Throughout the course of the research project, the PI may also plan periodic visits to off-site collaborators, randomly select intervention visits on which to accompany research assistants, and spot-check research files and coding procedures for accuracy and comprehensiveness.

21. How often should the research team meet?

The answer depends on the stage in the research process and how well it is going. Typically, a research team meets more frequently (perhaps weekly) as the project is getting off the ground, because many methodologic, data collection, and sample recruitment issues need to be addressed. As the project progresses, data collectors have been trained, and code books have been established, team meetings may occur less frequently. However, effective research teams often report a pattern of "fits and starts"; that is, they may meet several times in quick succession when annual reports are due or when the team is preparing a presentation or poster for a national conference and then postpone meetings during periods of relative calm as long as the research objectives are being met. In any case, ongoing communication among research members is essential.

22. What factors contribute to retention of research team members?

Ideally all team members feel invested or "buy into" the project and its importance to improving quality health care. It also helps if team members feel rewarded for their contributions. Rewards can take many forms, including the opportunity to present findings at important regional, national, or specialty society meetings and authorship for publications related to the research project. Other forms of public acknowledgement, such as media releases and newspaper stories about the project, should include the contributions of all team members. Finally, letters to deans or hospital administrators that can be entered into personnel files are always welcome as a tangible sign of the value of a particular team member. The PI should make an effort to acknowledge and thank all research team participants personally and to celebrate their accomplishments and important milestones, such as birthdays or graduations, with a party or card signed by all team members at the end of a research meeting. One of our multisite projects had an associated research newsletter, which afforded an opportunity to highlight the contributions of various team members in a "Research Spotlight" column.

23. How can I increase research team membership when budgetary constraints are a problem?

Several strategies may allow the research leader to increase the size and diversity of team membership despite limited finances. For example, if the expertise of a physician is required for the research project, rather than hiring an MD as a consultant whose hourly rates may be out of range of the grant budget, consider contracting with a resident whose fees are probably less and who may be eager for the research experience. Students make excellent members of the research team as well as volunteers. In one of our projects on family caregivers, a retired RN who had been the primary caregiver for her mother for many years volunteered because she was so passionate about what we were trying to accomplish through our research project. As it turned out, her insight and compassion as a former caregiver added an important dimension to the research team. Another way to save money, especially with multisite studies, is to have team meetings at events such as national meetings, where the majority of researchers will already be in attendance.

24. Does the statistician really need to come to research team meetings before all of the data are collected and ready for analysis?

Absolutely. The statistical consultant should have input from the beginning, as the project is conceptualized, into such factors as outcome measures and design. The statistician can also conduct preliminary data runs to check for outliers and to uncover miscoding of data and disparities among data collection sites or individuals. Moreover, he or she can report preliminary data to the research team, giving members a sense of progress and accomplishment, which can be especially important in a longitudinal study.

25. Is it acceptable to bring new members into the research team midway through a project?

Membership on the research team should be fluid, especially if the team desires to continue to function past an initial project. Many effective teams have a core of key investigators with common research interests. This core is then augmented by other team members with particular areas of expertise. Other members may join the team for a designated purpose and period (e.g., a postdoctoral student working with one of the core investigators to enhance qualitative analysis skills for one semester on a specific research project). It is essential that expectations for role performance and length of association with the research project be negotiated before members join the team to avoid misunderstandings and conflict.[2]

26. How can research teams maximize their productivity?

The research team can increase the visibility of scholarly efforts and maximize the number of publications and presentations related to the research project in a number of ways. For example, the team should consider whether the "state-of-the science" review of literature, prepared as part of a grant application, would make a contribution to the field and, if so, seek to publish it as a separate document. Similarly, interesting clinical observations or challenges may emerge during the course of the project before the findings are analyzed and ready for publication. For example, in one study we conducted with rural, in-home family caregivers, two unanticipated issues affected our relationship with study subjects and the veracity of data collected. We believed that other researchers might benefit from our quandary and chose to share our research experiences in the literature. The first issue was related to the discovery of elder abuse during our in-home data collection and the fact that, as nurses, we were first mandatory reporters and secondly researchers. We wrote a collaborative manuscript on how we approached and resolved this ethical dilemma in the research process. The second issue dealt with denial on the part of several caregiver respondents (e.g., "Oh, John doesn't have dementia—he's just hard of hearing"). As a team we pondered the reliability and validity of self-report data from caregivers who were in denial and chose to share this issue and our team approach with other researchers in the field. Another way to maximize productivity of the team, but only with prior agreement of all members, is to allow researchers to select a specific aspect of the project and to take the lead in analyzing and publishing or presenting it as their own. This strategy is particularly useful for interdisciplinary teams; members may wish to publish articles in journals specific to their own discipline or present at conferences among their colleagues.

REFERENCES

1. Thiele JE: Guidelines for collaborative research. Appl Nurs Res 2(4):150–153, 1989.
2. Tripp-Reimer T, Sorofman B, Peters J, Waterman J: Research teams: Possibilities and pitfalls in collaborative qualitative research. In Morse JM (ed): Critical Issues In Qualitative Research Methods. Newbury Park, CA, Sage Publications, 1994.

3. Stone KS: Collaboration. In Mateo MA, Kirchoff KT (eds): Conducting and Using Nursing Research in the Clinical Setting. Baltimore, Williams & Wilkins, 1991.
4. Walker PH, Baldwin D, Fitzpatrick JJ, et al: Commentary. Building community: Developing skills for interprofessional health. Nurs Outlook 46(2):88–89, 2001.
5. Gift A: Nursing research utilization. Clin Nurse Spec 8(6):306, 1994.
6. Titler M, Kleiber B, Steelman V, et al: Infusing research into practice to promote quality care. Nurs Res 43(5):307–313, 1994.
7. Titler MG: Research utilization: Necessity or luxury? In McCloskey JC, Grace HK (eds): Current Issues in Nursing, 5th ed. St. Louis, Mosby, 1997, pp 104–117.
8. American Psychological Association: Publication Manual of the American Psychological Association, 4th ed. Washington, DC, APA, 1997.

10. WRITING THE PROPOSAL

April Hazard Vallerand, RN, PhD, and
Rosemary C. Polomano, RN, PhD, FAAN

1. What are the key elements of a research proposal?

Research proposals should include three major elements:

- The **statement of the problem and significance** provides an opportunity to describe the problem that you hope to study and why you think it is important. It should be a short, concise section that emphasizes the importance of the problem and ends with the identification of the purpose of the study. Your hypotheses or research questions should also be included in this section.
- The **literature review** should be comprehensive but limited to studies pertinent to the proposal. The literature review should systematically build a case supporting the need for your study. The theoretical framework or conceptual model guiding the study should also be discussed in this section.
- The **methods** section describes how you plan to conduct the study. It includes the research design; the sample, sample size, and how you will recruit the participants; the procedure and steps of the research and data collection; and data analysis methods.

2. Where do I start when writing the proposal?

The most important part of the research proposal is the research question. Research questions originate from a variety of sources. Usually a problem emanating from the experience or clinical practice of the investigator is the stimulus that initiates the question. Other potential sources for research questions are previous research studies described in the literature that identify the need for further study and problems derived from theory or conceptual frameworks. Replication (duplication of research studies) is another source of research questions that provides the opportunity to confirm or refute the results of previous studies. Identify a well-delineated question that is simple and has the potential for achieving the purpose of the research study. Once the research question is identified, the other elements of the proposal describe the need for the question and how it will be answered.

3. What should be included in the title and introduction?

The title should be short and concise and include the major variables to be studied. Many grant applications have a word limit for the title. The introduction should describe the problem in general terms and discuss the significance of the research problem. Then it should identify the purpose of the study.

4. How do I write my problem statement?

The problem statement should begin with a strong, factual statement about the problem to be studied. It should give general details about the problem and then move to specific information to justify the research question and guide the study design. The hypotheses or research questions should be listed. The potential contributions of the study to practice or theory should be described. The problem statement should end with the specific aims or purpose of the proposed research study. In most proposals, the problem statement should be no more than 1–2 pages in length.

5. How do I support the significance of the problem?

The problem to be studied should have the potential for contributing to nursing's body of knowledge in a meaningful way. The significance of the problem is supported by other research studies that have studied the problem or the relationships among the concepts of the problem. These studies should be cited in terms of background information that supports the need for the study and potential contributions that the study will make to theory or clinical practice. The studies should be presented in a logical manner, addressing each element of the problem and justifying the purpose for the proposed study.

6. What is the best way to write the purpose of the research?

The purpose is a single statement that identifies why the problem is being studied. It should describe the overall goal of the study and discuss what knowledge will be gained. The purpose should be written in a straightforward and concise manner, including the intent of the research, the key variables and possible interrelationships, the setting for collection of data, and the subjects. It should be stated as simply as possible, without jargon or abbreviations that might distract the reader from understanding the study's purpose.

7. How do I organize the literature review?

The literature review should systematically discuss what is known about the topic of the study and each variable or concept in the research question, describing the relevant research. Preparing an outline of the concepts to be included in the literature review is helpful in organizing the content. The literature review should begin with an introduction, present relevant studies, and provide a summary of the current knowledge. Headings and subheadings may be used to organize the literature to reflect the concepts of the study. The literature review may be organized chronologically, describing the history of the research on the topic, or in terms of general-to-specific information, building a case for the proposed study. Studies should be described in terms of what questions they answer and which questions are left unanswered. References should be paraphrased or summarized in the author's own words rather than using multiple quotes. The review of each study should include the purpose, sample size, design, and specific findings. A sentence or two should be used to summarize the findings of each study.

8. What types of articles are the most important to include?

Articles included in the literature review should contain similar research questions or research questions that address the variables or concepts in the proposed study. Theoretical articles may be used to support the general premises of the proposal. Research studies should support the relationships among the variables to be studied and the concepts of the study.

Sources are divided into two categories: primary and secondary. A **primary source** is written by the person or persons who conducted the research or developed the theory. A **secondary source** is a summary of research conducted by someone other than the original author. A literature review should contain a majority of primary sources, using secondary sources only when necessary.

9. How do I summarize the review of the literature?

The literature review should conclude with a section that summarizes current knowledge about the research problem being addressed. The adequacy of the previous investigations related to the topic should be discussed. Finally, any gaps in the literature should be identified. Some of the gaps or unanswered questions are then identified as those that the proposed study attempts to answer.

10. Is a theoretical/conceptual framework necessary?

A framework is the conceptual foundation of a study that guides the research process. A theory is often the stimulus for the research question. In addition, research findings may be used for theory development. In many studies, the framework is implicit and, therefore, not described by the researcher. Whether or not the theoretical or conceptual framework is explicitly described, the concepts of the study must be clearly defined. Research is used to build and test theories, but this goal can only be accomplished with a clear understanding of the concepts and relationships among them.

Not all research studies need to have a theoretical framework. Descriptive studies may be used to describe phenomena that will later be incorporated into a theory. The addition of a theory that does not fit the study is awkward and distracts from the significance of the study. The theoretical/conceptual framework should be chosen carefully for its fit with the research concepts.

11. How do I select a theoretical/conceptual framework?

Theories may be borrowed from other disciplines, such as the Health Belief Model or Lazarus and Folkman's Theory of Stress and Coping, or developed from the discipline of nursing, such as the Roy Adaptation Model or Orem's Self-Care Model. The researcher should relate the concepts in a logical manner. The framework chosen should be the one that best describes and explains the relationship among the variables. A review of multiple theories may be necessary to identify the one with the best fit.

12. What are the pitfalls of integrating a theoretical/conceptual framework?

Generally, your research questions will evolve from practice, and sometimes a framework helps to establish a basis for your research. If you select a theoretical or conceptual framework for your study, it must fit the research. A framework is intended to guide, explain, explicate relationships, and support the research; often a framework helps to generate testable hypotheses. However, even the most thoughtfully constructed framework has pitfalls. The following points outline the potential barriers:

- The theoretical/conceptual framework does not fit the research. There is a mismatch between the researchable problems and the framework.
- The researcher is not familiar enough with the framework and is unable to describe how the framework guides the research. The discussion may be so conceptual that it is not clear how it relates to the research.

- A framework is inserted into the research proposal and never mentioned again. In such cases, the researcher has not linked the framework to the research or the research findings to the framework. The framework becomes irrelevant.

If you are not sure whether a theoretical/conceptual framework is appropriate for your research, do not use one—or consult a senior investigator or faculty member to help you decide. It is acceptable to conduct research without a theoretical/conceptual framework. Sometimes a logical discussion of the rationale for your study that is well substantiated with findings from other research or documented evidence is sufficient.

13. What belongs in the methods section?

- The **design** describes the plan for answering the research questions or testing the study hypotheses. It outlines the fundamental strategies used by the investigator. Therefore, the design is one of the most important elements of the proposal.
- The **sample** allows the researcher to gain information about a small group that may be generalized to a larger group. The sample must be representative of the larger group to achieve meaningful results. The sample section should also include the size of the sample and describe the methods used to recruit subjects. The **setting** should describe the type of area from which the subjects will be recruited (hospital, clinic, community) and include other descriptors, such as location, that will help with generalization of the sample.
- The **instruments** section should describe each instrument to be used in the study. The type of instrument, the number of items, how long it takes to complete the instrument, the developer of the instrument, previous use of the instrument, and the reliability and validity of the instrument are usually included in the description.
- The **procedure** outlines what exactly will be done in the study (e.g., how the subjects are contacted and informed consent obtained, what is entailed in the participation of each subject and when, and how the instruments will be used in the study).
- The **analysis** section describes the methods used to analyze the findings of the study. The chosen statistical measures should be justified for each finding.

14. How do I describe the sample?

Clinical populations are diverse, whereas research questions are often specific. Therefore, you should clearly define who is eligible to participate in your study. Start by describing demographic variables and whether you are interested in sampling subjects based on age, gender, race, ethnicity, educational level, or social variables. If there are no restrictions on these variables, simply say so. However, you probably need to establish age limits for the sample. Many external funding agencies/organizations require investigators to be familiar with their geographic or reference population demographics (e.g., age, race, ethnicity). If you plan to preselect subjects, excluding or including them based on race or ethnicity, you may need to justify the reasons for doing so.

You can organize your discussion of sample characteristics by listing inclusion and exclusion criteria and address the following information.

- Number of subjects for the study. The number of subjects is usually determined by the study questions, research design, and number of dependent or outcome variables. Applications for human subject approval and funding often require justification of the sample size either by a power analysis or calculation based on previous studies. Seek help in conducting a power analysis to ensure that the proposed number of subjects will provide adequate statistical power to detect differences between groups or to find statistical differences between other variables. Typically, pilot studies do not require a power analysis, but you may need to explain how your results will yield the necessary information to design a larger study.

- Age range of population of interest. If subjects are excluded based on their age, you should explain why they are not eligible.
- Gender, race, ethnicity, and socioeconomic status. Specify whether any of these variables will influence subject selection and provide a rationale.
- Factors dependent on participation and completion of the study. Your study depends on subjects' abilities to participate; list all of the necessary attributes, characteristics, and situations that must be present in your sample. For example, subjects must be able to understand and read English if they are to complete a questionnaire written in English. For repeated or serial measurements, you must have access to subjects; they must be available for follow-up visits, accessible at home or by phone, or willing to complete and return mailed information.
- Condition of subjects. Will subjects be healthy volunteers or have a specific illness, disease, or condition? If the latter is the case, you must provide criteria for determining subject eligibility (e.g., known diagnosis documented in the medical record; diagnostic criteria; degree of severity of the illness, disease, or condition; treatment status). If your study targets subjects during a phase of their illness or treatment, explain why it is necessary to exclude other subjects or limit confounding variables (also called extraneous or uncontrolled variables) that may have an effect on your dependent variables.

15. Why is it necessary to describe recruitment strategies?

Offices of Human Protection and institutional review broads (IRBs) at colleges, universities, and health care organizations (e.g., hospitals, medical centers) require a detailed plan of how investigators or designees (i.e., data collectors) will select and recruit research subjects. External funding agencies and organizations also ask that this information be included in your grant application. It is also necessary to comply with recent federal mandates, such as the Health Insurance Portability and Accountability Act of 1996 (HIPAA), which imposes numerous measures to protect the confidentiality of patient information. First, state the type of sampling that will be used. Nonprobability samples include convenience sampling, which allows the use of readily accessible subjects, purposeful sampling, judgment or expert sampling; and quota sampling. Probability sampling refers to random selection of subjects. You should describe your plans for subject recruitment by including the following information:

- How do you plan to identify eligible subjects for your study? For example, do you plan to use a mailing list, outpatient clinic schedule, diagnostic or procedure codes, or another list to select subjects? Will you rely on health professionals to identify eligible subjects?
- How will you approach subjects for permission to participate? Will you ask the patient's physician for permission before you review medical records and

approach patients to ask for their participation? If you are studying a discrete population, it may be possible to meet with physicians or the health care team ahead of time to explain the study and ask permission to recruit all eligible subjects.

- Where will you recruit subjects? All sites where subjects will be recruited must be named and described (e.g., outpatient clinic waiting areas, inpatient units at the bedside).
- Who will be recruiting subjects? Persons recruiting subjects must be identified along with assurance that they will be properly trained to obtain informed consent and execute all study procedures.
- Duration of the study. The exact dates from initial subject recruitment to the completion of the study must be provided.

16. What should I include about human subjects protection?

Obtain your institution's guidelines for human subject protection and the application for your institutional review board (IRB), which provide a template for addressing all pertinent information for protecting human subjects. Because you will be expected to include a section on human subjects' protection in your proposal, much of the same information can be used in the written consent for human subject participation in clinical research. Guidelines vary among institutions, but most provide explicit terminology and wording to guide proposal writing. Several key areas that must be addressed to comply with ethical conduct and federal mandates are summarized in the table below.

Ethical Conduct and Federal Mandates

KEY ELEMENT	DESCRIPTION OF GUIDELINES
Statement of the purpose or intent of the study	This statement is typically part of the consent for clinical research or informed consent form. It answers the questions, "What is being studied?", "Why am I selected?", Who are the investigators?", and "What will this study do?"
Procedures to be followed	Outline exactly what subjects should expect as study participants in terms of time-sequenced events and subjects' expectations. Describe each phase of the study with a detailed description of all procedures, administration of questionnaires, and contact with the investigators and/or data collectors. Be sure to provide information about where and when study procedures will be implemented and an estimate of the time that is required to participate.
Risks and discomforts	Subjects must have a clear understanding of all risks and any discomfort that are expected during the study. These risks include physical (e.g., pain or discomfort with procedures), psychological (possibility of emotional upset or distress associated with eliciting sensitive information from questionnaires), social (inconvenience, additional travel or costs), or legal implications. Possible risks or discomforts that are serious or commonly noted in similar studies must be addressed.
Benefits	An unbiased assessment of the benefits to subjects and society must be clearly explained. If there is no immediate benefit to subjects but the information gained from the study will help others with similar medical problems or in similar situations, include a statement to this effect. Any reimbursement or compensation to subjects is not considered a benefit to participation.

(Table continued on next page.)

Ethical Conduct and Federal Mandates (cont.)

KEY ELEMENT	DESCRIPTION OF GUIDELINES
Alternatives	Explain the therapeutic or treatment alternatives if subjects decline participation. Subjects should be given the right to refuse participation, which should be addressed in the consent form for clinical research. You must add a statement that you will reassure subjects that refusal to participate will not affect or compromise their health care.
Time and duration of the study	Specify the exact time frame, including the day, month and year, for the entire study and how long each subject will be required to participate in the study.
Compensation	If no compensation for participation will be offered, simply state so. For studies involving financial payment to subjects, provide the amount, when the payment(s) will be made, and other conditions for reimbursement. For example, will full compensation be provided if subjects drop out of the study? IRBs usually require a statement that neither financial compensation nor free medical care will be provided in the event of physical injury resulting from the study. In other words, the institution is not responsible for any physical harm from study participation; but this statement should not infer that subjects waive their rights to compensation if harm results from negligence of any person or institution.
Statement of Confidentiality	Discuss how you will protect subjects' rights to confidentiality. List any subject identifiers (e.g., medical record number, date of birth, date of admission, discharge or clinic visit) that alone or in combination could disclose the identity of the subject. Describe how you will keep all records, data, or information about a subject confidential. For example, you will store all information in a locked secure place, limit access of the data to authorized personnel only, and remove the medical record number or other identifiers if data are released for analysis or published. You may be required to list the phone number of a patient representative who can be contacted by subjects for assistance and support.

17. How much detail should I include in the procedure?

The more detail that you provide, the easier it is for IRB members and grant reviewers to appraise the scientific merit of your study, appropriateness of your procedures, concerns over safety and confidentiality, and burden to the subjects. First, indicate whether training or education of staff or data collectors, pilot testing of instruments, and other preparation are necessary before you execute the study. Second, include the consent process. Third, detail every step of your study, including interventions or treatments that you plan to implement, all encounters with study participants, and what is expected of subjects during those sessions or visits. Refer to recruitment strategies to provide the level of detail that will probably be required.

18. What information should I include about data collection forms and instruments?

A complete description of all instruments and their psychometric properties should be included in your proposal. You must find out whether you need to obtain permission or a licensing agreement to use published instruments. If you plan to use an instrument that is not published or that you have developed your own, you should address how you will test the instrument in the context of your study. You will jeopardize your findings and the likelihood that your proposal will be approved by the IRB or funded if your instruments are not reliable and valid. All data collection forms used to obtain information about demographic variables, social history, or health history must be included in the appendix of the research proposal. This section should include the following:

- State the name of all instruments with original citations that reference the development and testing of instruments. A copy of all instruments should be included as an attachment with your proposal. If permission for use or licensing agreement is required, attach a copy of the agreement contract or letter from the author/group granting permission.
- Include citations from other studies that support the utility and appropriateness of selecting your instruments.
- Indicate the number of items for all instruments, the anticipated time that it takes to complete the forms, and any special instructions or assistance that will be provided to respondents.
- Include information about the psychometric properties (reliability and validity) of the instruments and the structure, describing the items, how they are measured, and subscales to measure specific domains or concepts.
- Discuss plans to modify an instrument or use it in a way that is different from the way it is intended to be used.
- Describe how all instruments will be scored.

19. Are consultants necessary?

Consultants can provide expertise that may not be available from your coinvestigators. Decisions to include consultants in a research plan depend largely on whether you need expert advice in designing your study, executing procedures, analyzing and interpreting your data, or preparing a manuscript for publication. Whether you can compensate a consultant for work on your project is a major factor in deciding if you need help. If no research funds are available to pay a consultant, you can ask a consultant to be a coinvestigator or offer authorship on any publication resulting from your study.

20. How should consultants be utilized?

Study consultants provide advice, guidance, and sometimes resources to support the research effort (e.g., statistical support). It is best to anticipate whether you will need a consultant while you are developing your proposal. Early involvement of the consultant can circumvent unforeseeable problems. Do not overwork consultants, especially if you are not offering compensation. Keep in mind that their involvement should be peripheral to the ongoing work of the project; they should be consulted only when expert input is needed.

21. How many consultants should I have?

There is no rule for deciding the number of consultants that are necessary for a research project. You must consider the following:

- What advice and expertise do you need to conduct this research?
- What expertise do coinvestigators bring to the project?
- How will a consultant strengthen your program of research and improve your chances for funding?

New investigators may require help in launching their research and should partner with a senior investigator who can guide the project from start to finish. You may not know if you need a consultant; ask a senior colleague. Too many consultants may spark confusion and disagreement about how the study should proceed. It is always a good idea to have a statistical consultant, if you need one, to help with data management and statistical analyses.

Choose your consultants carefully. If you are a new investigator, you may want to use a consultant from your own institution or nearby so that assistance is readily available. When you apply for external funding, a nationally recognized expert in the field can add credibility to your research and strengthen your proposal application. Many established researchers are eager to help new investigators, especially if you plan to use their instruments or study an area of similar interest.

22. How should I contact consultants?

Do not be afraid to ask a consultant for help with your research, even if you do not know the consultant. Many expert researchers are frequently asked to provide expert advice and are probably flattered. Before you contact a consultant, you should have a clear idea of what you plan to study and what you are asking of the consultant. Regardless of whether you know the consultant, you should have a written draft of your plan of study and be clear about what help you need. Helpful hints in contacting an external consultant whom you do not know:

- Try to find someone in your institution who knows the consultant. It is always helpful to ask about the person ahead of time.
- Be familiar with the person's work, including research publications in your area of research.
- Contact the consultant by phone or e-mail, introduce yourself, state the reason for the call, and ask if you can arrange a convenient time to discuss your research. If the consultant says that he or she is too busy, ask him or her to recommend someone who may be able to help you.
- When you have the opportunity to discuss your research plan, first tell the consultant about your clinical and research experience and the experience of your coinvestigators.
- Describe the project and indicate whether you will be applying for funding and the amount of funding you hope to obtain.
- Discuss how you think the consultant can be of help. Be clear about whether any compensation is involved. If you have or are applying for funding, ask the consultant about a reasonable fee for service given the limitations of your research fund. If no funding is available, you should agree to pay for phone calls, mailing expenses, and other miscellaneous expenses.
- If the consultant agrees to assist you, send a letter outlining the time line for the project and terms of the agreement. Of course, be sure to express your appreciation.
- Even if the consultant declines to participate, follow up with a letter of thanks.

23. Do all research proposals include a timetable?

It is not necessary to have a timeline; however, most investigators find them useful. First, a timeline that outlines the sequence of events from the start to completion of the study enables investigators to decide whether the time frame for the study is realistic and the study is doable. Second, a timeline helps to keep a project on schedule. Third, a timeline assists the principal investigator with mobilizing the necessary resources to complete the study. If you are applying for funding, you must read the Request for Proposal Application (RFA) guidelines carefully to determine whether one is required.

A timeline includes the anticipated time frame for various phases of the investigation, such as proposal development, IRB approval, training and education of research staff, purchase of equipment and supplies, recruitment of subjects and data collection, data entry, interim data analysis, final data analysis, interpretation of the data, and preparation of the final written report or manuscript for publication.

24. What details should be addressed in the budget?

All research budgets should include an itemized account for all study expenditures. A budget justification may be required if you are applying for funding. You must substantiate the need for each item in the budget and show how these expenditures are critical to the execution of your research plan. Budget categories generally include:

- **Personnel**. Direct salary support for the principal investigator, coinvestigators, data collectors, and other support staff with fringe benefits, if allowed. Add a cost-of-living increase based on the institution's projection for year-to-year budget requests.
- **Equipment**. Equipment that you need to purchase or lease, such as a computer or any piece of technology, should be listed. If you are applying for funding, the RFA should provide criteria for determining whether an item is considered equipment or a supply.
- **Supplies**. Include licensing costs for questionnaires, costs associated with interventions or treatments, computer software such as databases or statistical programs, envelopes, and stamps.
- **Consultants**. Establish an agreed-upon fee for their involvement.
- **Miscellaneous**. Include costs of reproducing surveys, questionnaires and data collection forms, phone calls, travel, and any other items not included in the above categories (e.g., payment to participants).

25. How do I estimate the costs of conducting my research?

Every attempt should be made to estimate all budget line items and resources needed to conduct your research. If you are not applying for funding, estimate costs and negotiate with your manager or administrator for the support that is needed. It is wise to get any agreement in writing. If you are not careful, you may start your research with insufficient funds and support from your institution to complete the project.

When applying for funding, consult a grant administrator or someone from your office of research affairs, if available, to provide needed information, such as salaries for personnel. Estimate all items that must be purchased or leased. For year-to-year budgets, you are permitted to add an inflation cost in subsequent years of the study. Be sure to check the RFA to see whether administrative or indirect costs are allowed. This item is a percentage of the grant budget added to your overall budget request; it is intended to compensate the institution for overhead expenditures. Usually a set amount is assessed for full recovery of administrative costs. Most small grants do not permit inclusion of administrative costs in your budget or use a lower rate then your institution's full indirect allowance.

26. How do I describe the methods of analysis of the study?

All data analysis techniques that you plan to use should be outlined in the proposal. First, describe how you will report information about your sample and demographic variables. For example, descriptive statistics can be used to calculate the mean age and standard deviation and frequencies for all categorical variables (e.g., gender, educational level, socioeconomic status). Second, discuss whether you will conduct test for reliability and validity on the instruments using your sample data and specify the psychometric tests that will be used. Third, indicate which tests will be applied to your dependent variables to answer your research questions. It is best to organize this section by listing each research question/hypothesis and stating what statistical tests will be used to answer research questions or test hypotheses. It is important to reference the statistical software that you plan to use including the name of the statistical package and company's location. If you have enlisted the help of a statistician, you should provide the person's name, credentials, title, and institutional affiliation.

27. What should go into the conclusion of the proposal?

The conclusion should reiterate the importance of the study. A short, concise section, reviewing the goals of the study and the impact that the results may have on nursing, emphasizes the need for the study. The conclusion should also describe potential future research that may be identified from the study.

BIBLIOGRAPHY

1. Brink PJ, Wood MJ: Advanced Design in Nursing Research, 2nd ed. Thousand Oaks, CA, Sage Publications, 2001.
2. Burns N, Grove SK: Understanding Nursing Research, 3rd ed. Philadelphia, W.B. Saunders, 2001.
3. Fain JA: Reading, Understanding, and Applying Nursing Research. Philadelphia, F.A. Davis, 1999.
4. Gillis A, Jackson W: Research for Nurses: Methods and Interpretation. Philadelphia, F.A. Davis, 2002.
5. Munro BH: Statistical Methods in Health Care Research, 4th ed. Philadelphia, Lippincott Williams & Wilkins, 2001.
6. Nieswiadomy RM: Foundations of Nursing Research, 3rd ed. Saddle River, NJ, Prentice Hall, 1998.
7. Pagano M, Gauvreau K: Principle of Biostatistics. Belmont, CA, Duxbury Press, 1993.
8. Polit DF, Hungler BP: Nursing Research: Principles and Methods, 6th ed. Philadelphia, Lippincott, 1999.
9. Wilson HS: Introduction to Nursing Research, 2nd ed. Redwood City, CA, Addison-Wesley Nursing, 1993.

11. ETHICAL CONSIDERATIONS: PROTECTING HUMAN SUBJECTS

Lisa Marie Bernardo, RN, MPH, PhD, and
David D. Shackelford, RN, BSN

1. What principles guide ethical and legal considerations of research?

Three ethical principles guide research involving human subjects: respect for persons, beneficence, and justice. These principles guide research from formulating the research question through study design, subject recruitment, protocol initiation, statistical analysis, and discussion of findings. They are explained in detail in *The Belmont Report: Ethical Principles and Guidelines for the Protection of Human Subjects of Research.*

- **Respect for persons** has two aspects: autonomy (the ability to act independently) and additional protection to people with diminished autonomy (e.g., children, prisoners). The Belmont Report defines an autonomous person as "an individual capable of deliberation about personal goals and of acting under the direction of such deliberation." In other words, if a person is capable of making up his or her own mind and making decisions of his or her own free will, the researcher must let the person do so.
- **Beneficence** is an obligation from the investigator and society. The two beneficent actions documented in the Belmont Report are: (1) "do no harm" and (2) "maximize possible benefits and minimize possible harms." The researcher must construct the research protocol in such a manner that the benefits of participation outweigh the risks. Keep in mind that the subject may not always directly benefit from participating in a study. The beneficiary of the study may be society if more knowledge about a particular disease, drug, or device is gained.
- **Justice** addresses the issue of who participates in clinical research. Subjects should not be chosen simply on the basis of easy availability; rather, subjects are chosen to represent the broad spectrum of society. For example, a researcher would not recruit from a minority population when the research leads to new drugs or devices that minorities would not be able to afford. In other words, subjects should be able to benefit from the outcome of the research once it has been concluded.

2. What are the highlights of current human subjects protection?
1948: Adoption of the Nuremberg Code
- Developed in response to the human experimentation done by the Nazis during World War II. During the Nuremberg Military Tribunal, the Nuremberg Code was regarded as the standard for human subject treatment.
- Key feature: "the voluntary consent of the human subject is absolutely essential."
1964: Adoption by the World Medical Association of the Declaration of Helsinki: *Recommendations Guiding Medical Doctors in Biomedical Research Involving Human Subjects*

- Key feature: The distinction between therapeutic and nontherapeutic research. Therapeutic research is generally experimental research on people suffering from an injury or illness, and the expected outcome is an improvement in their condition. In nontherapeutic research, healthy subjects participate in an experiment as controls; they are neither ill nor injured and gain no benefit from participation.

1974: Passage of the National Research Act
- The National Commission for the Protection of Human Subjects of Biomedical and Behavioral Research was established. This commission met from 1974 to 1978.
- Key feature: Release of the *Belmont Report: Ethical Principles and Guidelines for the Protection of Human Subjects of Research.*

1980s: Revision of federal regulations regarding human subject research
- Based on the National Commission's reports and recommendations, the Department of Health and Human Services (DHHS) and the Food and Drug Administration (FDA) significantly revised their regulations regarding human subject research.
- Key feature: The DHHS and FDA regulations have undergone several revisions to include increased protection for vulnerable populations and increased regulations for the study of investigational drugs and devices.

1991: Adoption of the Common Rule
- The Common Rule or 45 CFR 46 Subpart A is the Federal Policy for the Protection of Human Subjects. It originated on June 18, 1991 in the DHHS regulations that govern human subject research.
- Key feature: Until 1991, federal departments that conducted or supported human subject research did not have a uniform set of regulations. The FDA has adopted parts of the Common Rule and made changes to the regulations concerning the function of an institutional review board (IRB) and regulations concerning informed consent.

3. What is the International Conference on Harmonization (ICH) guideline for good clinical practice? Why should I follow it?

The United States, European Union, and Japan (the ICH) created guidelines for good clinical practice (GCP) that help to establish standards and ethics for international research. Simply stated, the ICH guideline for GCP is much easier to understand than the federal regulations from the DHHS and the FDA. Although it is imperative that the appropriate federal regulations are followed, the ICH guideline for GCP is quite descriptive about practices necessary within the scope of a clinical trial. There is little room for interpretation in the ICH guideline for GCP. Pharmaceutical companies may require the investigators to certify that they follow the ICH guideline for GCP because in some ways they are more stringent than the federal regulations. It should be noted that the FDA has taken quite an interest in these guidelines, and in 2001 the FDA's Office for Good Clinical Practice (OGCP) was established.

4. What are the major differences between the human subject research regulations from the FDA and DHHS?

The differences are outlined in the following table.

Comparisons Between the DHHS and FDA

DHHS	FDA
Allows the institutional review board (IRB) to grant a waiver of signed consent for research if certain criteria are met and if the greatest risk to the subject is a breach of confidentiality.	Has no provisions for permitting a waiver of signed consent.
Does not recognize research in emergency situations.	Provides explicit guidance on obtaining an exemption from informed consent requirements in an emergency situation.
Allows research on behavior or characteristics of individuals or groups to qualify for expedited review under certain circumstances.	Does not regulate research on behavior or characteristics and, therefore, does not recognize expedited review for this type of research.
Under certain circumstances, some elements of the informed consent may be altered or waived.	Consent forms must contain all required elements without being altered.
The DHHS has the right to inspect a subject's research and research-related medical records if the research falls under the jurisdiction of the DHHS. However, this fact does not need to be disclosed to the subject in the consent form.	The FDA also maintains the right to inspect a subject's research and research-related medical records if the research is regulated by the FDA. Unlike the DHHS, the FDA requires that the subjects are informed of this fact, and such a statement must be included in the research consent form.
If IRB membership changes occur, the DHHS requires notification.	The FDA does not require notification of IRB membership changes because they do not maintain files on individual IRBs.

5. Who are vulnerable populations in research? What can be done to protect them?

Vulnerable populations may not be able to give informed consent because of their age, mental status, or other attributes. Typically, vulnerable populations include infants, children, and adolescents; institutionalized children and adults; prisoners; and pregnant women.

The DHHS has provided additional protections to vulnerable populations. These regulations can be found in 45 CFR 46 Subpart B (Additional Protections for Pregnant Women, Human Fetuses and Neonates Involved in Research), 45 CFR 46 Subpart C (Additional Protections Pertaining to Biomedical and Behavioral Research Involving Prisoners as Subjects), and 45 CFR 46 Subpart D (Additional Protections for Children Involved as Subjects in Research). Detailed information describing these protections are found at <http://ohrp.osophs.dhhs.gov/humansubjects/guidance/45cfr46.htm>.

The FDA has also provided additional protections to children involved in clinical trials that are regulated by the FDA. These regulations can be found in 21 CFR 50 Subpart D (Additional Safeguards for Children in Clinical Investigations of FDA-Regulated Products). Detailed information describing these protections are found at <http://www.fda.gov/ohrms/dockets/98fr/042401a.htm>.

6. What is the institutional review board (IRB)? What is its role in research?

The IRB is responsible for reviewing the scientific merit and ethical conduct of research involving human subjects. This review process is to protect the rights and welfare of human subjects by selecting them equitably; obtaining informed consent; minimizing risks; and ensuring privacy and confidentiality (http://obssr.od.nih.gov/ IRB/protect.htm). No study should begin until IRB approval to conduct the proposed research study has been secured. Once approved, the IRB reviews the research study at least annually and whenever changes are made to the research protocol. Hospitals and institutions receiving federal funds for health care are required to have an IRB. Institutions generally have a separate board for review of animal research. Federal regulations require that IRBs be composed of at least five members. Membership must include individuals who have interests in nonscientific areas as well as individuals with expertise in scientific areas. Additionally, the IRB must have one member who is not affiliated with the institution and is not an immediate family member of a person affiliated with the institution.

7. When do I need IRB approval to conduct research studies?

IRB approval is needed for all studies involving human subjects. The process can be a full-board, expedited, or exempt review. A **full-board review** is required when human subjects receive a treatment or other intervention that involves more than minimal risk. Approval is obtained by majority vote. In an **expedited review**, human subjects receive a treatment or intervention that involves minimal risk and fits into one of the specific categories outlined by DHHS (see question 4). In an **exempt review**, the research involves human subjects' existing data or specimens that are publicly available and the information obtained cannot be linked to the subjects. A researcher cannot, however, declare his or her research to be exempt. Exemption is determined by the IRB. When in doubt about the need for IRB review and approval, contact your IRB chairperson for clarification.

8. What is HIPAA? How does it affect my research?

HIPAA is the acronym for Health Insurance Portability and Accountability Act. HIPAA regulations afford more protections to patients in the sense that their personal information will be guarded even more than it is now. There are also implications concerning consent, chart reviews, and recruitment. HIPAA regulations went into effect on 14 April 2003. For more information, refer to <http://www.hhs.gov/ocr/hipaa/>.

9. Define informed consent.

Informed consent means that a subject has sufficient knowledge and information to make a decision about participation in research. The general standard is that the information to be included should be what an ordinary reasonable person would want to know about the study. There are eight minimal requirements for informed consent according to the Common Rule. Individual IRBs may require additional elements of informed consent; check with your IRB to find out its specific requirements.

Minimal Elements of Informed Consent

ELEMENT	DESCRIPTION	CITATION FROM THE FEDERAL REGISTER
Study purpose and procedures are described	The reason for the study is stated. The procedures that will be done during the study are listed. The length of time that subjects are required to participate is identified.	"A statement that the study involves research, an explanation of the purpose of the research and the expected duration of the subject's participation, a description of the procedures

(Table continued on next page.)

Minimal Elements of Informed Consent (cont.)

ELEMENT	DESCRIPTION	CITATION FROM THE FEDERAL REGISTER
		to be followed, and identification of any procedures which are experimental" 45 CFR 46.116(a)(1).
Potential risks, and measures to modify the risks, are described	Any risks from the medications, procedures or other aspects of the research are described. The chances of having a risk factor are stated. Measures to minimize these risks are outlined.	"a description of any reasonably foreseeable risks or discomforts to the subject" 45 CFR 46.116(a)(2)
Potential benefits are described	Any benefits from participating in the research are described. If the subject derives no direct benefit from study participation, this should be stated.	"A description of any benefits to the subject or to others which may reasonable be expected from the research" 45 CFR 46.116(a)(3)
Alternative treatment, or procedures, are listed if appropriate	Subjects should be informed of options for treatment or procedures other than the research.	"A disclosure of appropriate alternative procedures or courses of treatment, if any, that might be advantageous to the subject" 45 CFR 46.116 (a)(4)
Assurances of confidentiality and/or anonymity are assured	*Anonymity* means that the subject cannot be identified. If the researcher can link subjects' names and their data, then anonymity is not assured. However, anonymity can be assured by not disclosing subjects' names or identifying data when the research is published. *Confidentiality* is protecting subjects' data and identities by locking and storing data appropriately. At times, the OHRP, FDA, or IRB can inspect research records, and subjects' data will be reviewed. Also, IRB members may contact subjects, but subjects are not obligated to speak with IRB members about their research participation.	"a statement describing the extent, if any, to which confidentiality of records identifying the subject will be maintained" 45 CFR 46.116(a)(5)
Compensation for injury	Monetary or other compensation for research-related injury is described, as well as who should be contacted if a research-related injury occurs or is suspected.	"For research involving more than minimal risk, an explanation as to whether any compensation and an explanation as to whether any medical treatments are available if injury occurs and, if so, what they consist of, or where further information may be obtained" 45 CFR 46.116(a)(6).

(*Table continued on next page.*)

Minimal Elements of Informed Consent (cont.)

ELEMENT	DESCRIPTION	CITATION FROM THE FEDERAL REGISTER
Right to refuse partici-pation; right to withdraw from the study without penalty is addressed	Subjects' participation must be voluntary, without coercion or fear of reprisal. If subjects withdraw from the study, they should continue to receive the same quality of treatment as other patients. Subjects must know that they can withdraw their participation at any time for any reason.	"A statement that participation is voluntary, refusal to partici-pate will involve no penalty or loss of benefits to which the subject is otherwise entitled, and the subject may discon-tinue participation at any time without penalty or loss of benefits to which the subject is otherwise entitled" 45 CFR 46.116(a)(8)
Offer to answer all questions is addressed	Subjects must know that they can contact the researchers with any questions or concerns. If they have any questions about their research rights, they can contact the IRB or the institution's patient representative.	"An explanation of whom to contact for answers to pertinent questions about the research and research subjects' rights, and whom to contact in the event of a research-related injury to the subject" 45 CFR 46.116(a)(7)

10. For what type of research must I obtain informed consent?

Almost all research involving human subjects requires their consent. If in doubt it is best to check with your IRB office. After the HIPAA regulations are in place, re-search involving patient databases or medical record review may require subjects' written informed consent.

11. Under what circumstances can informed consent be waived?

FDA rules allow no provisions for waiver of informed consent. Researchers can request a waiver of consent if the following four DHHS regulations are met:

1. The research involves no more than minimal risk.
2. The waiver will not adversely affect the rights and welfare of the subjects.
3. The research could not be practicably carried out without the waiver.
4. Whenever appropriate, the subjects will be provided with additional perti-nent information after they have participated in the study.

HIPAA regulations impart more circumstances that must be met. Refer to the Office for Civil Rights website in question 8 for more information.

12. How is a subject's informed consent obtained?

The most important point for the researcher to know is that informed consent is a process. This process is ongoing, beginning with the first subject contact and con-tinuing with each interaction. The process does not end until the research is com-pleted. Having a subject sign the consent form provides an historical starting point.

A subject's written informed consent is obtained by having the subject sign an informed consent document. For a treatment study, the subject and the researcher meet in person to review the research protocol. The informed consent document is reviewed step by step. The subject asks questions, and the researcher answers them; conversely, the researcher asks the subject questions to ensure the subject's complete understanding of the research protocol. Once this process is complete, the subject and the researcher sign the informed consent document; the subject dates the consent form. The subject is given a copy of the document for future reference.

For a survey study using telephone interviews, the researcher sends a letter to the potential subject explaining the research and stating that the researcher will telephone the potential subject to explain the study further. The researcher speaks to the potential subject and describes the telephone survey. If the potential subject agrees to participate, the researcher mails an informed consent document to the subject, who then reviews, signs, and returns it to the researcher. Once the informed consent document is received by the researcher, the telephone interview with the subject can begin.

In minimal-risk survey research, when a written survey is mailed to potential subjects, a letter that addresses all of the elements of informed consent is included with the survey. In this instance, the subject gives consent by completing and returning the survey. Because no identifying information is on the survey form, such a design is likely to qualify for IRB approval for waiver of signed informed consent. IRB approval for the waiver is possible because the major risk to the subject is a breach of confidentiality.

13. How is informed consent obtained from non–English-speaking subjects?

According to 45 CFR 46.117, "informed consent shall be documented by the use of a written consent form approved by the IRB and signed by the subject or the subject's legally authorized representative. A copy shall be given to the person signing the form." In order to best carry out this process, the IRB-approved consent form should be translated into the subject's native language. The translated consent form should then be translated back to English by another party. This is done to compare the two English consent forms for consistency and accuracy. Once the IRB has approved the translated consent form, a person who is fluent in English and the subject's native language should discuss the study with the subject. One of the study's investigators should also be present during this process to answer any questions from the subject.

14. How is informed consent obtained from a subject who is decisionally impaired?

Most IRBs have a policy in place for addressing this issue. When this situation arises, the IRB should be consulted to ensure that proper institutional policies are followed. Also, although many states have statutes that permit surrogate consent for medical procedures by use of a "legally authorized representative," few states address consent for research in the statutory language. An institution's attorney should be consulted before surrogate consent is considered as an option. One of the ways that informed consent may be obtained from decisionally impaired subjects is the use of an independent witness. The independent witness should not be associated with the study in any manner to avoid a potential conflict of interest; however, the witness should have a background sufficient to understand the study, risks involved, and what is to be expected of the subject once he or she is enrolled in the study. The independent witness should also have a background in research ethics and should have completed training in the protection of human research subjects. Ideally, the subject, his or her legally authorized representative, an investigator, and the independent witness should all be present during the explanation of the study and the presentation of the consent form. Once an investigator has explained the study to the subject and his or her legally authorized representative and the independent witness is satisfied that the subject's rights have not been violated and that the study has been completely explained, the consent form should be signed by the investigator, the subject's legally authorized representative, and the independent witness. When it is not possible to have all parties present, a telephone conference with the legally authorized representative may take place. The study should be explained, the consent form read, and questions answered. The consent form is then faxed to the representative, allowing time for the person to read it. Any questions may be addressed on the phone. The legally authorized representative then faxes the signed consent form back to the investigator. During this process, it is paramount to keep the subject's wishes in mind. The subject should retain the ultimate right to withhold permission to enroll in the study and to withdraw at any time during the study.

15. What special considerations are required for obtaining informed consent from children?

For children who are capable of understanding the study protocol and its potential risks and benefits, including discomforts, assent should be obtained. Assent is the child's informed agreement to participate in the study.[1] The study protocol is explained to the child in terms that he or she can understand. The child is permitted to ask questions and receive answers. Both the child's assent and the parent's consent must be obtained before any research activities are undertaken. In general, a child's lack of assent to research means that he or she may not become a study subject. The exception is situations in which a child can receive a potentially life-saving therapy only through study participation.

Subjects who were children at the time of study enrollment may remain in the study for many years. When they reach the age of majority, they must give informed consent to remain in the study; otherwise, the researcher cannot continue to collect the subjects' data. If the subject declines continuation in the study, the data cannot be used. (Data collected under valid consent can still be used. The issue is ongoing data collection or ongoing use of a database or tissue bank).

Additionally, when children are subjects in a study that involves more than minimal risk and no direct benefit to the participating child, federal regulations require both parents to give their written consent. Exceptions to this regulation include single parents; incompetence; or inability to contact one parent after reasonable attempts have been made. Parental consent may not be needed in research on child abuse and neglect if the researcher believes that the parents will not act in the child's best interests. The IRB must make special provisions to protect the children's rights. Foster parents cannot consent for foster children's participation in research studies.

Adolescents may consent to participate in research involving treatment of sexually transmitted diseases, pregnancy, and reproductive counseling without parental consent if the IRB has granted a waiver of consent. The FDA has no mechanisms in place for an IRB to grant a waiver of consent; thus, a researcher conducting a study of oral contraceptives would need parental consent. This is a topic of debate within the research community.

16. What additional factors should I consider when obtaining informed consent or writing informed consent documents?

The language should be at a sixth-grade reading level to ensure comprehension. The use of medical jargon should be avoided or at least explained in layman's terms. Ethnic and cultural diversity should be considered and respected.

17. To enroll a broad range of subjects for my research study, I need to advertise. What rules relate to advertising?

The FDA requires IRBs to review and approve advertising campaigns to recruit human subjects. The advertisement must clearly state that the subjects are being recruited for research and must include the following features[2]:

- The wording in the advertisement must not confuse standard clinical health care and research participation.
- The benefits for participation must be commensurate with the research protocol and consent form
- The advertisement must disclose aspects of the study design that may influence enrollment, such as the use of placebos.
- The advertisement states that risks involved in study participation will be disclosed before subject enrollment.

18. What is a data safety monitoring plan (DSMP)?

A DSMP is required for all research supported by the NIH. However, a vast majority of the pharmaceutical research studies also use large, external DSMPs. The DSMP addresses the following:

- Who will be responsible for data monitoring
- Parameters that will be monitored
- Plans for reporting serious adverse events
- Frequency of monitoring
- Plans for submitting DSMP reports to the IRB

DSMPs further protect human subjects. Depending on the type of research and the risk to study subjects, DSMPs can be either internal or external. Internal DSMPs are overseen by those directly involved with the research. External DSMPs are overseen by individuals with no direct ties to the research protocol.

19. Define adverse event (AE).

Most researchers recognize two types of AEs: a serious adverse event and an unexpected adverse event.

If the AE results in a fatal or life-threatening condition (or causes disability through blindness, deafness, loss of limb, miscarriage, or fetal defects) the AE is classified as a serious adverse event (SAE). SAEs also encompass such outcomes as disability, congenital anomaly, birth defect, or requirement or prolongation of hospitalization.

An unexpected AE is not normally associated with the study intervention and is not a common condition in the population enrolled in the research. For example, alopecia is considered an adverse event in oncology studies; however, this type of AE is expected. If a healthy subject enrolled in a hepatitis B vaccine trial experiences alopecia, it is considered an unexpected AE. This type of event should be reported to the study sponsor and the IRB, but, by definition, it is not a serious adverse event.

20. What is an investigational new drug (IND)?

An IND is a pharmaceutical agent that is tested in human subjects with permission from the FDA, as evidenced by obtaining an IND number. This new drug has yet to be proved safe and effective for a particular use in the general population and has not yet been given a license to be marketed in the United States. An IND number can be obtained only after an application is filed with the FDA and given approval.

According to 21 CFR 312.2(b)(1), the clinical investigation of an approved, marketed drug, however, does not require an IND application to be filed if it meets all of the following criteria:

- It is not intended to be reported to the FDA in support of a new indication or any other significant change in the labeling of the drug.
- It is not intended to support a significant change in the advertising of the product.
- It does not involve a route of administration or dosage level, use in a subject population, or other factor that significantly increases the risk (or decreases the acceptability of the risks) associated with the use of the drug product.
- It is conducted in compliance with the requirements for IRB review and informed consent.
- It is conducted in compliance with the requirements concerning the promotion and sale of drugs.

21. What are the differences among phase I, II, III, and IV drug trials?

When pharmaceuticals are tested, they undergo different stages, from limited use in humans to larger clinical trials then to postmarketing studies. The phases are as follows:

- **Phase I**. Phase I studies are dose-escalating trials designed to test the pharmacologic and metabolic actions of the drug in a human population. The maximum tolerated dose of a new drug is also determined, and side effects with increasing drug doses are monitored. The number of subjects for a phase I drug trial ranges from 20 to 100.
- **Phase II**. In this phase, the drug's effectiveness in subjects with the disease is evaluated in controlled clinical trials. Short-term side effects are monitored; toxicities are more clearly defined. Several hundred subjects may be enrolled.
- **Phase III**. Phase III studies compare a promising new drug treatment with established therapy in clinical practice to determine whether one is superior for treating a particular disease. In this phase, the drug is used as it would be administered when it is marketed to health care providers. At the completion of phase III, the pharmaceutical company can apply to the FDA for approval to market the drug. Several thousand subjects are enrolled, usually in randomized, blinded, controlled clinical trials.
- **Phase IV**. The final phase of testing may be required by the FDA to determine the drug's risks, benefits, and use. The drug may be administered to other populations; patients with other stages of disease; or over a longer period. Often phase IV trials are postmarketing studies.

22. How can I keep up with changes in regulations and rules so that my research is not affected?

Since October 2000, the NIH requires education on the protection of human subjects for all researchers receiving federal or other funding for research. Most, if not all, hospitals and institutions who have IRBs require all investigators, funded or not, to receive an education program on human subjects protection. Most often, this education is on-line and requires at least one hour's time to complete. Check with your IRB to learn about its education requirements for researchers.

23. What websites and list-serves provide updated information about human subjects rules and regulations?

- **IRB Guidebook**. Protecting Human Research Subjects: Institutional Review Board Guidebook. Available at <http://ohrp.osophs.dhhs.gov/irb/irb_guidebook.htm>.
- **FDA Information Sheets.** Guidance for Institutional Review Boards and Clinical Investigators. Available at <http://www.fda.gov/oc/ohrt/irbs/default.htm>.
- **OHRP.** Website for the Office for Human Research Protections. Available at <http://ohrp.osophs.dhhs.gov/>.
- **FDA.** Website for the Food and Drug Administration. Available at <http://www.fda.gov>.
- **FDA's Office for Good Clinical Practice**. Available at <http://www.fda.gov/oc/gcp/default.htm>.
- **CDER**. Website for the Center for Drug Evaluation and Research. Available at <http://www.fda.gov/cder/>.
- **Belmont Report**. Available at <http://www.fda.gov/oc/ohrt/irbs/belmont.html>.
- **Declaration of Helsinki (1989 Version)**. Available at <http://www.fda.gov/oc/health/helsinki89.html>.
- **The Nuremberg Code**. Available at <http://www.dallasnw.quik.com/cyberella/Anthrax/Nuremberg.htm>.
- **ICH Guideline for Good Clinical Practice (PDF Format)**. Available at <http://www.ifpma.org/pdfifpma/e6.pdf>.
- **45 CFR 46**. (DHHS) Protection of Human Subjects. Available at <http://ohrp.osophs.dhhs.gov/humansubjects/guidance/45cfr46.htm>.
- **21 CFR 50**. (FDA) Informed Consent Regulations. Available at <http://www.fda.gov/oc/ohrt/irbs/appendixb.html>.
- **21 CFR 56**. (FDA) IRB Regulations. Available at <http://www.fda.gov/oc/ohrt/irbs/appendixc.html>.
- **21 CFR 312**. (FDA) Investigational New Drug Regulations. Available at <http://www4.law.cornell.edu/cfr/21p312.htm#start>.
- **IRB Forum**. The Institutional Review Board—Discussion and News Forum. Available at <http://www.irbforum.org>.

REFERENCES

1. Conrad B, Horner S: Issues in pediatric research: Safeguarding the children. J Soc Pediatr Nurses 2(4):163–171, 1997.
2. Miller F, Shorr A: Advertising for clinical research. IRB Rev Human Subjects Res 21(5):1–4, 1999.

BIBLIOGRAPHY

1. Amdur R, Bankert E (eds): Institutional Review Board Management and Function. Boston, Jones & Bartlett, 2002.
2. Code of Federal Regulations, Title 45, Part 46.
3. Code of Federal Regulations, Title 21, Part 50.
4. Code of Federal Regulations, Title 21, Part 56.

5. FDA Information Sheets, Guidance for Institutional Review Boards and Clinical Investigators. Bethesda, MD, Food and Drug Administration, 1998.
6. Penslar RL: Protecting Human Research Subjects: Institutional Review Board Guidebook. OPRR, 1993.
7. Protection of Participants in behavioral and Social Sciences Research. Available at <(http://obssr.od.nih.gov/IRB/protect.htm)>. Accessed December 8, 2001.
8. Russell-Einhorn M, Puglisi T (eds): Institutional Review Board Reference Book. Pricewaterhouse Coopers LLP, 2001.
9. Sugarman J, Mastroianni AC, Kahn JP (eds): Ethics of Research with Human Subjects, Selected Policies and Resources. University Publishing Group, 1998.

III. Designing the Study

12. DESIGN OVERVIEW

Katherine N. Bent, RN, PhD, CNS

1. What is a research design?

A research design is a plan for how the researcher will study and ultimately answer the questions at hand. We plan and design studies to guide us in generating and analyzing data so that we can be more confident in the results. Research designs give us information about:

- **What** is being studied, known as the study variables, which the investigator may measure. In nursing we usually attend to more than one variable at a time. For example, we may measure the variables of age and sex of the patient, location or timing of a nursing intervention, or severity or change in patients' health concerns before and after implementing a nursing intervention.
- **Who** the study participants are. The participants may be individuals, families, or communities. Participants may be grouped according to an important variable, such as pain or no pain. Participants may be large numbers of people who enter the study in waves (called a *cohort*), based on a common characteristic, such as year of birth, type of treatment they received in the past, or exposure to a statewide policy change. Participants may be patients or health care providers. Describing the participants identifies the *unit of analysis*—that is, whether the study will report findings about individuals, an entire ethnic population, or an entire geographic community.
- **When** (how often and in what order) the researcher will observe the variables. The researcher may look back in time to measure past events—for example, the rates of leukemia in a community near an oil refinery. This approach is known as a *retrospective study*. Or a researcher may wish to measure what happens in the future after a new intervention is implemented to reduce anxiety. This approach is known as a *prospective study*.
- **Where** the study is conducted. Much of nursing research is done in the natural or clinical setting, not in the laboratory. It is particularly important for the design to describe the setting so that readers will know whether the findings of the study are likely to be similar in their own practice environment.

2. What are the types of research designs?

- **Level I** designs (exploratory-descriptive designs) identify or describe a concept, event, or experience that is important to nursing practice.
- **Level II** designs (survey designs) study how concepts, events, or experiences are related to or different from each other.
- **Level III** designs (experimental designs) explain or predict how a person will respond or predict events or experiences.

Each category contains several well-known and emerging study designs that are described briefly in the next questions and in greater detail in other chapters. Although these categories are assigned a numerical order, no level of design is better than another. Each research design has a distinct purpose and uses various methods to answer specific research questions. Research conducted using any design needs to be of the best quality, done accurately and with attention to detail and ethics.

3. How do I choose a design?

The best design is the one that answers the research question. Your question will be informed by what is already known about a topic. If not much is known, you want to explore or describe the issue. If more is known and a theory already explains how aspects of the problem are related to one another, you may want to use an experiment or quasi-experiment to predict what will happen if you change nursing care.

You should also take into consideration practical questions, such as cost and resources. Studies that collect data once or over a short period are generally less expensive than those extending over a long period. Available resources can influence the ability to conduct a study effectively. For example, if you have access to only one type of data, such as a medical record or a dataset collected for another purpose, you may be limited to descriptive, correlational, or comparative designs.

4. What level I designs are commonly used to describe concepts, events, or experiences?

Level I designs may be exploratory, descriptive, or historical. The purpose of **exploratory** research is to study a problem or issue that has not been studied before. Examples include studying well-known nursing concerns in a new population or a new concept, event, or experience in a population that has been studied in other ways. Although exploratory designs have become synonymous with qualitative research, quantitative methods may be used to answer certain exploratory questions. **Phenomenology** is the design selected by researchers who want to know what an experience is like, how it feels, and what it means from the perspective of people who have had the experience. A **grounded theory** research design is used when a researcher wants to investigate and generate theory about a process or social interaction. In **ethnography**, the researcher is concerned with understanding not only what is happening, but also how the norms and expectations of a culture contribute to the event, concept or experience. Ethnographic research may also yield a theory.

Descriptive research is used to describe an event, experience or concept accurately, thoroughly, and completely. Such designs give researchers an opportunity to confirm and validate what they may have started to see in an exploratory study. Descriptive designs can be either qualitative or quantitative; frequently a descriptive study includes methods to generate both qualitative and quantitative data. A descriptive study often has no theory guiding it. In such cases, the researcher faces the challenge of ensuring that a study is not only interesting but also adds to what we already know and can be applied to practice or further research.

As researchers use data from a study to describe an event, experience, or concept thoroughly and accurately, they may start to see how pieces of the puzzle are related to or different from one another. A descriptive study can describe what seems to be a relationship but cannot support a prediction about cause and effect in how the relationship works—nor can cause and effect be tested with a descriptive study.

The **historical design** is used to answer the question "why" about historical events or persons by reviewing data that already exist and to interpret why past events are important to current or future nursing practice. Findings from historical research studies illuminate the broader context in which nurses and nursing are located.

Pilot studies are generally conducted to determine whether and how to conduct a large study. A pilot study may be used to test and improve the ways in which data will be generated, the steps that will be followed to carry out the study, and the techniques that the researcher expects to use to analyze the study data. The inclusion of the pilot study as a research design is somewhat controversial, because a pilot study may or may not yield results that can be published or are useful to anyone but the researcher. However, it is important to complete a pilot study before applying for research funding, because agencies with money want to know that any serious flaws or unanticipated challenges can be addressed in the larger study, thereby saving time, energy, and their money. Pilot studies can be a valuable way to communicate "lessons learned" to other researchers.

5. What level II designs are commonly used to analyze relationships or differences?

After you or your colleagues have thoroughly explored an event, concept or experience, you may be able to publish your work. Next, you may want to ask questions about how the aspects of the phenomenon you have described are related to or different from one another. An important feature shared by level II designs is that the researcher is looking at phenomena exactly as they exist—the researcher does nothing to try to change the order or outcome of events.

A **correlational design** is a good choice if you believe that the variables are related and can support your belief with professional literature or other research. This approach is different from a descriptive study, because the researcher is not looking at all variables equally but has at least some reason or some theoretical framework for believing that the selected variables are the right ones to investigate. The data from a correlational study are quantitative and support conclusions about whether there really is a relationship between or among variables, how strong the relationships are, and how the relationships work. Is one variable influenced by another, or does it influence the other? The researcher also uses the conclusions drawn after analyzing correlational data to propose a theory about how and why variables are related.

A **comparative design** answers research questions about differences in concepts, events, or experiences (phenomena) of interest by contrasting groups that are as much alike as possible except for the focus of the research. An example is a study of smokers vs. nonsmokers. That the groups are alike in every other way is important, because the researcher can be more certain that any difference in health status is related to smoking rather than another variable, such as the patient's age. Before starting a comparative study, the researcher must have a strong theoretical framework that suggests how and why the variables are related. This theory is based on earlier exploratory, descriptive, and correlational research about the concept, event, or experience of interest. Using this framework, the researcher commits to a "best guess" of what he or she believes that the study will show or not show. This best guess is called an **hypothesis**, and the goal of the study is to test the researcher's hypothesis about what will happen.

Epidemiologic research investigates patterns of health or disease in an entire population. When the pattern is described at one point in time, the study is known as a **cross-sectional** study. When the pattern is described over time, it is known as a **longitudinal** study. Generally, epidemiologic designs use elements of other designs, such as correlational studies, although it is possible to have an experimental epidemiologic study. The results from epidemiologic studies are used to develop interventions, but because the focus is an entire population, the intervention is usually a program rather than individual treatment.

For some researchers, the **case study** is a research design; for others, it is simply what the researcher has chosen to study. The researcher may study an individual person, hospital unit, geographic community, clinic, or state, but she or he is ultimately interested in how and why this single case can instruct about and illustrate the phenomenon of interest. If you read case study reports, you can expect also to learn about the historical background of the case, the context of the case and how it relates to other cases, and the persons who were part of the study.

In a **methodologic study**, a researcher develops and tests new instruments, such as standardized tests or surveys, that will be used to gather data in research or practice. Any tool has to measure what we think it measures (known as **validity**) and must do so time after time (known as **reliability**) in a precise manner (known as degree of measurement error). Less measurement error results in better reliability and validity. Much of the effort a researcher puts into methodologic work is designed to reduce the amount of measurement error in a tool.

6. What level III designs are commonly used for explaining cause and effect or for making predictions?

An **experimental design** is used to test a theory by predicting what will happen to one variable if another variable is changed. One group of subjects receives an intervention or treatment and another group does not; which group an individual subject is assigned to is completely random. The researcher maintains tight control over what happens to each group, ensuring that the group that is not supposed to get any treatment in fact does not. Although this tight control allows the researcher to know that the intervention or treatment resulted in the observed effect, such control is difficult to maintain in the real world of clinical nursing. Experimental designs may test the effect of one independent variable on one dependent variable (classic) or the effects of several independent variables on several dependent variables. They also may test the ways in which the independent variables may influence each other in addition to the dependent variable.

The goals of a **quasi-experimental design** may be the same as those of an experiment, but the researcher has less control over some of the independent variables that are expected to have an effect. This design is particularly useful in the real world of nursing practice, where ethical or other practical concerns prohibit the researcher from randomly assigning study volunteers to different groups.

7. How are research questions formulated based on study design?

The table on the following page summarizes the major levels of research designs and gives examples of research questions that might be asked with different designs.

Common Research Designs

LEVEL	GOAL OF THE RESEARCH	DESIGN AND POSSIBLE RESEARCH QUESTION
Level I: exploratory-descriptive designs	Identify or describe a concept	Grounded theory: What is the process of decision making around moving to a nursing home? Ethnography: Is the experience of transition to a nursing home different for rural and urban populations? For Anglo and Hispanic populations? Phenomenology: What is it like to move to a nursing home? Historical: How have processes and experiences of transitions to nursing homes changed since nursing homes were first created? Pilot: Will this study of an intervention to improve sleep disruption by staging transition to a nursing home actually work?
Level II: survey designs	Compare similarities or differences in phenomena, predict a relationship	Correlational: Is there a relationship between moving to a nursing home and sleep disruption? Comparative: Does transition to a nursing home create or increase sleep disruptions? Epidemiologic • Cohort (looking forward from today): How many nursing home residents will develop sleep disruption in their first month in a new nursing home? • Case-control (looking back in time): How many nursing home residents with a sleep disruption have moved to the nursing home in the past month?
Level III: experimental designs	Test theory or prediction to explain a phenomenon	Experiment: Does a staged transition into a nursing home decrease sleep disruption in the first month? Quasi-experiment: Does a staged transition into a nursing home decrease sleep disruption in the first month?

8. Explain manipulation and control.

These terms refer to how well a particular research study will be able to explore cause-and-effect relationships in phenomena. When a researcher has total **control** over the intervention or treatment in a study and can **manipulate** the study so that some subjects receive the intervention or treatment and some do not, the researcher is better able to use the results of the study to predict what will happen if a patient receives or does not receive the intervention or treatment. Research has its own language; most research texts include a glossary of terms to which you can refer as often as needed.

9. What if different parts of more than one design seem to make sense for the question that I plan to ask?

Often you can successfully mix and match elements of various designs. The epidemiologic study may ask questions about how variables are related (correlational) and how they are different (comparative). The descriptive study not only studies the meaning and nature of a health experience but also identifies how many people have had this experience to makes a case for why we should be doing more research. A pilot study is an excellent opportunity to do a test run of your design, and you should plan to include the pilot within your overall study design. It is also not unusual for a researcher to combine elements of designs in ways that increase the rigor of the study and improve the results while also making it more doable. The key to successful research is that the design will answer your research question and make the best use of what we already know about a concept, event, or experience.

10. Which of these designs are commonly used in nursing research?

Nurse researchers have been instrumental in efforts to expand the definition of research to mean more than just experiment. Because of our interest in human health experiences, events, and phenomena, nurses are able to conduct many kinds of studies to answer questions about such issues. Nurse researchers who wish to understand the context of an event, experience, or phenomenon or the meaning of an experience or phenomenon are likely to use exploratory, descriptive, epidemiologic, or other designs that are not experimental.

There are also important new designs that nurse researchers are developing or refining to study the complex concepts of health, person, environment, and nurse caring. These designs may be based on important philosophies and conceptual frameworks, such as feminism, complexity science, critical theory, ethics, and post-modernism.

Nurse researchers who wish to make predictions about health experiences or explain the cause-and-effect relationship between events or experiences are likely to use quasi-experimental designs for research. Experimental designs are used infrequently in nursing, because in the natural setting of nursing practice and care, it is difficult or unethical to achieve the necessary level of control. Control is often limited in the world of practice; the researcher examines the variable or phenomenon as it exists.

It is common for nurse researchers to combine designs in a study. This approach is known as **triangulation**. Although it seems to offer the best of both worlds, it can be controversial. On the one hand, we get a better understanding of the phenomenon of interest. On the other hand, the basic philosophy of "understanding" is quite different from the basic philosophy of "controlling." Some researchers believe that the two cannot be mixed in a single study.

11. How is design different from methods?

The design is the plan; the method is how the design is implemented to learn about the research question. Methods are the ways in which the researcher generates data (e.g., interviewing, observing, performing health assessments, administering surveys or questionnaires), and uses data that already exist (e.g., medical records, Geographic Information Systems [GIS] measures, newspaper reports).

12. What is the difference between qualitative and quantitative?

The terms *qualitative* and *quantitative* are used in many different ways and can confuse a new researcher. They refer to the type of data generated and analyzed in a study. Quantitative data are numerical and are generated in research designs at all levels, whereas qualitative data may be verbal or esthetic (e.g., photos, murals) and are generated primarily in descriptive or exploratory studies. Both qualitative and quantitative data are based on the general belief that a human experience can be communicated to others, whether by rating an experience on a scale from 0 to 10 or describing the experience with words or other artistic expressions. We accept that the numbers and words are a substitute for the experience and not the experience itself. Some designs, such as ethnography, grounded theory, phenomenology, or narrative inquiry, rely on methods that yield qualitative data and are known as qualitative designs.

It is less correct to refer to a method of gathering data as qualitative or quantitative. For example, interviews are not qualitative, but the answers to interview questions may be qualitative. Although people generally associate interviews with qualitative data, a subject could be asked to list the number of times that she or he ate green vegetables in the last week. Such answers are quantitative data. Observations about whether the person was uncomfortable answering the question, avoided eye contact, took a long time to answer, or answered quickly are qualitative data.

13. Do I need a design if I simply want to do a few statistics?

Certainly you can collect data, enter them into a computer, and run statistical tests without developing a design; this may be the extent of what you need for a quality improvement project. You have to know what you give up, however. When you run statistics without linking your questions to existing theory and knowledge, the numbers that you get after running statistics will not have much meaning outside the current project. For this reason, such data may be appropriate for quality improvement but not for research. This is not to say that the data and results are worthless. On the contrary, they may give you important information about a clinical or process problem in your practice. But it is unlikely that someone else with a similar problem will be able to apply your data directly to their own practice. They may be able to learn about what steps to take to make a problem visible to others in their agency, but they will need their own data to make conclusions about issues in their own setting. Furthermore, unless a project has been reviewed by an institutional review board (IRB), the data that you collect and analyze cannot be published. Many scholars advocate for a skillful and knowledgeable blend of quality improvement strategies with research principles to facilitate better and easier utilization of research in practice and improved program evaluation.

14. Do I have to be concerned with ethics when selecting a research design or only when conducting the study?

Ethical considerations underlie any choice of research design. Some studies are unethical in any situation, such as those that actively deprive participants of necessary health care or nutrition. A study about the health effects of keeping children out of school can be conducted only if children did not attend school for some other reason; we cannot keep children out of school for the sake of an investigation. Any design should adequately protect the rights of the participants, including but not limited to the right to choose to participate and to understand fully what that choice is about, the right to privacy, the right to confidentiality or anonymity, and freedom from feeling forced to participate.

15. How are research and theory related?

When a phenomenon is new or not well understood, we use research to identify what is going on and to describe it carefully and with as much precision as possible. After we describe what we are looking at, how often it happens, how serious or important it is, and whether it always happens in the same way, we can start to ask and answer questions about how elements of the phenomenon are related and how the phenomenon is related to other phenomena that we know about.

Theories are simply our ideas about how concepts (the phenomena of experiences, ideas, and events) are related. Early research describes the concepts that become the building blocks of theory and how the concepts might fit together or be related, and later research aims to test these ideas to see whether they are correct. With enough research, we may come to accept a theory or decide that we need to do a better job describing the details of how the concepts are related and how the blocks fit together. Then we do more research to test the modified theory. Without theory, we do not know what to research; without research, we do not know whether our theories are correct or helpful.

16. Do I need to write down the design?

You need to describe and document your design for several reasons. Most importantly, you can use it as you would use a map. It helps guide your research. You also need to document the design if you apply for funding, when you apply for human subjects approval, and when you submit results for publication. You provide everyone who reads your proposal or report with the information necessary to determine whether the study was well designed to answer the research question, whether you have minimized the problems with the study, and how to use the results in practice.

17. Does the design ever change in the middle of the research project?

If you are conducting a study with an exploratory design, you may expect certain elements of your plan to change as you progress. Examples may include the people to whom you talk or the situations that you observe. For example, the more you explore a topic, the more you believe it is important to observe a particular situation. In exploratory studies, the researcher is considered the instrument of gathering data. And as a human, you are more than a survey. Although a survey does not change while someone is answering the questions, the researcher may change the questions in an interview in response to the context of the interview, other people, or the researcher's own situation.

Other types of investigations, no matter how much thought you put into designing your study, will raise questions or issues that you did not expect. One of the primary reasons for conducting a pilot study is to identify such problems in design and methods in advance and to test whether the study is really doable. By conducting a pilot study, the researcher in essence gives him or herself permission to modify the design early rather than struggle with problems that are costly and time-consuming later during the investigation.

Occasionally, despite a researcher's best efforts, the design may change in the middle of a study. Perhaps the researcher does not have as much control over the setting as expected. Some studies have been stopped for ethical reasons. It is also possible that you design a study and plan a certain kind of statistical test to analyze the data. But, because of the rules of statistics, the data that you gather may not be useable for the analyses that you wish to do. Usually you can do other statistical tests with the data that you have, but the change in data and analysis may change the conclusions that you can reach about the topic. What was to be an experiment may become a descriptive study.

18. Is there such thing as a wrong design?

A design is considered "wrong" if it is unethical or will not answer the research questions. For example, a survey that asks participants to rank twenty events from the most to the least stressful may provide information for the nurse seeking to modify stressful situations in the practice area, but it will not answer questions about coping with stress.

19. Where can I get help in designing a study?

Many helpful resources may be available to nurses interested in research. Examples include nurse researchers and other researchers who work where you work. They may have clinical responsibilities or work exclusively in research. Nurses interested in research frequently attend and are active in professional organizations; when you join and participate in your professional organization, you develop relationships with them and benefit from their presentations to your group or other groups. Professional organizations frequently bring in speakers who present research in membership programs.

Other people in organizations where nurses work may not be researchers, but they generally possess good analytic skills and can help you think about data. They may work in the business office, quality improvement program, information department, or epidemiology division of a public or community-focused care setting. If journal clubs are available where you work, they are a great way to learn about research, as are nursing research committees or practice committees that explicitly address evidence-based criteria.

You can find resources not only in the school of nursing, but also in other departments of a local college or university. Many faculty conduct and teach research and have or can recommend resources for interested nurses. Colleges and universities have reference librarians who can help you find research journals and texts in their collection and access resources from other places. Librarians can also help you with online resources. The sheer volume of information available online can be overwhelming, and a reference librarian can help you use your time online wisely and evaluate the quality of what you find online.

BIBLIOGRAPHY

1. Brink P, Wood MJ: Advanced Design in Nursing Research, 2nd ed. Thousand Oaks, CA, Sage, 1998.
2. King KM, Teo KK: Integrating clinical quality improvement strategies with nursing research. West J Nurs Res 22:596–608, 2000.
3. Playle J: Research designs: The survey. J Comm Nurs 14(6):17–18, 2000.
4. Polit DF, Beck CT, Hungler BP: Essentials of Nursing Research: Methods, Appraisal and Utilization. Philadelphia, Lippincott Williams & Wilkins, 2001.
5. Van-Teijlingen ER, Rennie A, Hundley V, Graham W: The importance of conducting and reporting pilot studies: The example of the Scottish Births Survey. J Adv Nurs 34:289–295, 2001.

13. EXPERIMENTAL DESIGNS

Sandra G. Funk, PhD

1. What is the purpose of experimental designs?

The goal of most nursing and health-related research is to find ways to improve health outcomes—to devise new interventions and care-delivery systems that maximize health and quality of life. But before implementing innovations in practice, we need some assurance that they work. Are they having the desired effect? Is the effect large enough to be meaningful? Studies are needed to evaluate the impact of the interventions and rule out alternative explanations for any changes that occur. This is what experimental designs are intended to do —to determine cause and effect. They evaluate whether changes measured in patient outcomes can reasonably be attributed to the experimental manipulation (i.e., the intervention) and not to other causes.

2. What conditions need to be met before causation can be determined?

For cause and effect to be determined:
- There must be a relationship between the potential cause (the intervention) and the potential effect (patient outcomes). This relationship must be supported by more than just the investigator's belief that it exists. Ideally, one will have both empirical evidence from the literature and a theoretical basis to help explain how the causal variable impacts the outcome.
- There must be an appropriate time order—the cause must precede the effect.
- Plausible alternative explanations for the observed outcomes must be ruled out. A change may be noted in patient outcomes, but was the change due to the intervention? Can other factors explain how the change came about?

3. How do experimental designs meet these criteria?

Experimental designs meet these criteria through:
- Manipulation
- Inclusion of control groups
- Random selection
- Random assignment
- Measurement over time
- Strict adherence to the established research protocol
- More advanced techniques, such as statistical controls, are addressed in texts such as Pedhazur and Schmelkin.[1]

The control provided by these approaches enhances the probability that changes observed in patient outcomes can be attributed to the presumed cause (the intervention) and not to other factors. This characteristic is known as **internal validity**. Approaches such as random selection enhance the ability to generalize the study's results to the population of interest, increasing its **external validity**.

4. What are the main threats to internal validity?

Most major research texts review the threats in detail (e.g., Polit and Hungler,[2] Pedhazur and Schmelkin[1]), but for the seminal work in this area refer to Campbell and Stanley's book[3] about experimental and quasi-experimental designs and Cook and Campbell's book[4] on quasi-experimentation. Key factors that might hinder one's ability to determine cause and effect include:

- **Maturation**. Humans change all the time—aging, getting more or less physically fit, perhaps getting sicker. Such changes occur as a function of time and may affect outcomes in the study or interact with the intervention.
- **History**. During the course of the study, new events occur in the world and subjects' lives that may alter outcomes. For example, if your study focuses on prostate cancer screening for older men and a major national initiative in this area is undertaken at the same time, it may become difficult to distinguish the effects of the study intervention from those of the national initiative.
- **Diffusion of treatment**. This threat occurs when control-group subjects unintentionally receive the intervention. Perhaps experimental subjects share their experiences with those in the control group, or perhaps health care providers become enamored of the intervention before the conclusion of the study and begin to implement it in practice.
- **Selection**. This threat occurs when the process of assigning subjects to study groups introduces bias, resulting in groups that differ at the outset of the study.
- **Mortality**. This threat results from differential attrition of subjects between the experimental and control groups over the course of the study. Attrition occurs for many reasons (lack of interest, moving away, change in health status, negative reaction to the intervention, or even death). When subjects leave the study groups at different rates, the groups that you wish to compare can no longer be considered comparable.
- **Testing**. When subjects are measured repeatedly over time, their later responses may be affected by their earlier responses—perhaps from remembering how they responded earlier, from "learning" the instrument, or being sensitized to a topic they had not previously thought much about.
- **Instrumentation**. If, over the course of a study, changes occur in the tools that are used, in their calibration, or in how subjects are observed or scored, changes in subjects' outcomes may be an artifact of instrumentation changes rather than the result of the intervention.

5. **What are the main threats to external validity?**

Many factors may influence the ability to generalize to the larger population, but two key threats are:

- **Systematic bias in selecting subjects to participate in the study**. To generalize from the study to the larger population, the subjects must be representative of that population. As discussed below, random selection is the most accepted approach to eliminating bias.
- **Artificiality of the experiment itself**. The characteristics of the experiment itself have an impact on the outcomes—outcomes that may not occur outside the confines of the study situation. For example, one usually tries to control as many extraneous factors as possible to determine cause and effect. But in the real world, all of these factors come into play; the results in the refined environment of the experiment may not be found in a more real world situation.

6. What is meant by manipulation?

Manipulation refers to the fact that the investigator alters something about the environment or care that some of the study participants receive. Typically, the alteration is an intervention that the investigator has designed and wishes to assess. Subjects receiving the intervention form one or more groups in the study design. If there is only one form of intervention, there is only one experimental (i.e., intervention) group. However, sometimes the investigator wishes to test variations in the intervention—perhaps comparing an intervention for the patient alone with an intervention for both the patient and his or her family. Thus, the number of experimental groups depends on how many different manipulations the investigator wishes to test. The more groups you have in your design, the more subjects you need in your study. But remember, the groups formed by the experimental manipulations, along with the control group, form the independent variable for the study.

7. Why are control groups important?

The inclusion of control group(s) is the hallmark of the strongest experimental designs, for it is through comparison of the experimental and control groups that one learns whether the intervention makes a difference. The control group (or groups) consist of subjects who do *not* receive the intervention. They provide the best estimate of what would have happened to the experimental subjects if you had not intervened. Without a control group, one must assume that no change would have occurred in the experimental subjects if they had not had your intervention. But humans are always changing, constantly bombarded by new information. Comparing experimental and control groups tells you how much more the experimental subjects changed than the control subjects, thereby reducing the threats of history and maturation.

The fact that the control group does not receive the intervention does not necessarily mean that control subjects receive nothing. Indeed, subjects in the control group most often receive usual care, whereas subjects in the experimental group receive the intervention in lieu of or in addition to usual care. Sometimes merely the extra attention received by experimental subjects can be expected to affect outcomes. To rule out this possibility, subjects in the control group are often given an "attentional" intervention—an equivalent amount of contact with study personnel in which they may be given an intervention unrelated to the study—for example, a general health information intervention.

8. What does random selection mean?

It is not always clear that there are two different kinds of randomization. The first is random selection—a strategy for selecting subjects to participate in the study. Because most studies are conducted to draw conclusions that will be applicable beyond the small group of subjects studied, the subjects must be selected in a way so that they represent the larger group (or population) to which one wishes to generalize. For example, if you wish to test an intervention for children with cystic fibrosis, you have to be careful to select study subjects that represent the range of children with cystic fibrosis. It is also important to minimize any biases that may be introduced if subjects are selected purposively. Random selection from the population being studied is the recommended strategy for subject selection. Random selection enhances the chance for representativeness, minimizes the chance for bias, and increases one's confidence that the results can be generalized to the larger population, thus increasing the study's external validity.

However, to randomly select study subjects, one must be able to enumerate all individuals in the target population so that each has an equal chance of being drawn to participate in the study. Unfortunately, all members of many study populations— for example, all women with breast cancer, all cardiac rehabilitation patients, or all patients experiencing pain—are rarely known. Therefore, they cannot be enumerated, and true random selection is not possible. In such cases, one typically draws a random sample from an accessible population, such as all the cardiac rehabilitation patients seen at one or two area facilities. Because the accessible population may differ from the larger population of rehabilitation patients, the investigator must collect and present data describing the characteristics of subjects so that similarities and differences from the larger population can be known. Although weaker than true random selection, this information gives the investigator and readers of the study a better sense of how representative the study sample is of the larger population.

Once selected for inclusion in the study, the subjects must decide whether they wish to participate. If refusal rates are high and some types of people are more likely to refuse than others (e.g., those who are older, those from minority ethnic groups), even the best drawn random sample is no longer representative of the larger population. The researcher must develop recruitment plans that are effective, noncoercive, and equally appealing to all members of the study population. It is also important to keep close track of study refusers so that they can be compared with those who choose to participate. This comparison helps determine whether any systematic bias has been introduced.

9. What is random assignment?

The second kind of randomization, random assignment, refers to the way that subjects are assigned to the study groups. The first goal is to rule out any bias that may be introduced by the investigator or others assigning subjects to groups. The second goal is to minimize preexisting differences between the groups. One does not wish for all males to be in one group and all females to be in the other or for all sicker or older patients to be in the same group. Although random assignment cannot assure the equality of the groups, it removes systematic bias and, with an adequate sample size, typically balances the group characteristics. Because equality cannot be assured, baseline measures of key subject characteristics are recommended so that the study groups can be compared for equality, the differences in the groups can be taken into account in drawing conclusions, and statistical control of preexisting differences can be included in the analyses.

In studying subjects over time, differential attrition in the study groups (mortality) can also result in nonequivalent groups. Careful record keeping is essential so that those who drop out can be compared with those who stay in the study and so that study groups can be compared to see whether both the rate of attrition and types of people who drop out are similar.

10. Why is it important to measure subjects over time?

In the simplest form of measurement over time, measures are taken before delivery of the intervention (baseline or pretest) and at least once after the conclusion of the intervention (posttest). As noted in the criteria for determining causation, cause must precede outcome. However, if the outcome (i.e., the dependent variable) is measured only after the cause (intervention), one will never really know whether differences observed between the experimental and control groups may be attributable to preexisting differences. Inclusion of a baseline assessment strengthens the ability to draw causal inferences by providing the data needed to examine the initial equivalence of the experimental and control groups in terms of the dependent variables. Baseline data also allow comparison of the magnitude of change (from baseline to posttest) in the experimental group with that of the control group. The comparison of these changes (either through analysis of change or analyses of covariance) provides the strongest test of causal effects.

11. Why is adherence to study protocols important?

Many texts do not address this aspect of control in experimental designs because it has more to do with conducting than designing the research. But the best planned study is of little use if the procedures and protocols are not followed carefully. If you plan for subjects to be randomly assigned to groups but abandon this approach in mid-study, you have compromised your ability to draw causal conclusions. If an intervention has been developed but is administered haphazardly, there is little chance that it will have the intended effect. If subjects in the experimental group have the opportunity to tell control subjects all about the intervention, both groups may benefit from the information, and the investigator may find no significant differences between the outcomes of the two study groups. Thus, the study design must be well specified and protocols and procedures for enacting each aspect of the design must be developed, written out, and followed. It is wise to keep a log throughout the study to document study activities and make particular note of any deviations from protocols. This information may be critical in interpreting results and in helping others to implement the protocol.

Another factor that can affect adherence to study protocols is the enthusiasm of the investigators, intervenors, data collectors, and even the subjects themselves. The goal is to deliver the intervention in a standardized way that can be replicated by others. You should guard against the study intervenor who goes the extra mile to help subjects, adding his or her own twists to the intervention. Data collectors want the study to succeed and may be susceptible to asking leading questions or interpreting subject responses favorably. Subjects often want to please the researcher and may give positive responses to "help" the study succeed. Such threats can be minimized in several ways. The most common is **blinding**. Ideally, subjects and data collectors should not know to which group the subject belongs—they are "blinded" to the subject's group assignment. Intervenors should also be blinded when possible. However, if the intervenors provide an alternate plan of care, an educational program, or some technique that clearly differs from standard treatment, they cannot be blind to what they are doing. In such cases, a detailed protocol must guide delivery of the intervention. To ensure that the intervention is not unintentionally delivered to the control group, intervenors should not also provide care to the control subjects.

12. What are true experimental designs?

Experimental designs are a family of designs that differ in the degree to which they use the above strategies to maximize control over rival explanations for changes in outcomes. True experimental designs are the most rigorous and provide the greatest control over rival hypotheses. The classic two-group design is depicted below. Once subjects are randomly selected from the populations, they are randomly assigned

(R) to the study groups. One experimental group receives the experimental intervention (X), and one control group does not. Each is measured at baseline (O_1 for initial observation) and after the conclusion of the intervention (O_2). This design controls threats to external validity (generalization) by random selection from the population and threats to internal validity (causal conclusions) through use of a control group, random assignment to groups, and pre- and posttest measures.

Pretest Posttest Control Group Design

ASSIGNMENT	GROUP	PRETEST	INTERVENTION	POSTTEST
R	Experimental	O_1	X	O_2
R	Control	O_1		O_2

However, this is but one of many experimental designs. The goal is to tailor the design to test the particular hypotheses in which you are interested without losing the control provided by the basic design. For example, if one wanted to compare two different versions of an intervention (perhaps an in-person and a phone-based delivery of a support intervention) with a control group, the design would be as follows:

Pretest Posttest Control Group Design with Two Experimental Condtions

ASSIGNMENT	GROUP	PRETEST	INTERVENTION	POSTTEST
R	Experimental (in person)	O_1	X_1	O_2
R	Experimental (phone)	O_1	X_2	O_2
R	Control	O_1		O_2

In some cases, the investigator may wish to follow study subjects for a longer period to see whether the effects found immediately after the intervention are sustained over time. In this case, the investigator adds additional measurement points to the design:

Pretest Posttest Control Group Design with Repeated Follow-up

ASSIGNMENT	GROUP	PRETEST	INTER-VENTION	IMMEDIATE POSTTEST	3-MONTH FOLLOW-UP	6-MONTH FOLLOW-UP
R	Experimental	O_1	X	O_2	O_3	O_4
R	Control	O_1		O_2	O_3	O_4

Neither of these tailored designs results in loss of control over alternative causes of the outcomes. Each is just as strong as the basic experimental design.

What if the investigator wanted to conduct the basic two-group experimental design but was unable to collect baseline data? In this case, a posttest-only design may be used but with some loss of control over rival explanations of what caused the effects. With no baseline (pretest) assessment, it is not known whether the random assignment to groups was successful in achieving equivalence between the groups in terms of the dependent variable. If differences are found on the posttest, one cannot entirely rule out the rival hypothesis that the groups were different from the beginning.

Posttest Only Control Group Design

ASSIGNMENT	GROUP	INTERVENTION	POSTTEST
R	Experimental	X	O
R	Control		O

Additional experimental designs that may serve your needs, such as factorial designs and the Solomon four-group design, can be found in the texts noted above.

13. What are quasi-experimental designs?

Real-world conditions do not always afford the investigator the luxury of the level of control required for a true experimental design. In such cases, quasi-experimental designs provide alternative, less rigorous means to examine cause and effect. Unfortunately, as the rigor decreases, so does the investigator's confidence that the effects are due to the intervention.

Perhaps, for example, you cannot randomly assign subjects to the study groups. Perhaps all of your experimental subjects must come from one clinic and all of the controls from another. These groups would be considered nonequivalent because of possible differences between patients at the two clinics or in the care provided. Although preexisting differences between subjects in the two groups cannot be ruled out as an explanation for changes in the dependent variable, confidence in causal conclusions can be enhanced by including pretest measures on which to compare the two groups for equivalence. This design is depicted much like the first experimental design, but without the R for random assignment to groups:

Nonequivalent Control Group Design

GROUP	PRETEST	INTERVENTION	POSTTEST
Experimental	O_1	X	O_2
Control	O_1		O_2

It is also helpful to obtain detailed information about the two clinic settings, the populations they serve, and the care they provide as well as demographic and health information about the subjects in your study so that you can describe and compare the groups for similarities and differences.

What if there is simply no way to obtain a control group? A one-group design is one of the weakest available—threats to internal validity, such as history and maturation, are substantial and you cannot be confident that any changes are truly a function of the intervention. Pretesting is critical for determining whether change has occurred.

One-group Pretest Posttest Design

GROUP	PRETEST	INTERVENTION	POSTTEST
Experimental	O_1	X	O_2

To help buttress your ability to conclude that the intervention created the change, the investigator should consider collecting data from the subjects about other experiences during the study period that may also have affected their outcomes. Knowledge of this information can help with interpretation of the results.

Just as with true experimental designs, quasi-experimental designs can be tailored to help strengthen one's confidence in the data and to test more complex hypotheses. An example is the one-group design with the addition of multiple pre- and posttest measures:

Time Series Design

GROUP	PRE-TEST 1	PRE-TEST 2	PRE-TEST 3	INTERVENTION	POST-TEST 1	POST-TEST 2	POST-TEST 3
Experimental	O_1	O_2	O_3	X	O_4	O_5	O_6

The multiple pre- and posttests show patterns of response over time—patterns that can provide a more complete understanding of the subjects' status before and after the intervention and that also may be of interest in and of themselves.

As with experimental designs, there are many other quasi-experimental designs, and the reader is referred to the texts above for a more comprehensive discussion.

14. How do I decide which design to use?

Select the design with the greatest amount of control that is feasible. Tailor the design to your particular needs (e.g., a second experimental group, long-term follow up assessments). When less control is possible, as with quasi-experimental designs, enhance your confidence in attributing study effects to the experimental manipulation by collecting ancillary data that enable you to compare nonequivalent groups and describe nonstudy experiences and events that may affect posttest scores. Describe these characteristics when presenting your findings so that others can reflect on them when interpreting your study results.

15. How do I go about designing the intervention?

An intervention is designed as a solution to a problem—if there were no problem, there would be no need to develop and test an intervention. The intervention should be derived from current knowledge—the literature, theory, and perhaps clinical knowledge. What have other people tried? What has worked? What has failed? Why did it fail? Just another intervention is not what is needed, but an intervention that has been informed by the answers to these questions—in other words, it is based on the literature. Ideally, the principles guiding the design of the intervention are theoretically based as well.

The intervention must also be strong enough to have the potential to make a difference. If you are interested in improving diabetic patients' self-care practices, a 10-minute lecture is probably not going to have much of an impact. Again, the literature can usually guide one regarding the approximate "dose" of the intervention that is needed and the style of delivery that is best for your population. The investigator must maintain tight control on the manipulation—ensuring that each experimental subject receives the intervention exactly as designed, using standardized, well-delineated procedures. Interventionists must be well trained to deliver the intervention consistently to all experimental subjects. It is equally important that the control subjects *not* receive the treatment during the course of the study, either from the investigator or by talking to subjects in the experimental group.

16. How do I go about conducting an experimental study?

Many additional decisions must be made in planning your study:
- Which settings should I use?
- What types of people do I wish to include in the sample?
- How should I approach subjects?
- Should I do anything special to encourage them to stay in the study?
- How many subjects do I need?
- Which instruments should I choose to measure the study outcomes, both in terms of conceptual fit and psychometric qualities?
- What are the most appropriate times to measure outcomes?

• How do I maintain quality control in data collection?

• How will I analyze the data?

The answers to most of these questions can be found in other chapters in this book. In addition, applied texts such as those by Brink and Wood,[5] Hulley et al.,[6] Issac and Michael,[7] LoBiondo-Wood and Haber,[8] and Friedman, Furbert, and DeMets[9] provide useful information about the "how-to's" of conducting experimental studies from the nursing, epidemiologic, and behavioral science perspectives. Most importantly, call on your own knowledge and common sense. Ask *yourself* the critical questions—you may just have the best answers.

REFERENCES

1. Pedhazur EJ, Schmelkin LP: Measurement, Design, and Analysis: An Integrated Approach, Student Edition. Mahwah, NJ, Lawrence Erlbaum, 1991.
2. Polit-O'Hara DP, Hungler BP, Polit D: Nursing Research. Principles and Methods, 6th ed. Philadelphia, Lippincott Williams & Wilkins, 1998.
3. Campbell DT, Stanley JC: Experimental and Quasi-Experimental Designs for Research. Boston, Houghton Mifflin College, 1966.
4. Cook TD, Campbell DT: Quasi-Experimentation: Design and Analysis Issues. Boston, Houghton Mifflin, 1979.
5. Brink PJ, Wood MJ, Brink PR: Basic Steps in Planning Nursing Research: From Question to Proposal, 5th ed. Sudbury, MA, Jones & Bartlett, 2001.
6. Hulley SB, Cummings SR, Browner WS, et al: Designing Clinical Research: An Epidemiologic Approach, 2nd ed. Philadelphia, Lippincott Williams & Wilkins, 2001.
7. Isaac S, Michael W: Handbook in Research and Evaluation : A Collection of Principles, Methods, and Strategies Useful in the Planning, Design, and Evaluation of Studies in Education and the Behavioral Sciences, 3rd ed. San Diego, EdITS Publishers, 1995.
8. LoBiondo-Wood G, Haber J: Nursing Research: Methods, Critical Appraisal, and Utilization, 5th ed. St. Louis, Mosby, 2002.
9. Friedman LM, Furberg C, DeMets DL: Fundamentals of Clinical Trials, 3rd ed. New York, Springer Verlag, 1998.

14. QUALITATIVE DESIGNS

Joan K. Magilvy, RN, PhD, FAAN

1. What qualitative research designs are used most frequently in nursing research?

Nurse researchers use a wide variety of qualitative research designs. The question or problem to be studied indicates the selection of the research design. Some of the qualitative research designs used most frequently by nurse researchers include:

- Qualitative descriptive
- Ethnography
- Grounded theory
- Narrative inquiry
- Phenomenology
- Hermeneutics
- Philosophic inquiry
- Life history
- Case study
- Action research
- Feminist inquiry
- Critical theory approach
- Historical research

The reader is referred to Munhall[1] and other references for information about designs not reviewed here.

2. When are qualitative designs used?

Nurse researchers use a variety of qualitative research designs to answer questions related to the nature of human experiences in health, illness, healing, and dying or phenomena related to environmental contexts of health and health care delivery. In the conduct of such studies, a variety of qualitative data generation and analysis methods are used to produce a rich description and in-depth understanding of the phenomenon of interest, the cultural or lived experience of people in natural settings.

3. Where can I read more about qualitative research?

Several recent texts are excellent sources of information about qualitative research designs and methods, such as those by Munhall,[1] Denzin and Lincoln,[2] and Creswell.[3] These texts provide overviews of design and methods, comparisons and critiques of the designs, and examples that are beyond the scope of this discussion.

4. Describe the philosophic underpinnings of qualitative designs.

Phenomenology is the philosophic approach that underlies much of qualitative research. Although some qualitative designs may be informed by other philosophic traditions (e.g., symbolic interactionism underpins the grounded theory design), phenomenology is the most widely known. Basic knowledge about the philosophic tradition of phenomenology is key to understanding qualitative research.

Phenomenology deals with the subjective nature of human experience. As summarized by Oiler[4] (p. 86) the phenomenological philosophic perspective focuses on:

> Phenomena as they appear, and recognizes that reality is subjective . . . Subjectivity means that the world becomes real through our contact with it and acquires meaning through our interpretations of that contact. Truth, then, is a composite of realities and access to truth is a problem of access to human subjectivity.

The qualitative researcher examines lived experiences as viewed from the perspective of the experiencing person. The qualitative nurse researcher is intimately involved in the research, and is, in fact, the instrument of research. The qualitative researcher uses many different modes of awareness to understand, describe, interpret, and express the findings, yielding a thorough and accurate description of the nursing phenomenon.[4]

5. What is meant by qualitative descriptive design?

The term *qualitative descriptive* refers to descriptive research studies that are informed or guided by a major qualitative design but are usually smaller in scale. For some research situations, the scope of a study may be limited by practical considerations such as small sample size, time limitations, or inability to conduct a full study true to the tenets of ethnographic, grounded theory, narrative inquiry, or phenomenologic designs. These situations may occur, for example, when students conduct small research studies within the constraints of a semester or an academic year or when a researcher has a more focused research question or obtains limited funding or logistic support that may preclude a more major investigation. However, when the methods are qualitative, philosophic in tradition, and descriptive in scope and methods, the term *qualitative descriptive* design can be applied.

Sandelowski[5] (p. 336) noted that qualitative descriptive studies provide a "comprehensive summary of an event in the everyday terms of those events" and that qualitative descriptive studies sometimes involve a "re-presentation" of events as researchers put "their own interpretive spin on what they see and hear." Data collection and analysis are highly descriptive of what is, congruent with the ideas of naturalistic inquiry[6] or the qualitative research orientation of studying a phenomenon in its natural state.

6. Is phenomenology a philosophy or method?

Both. Phenomenological research is informed by phenomenological philosophy. Building on the work of philosophers such as Husserl, Merleau-Ponty, Schutz, Spiegelberg, and Heidegger, nurse researchers have shaped phenomenological designs and methods used in nursing science to answer questions related to the meaning of lived experiences. A phenomenological study may focus on a specific health, illness, healing, and dying phenomenon or experience. Such phenomena are significant factors to nursing practice to help gain an in-depth understanding of the human condition. From phenomenologists of the second-generation[1] such as Georgi, Colaizzi, van Kaam, and van Manen, we see contrasting perspectives that guide the methods of phenomenological research, such as existential, hermeneutical, and transcendental phenomenology. These philosophies guide many of our nurse phenomenologists (e.g., Munhall, Oiler, Benner, Parse, Reeder, Ray).[1,4,7,8] Nursing phenomenological studies have contributed greatly to our knowledge about human experiences in health and illness, healing and dying (e.g., loss of an unborn child, recurrence of cancer), and the meaning of these experiences to patients, clients, and colleagues.

7. How are data generated in descriptive qualitative research studies?

Techniques used in generating data for qualitative descriptive studies include purposive or convenience sampling, semistructured interviews with open-ended questions, and sometimes observations of behavior and activities in the study setting and context. A descriptive analysis of data is informed by an approach to discovery in which ideas emerge from the data rather than from previously determined theoretical notions. As in many other qualitative designs, findings are presented descriptively in a narrative text illustrated with examples or quotations from the participants. Although many discount the importance of qualitative descriptive design, it is a viable and appropriate choice for many nursing research questions when the purpose of the study is exploratory.

8. Define ethnography. How commonly is it used in nursing research?

Ethnography is the study of people within the context of their culture. Based on the methodology developed in cultural anthropology, ethnographers study cultures and subcultural groups. Ethnography is commonly used in nursing research to study phenomena of health and illness within a cultural, community, or environmental context. In other words, the lived experience of health, illness, healing, and dying can be studied from the perspective of people informed by the lens of their culture. For example, rural dwelling Hispanic and Anglo older persons were the focus of a study of health care transitions in rural settings by two nurse ethnographers.[9] Community analysis studies conducted by public health nurses can also use ethnographic design.

Several characteristics of ethnographic design can be identified. First, ethnography is a holistic combination of the emic (cultural insider's) and etic (outsider or researcher's) perspectives that provides a cultural description of the lifeways and activities of people in their natural environments. Participants in ethnographic research are often viewed as coresearchers in this inductive approach to description. In some ethnographic investigations, categories and domains are identified, leading to descriptions of cultural themes, which then may lead to development of theory by participants and researchers. In other ethnographies, a critical theory lens can be used to provide critical ethnographic descriptions of the differentials in power, social status, or health care disparities.

The ethnographic investigator uses methods such as participant observations, unstructured or minimally structured interviews, examination of cultural artifacts, photography, and other visual techniques to understand the lived experiences of people within a culture. Through these techniques, the researcher can learn about what people in a culture know and what they do and about the things they use in everyday life.[10] Nurse researchers conducting ethnographic research identify a problem of study and select the appropriate sample. Ethnographic methods are used to analyze, interpret, and describe a clinically relevant problem in a cultural context, discovering important themes that may lead to development of culturally congruent health care interventions and outcomes.

9. What are the strengths of a grounded theory approach?

Grounded theorists study social processes in everyday human life and interactions. For nurse researchers, the grounded theory approach facilitates the development of mid-range theory grounded in the life and language of people living with health and illness conditions or the experience of providing and receiving health care. Grounded theorists have the goal of generating or discovering a theory to describe how people act and react to a phenomenon or process and propose theoretical propositions or models that illustrate and explicate the theory.[3]

Many phenomena of interest to nurse researchers involve a process rather than a focus on a moment in time. Grounded theory designs are well suited to the identification of basic social processes in health and illness. Examples of grounded theory include the discovery of theory about development of professional identity in nursing, the experience of low-income women living with HIV/AIDS, or transitions of older persons discharged from hospitals or moving into long-term care settings. Methods of theoretical sampling, participant observation and interview, and constant comparative analysis form the framework for this more tightly structured and focused qualitative research design. Although a grounded theory study may produce an initial theory, further study in different settings or populations focused on the same phenomenon or process can lead to the development of formal theory, such as the classic nursing research about dying conducted by Benoliel, Glaser, and Straus. A methodologic overview about grounded theory design and method can be found in Charmaz.[11]

10. Discuss the development of narrative inquiry.

Stories are a primary way in which people communicate their experiences to others. According to Witherell and Noddings:[12]

> Stories and narrative, whether personal or fictional, provide meaning and belonging in our lives. They attach us to others and to our own histories by providing a tapestry rich with threads of time, place, character, and even advice . . . offers us images, myths, and metaphors that are morally resonant and contribute both to our knowing and our being known (p. 1).

The use of narrative designs allows the researcher to elicit the stories of everyday life as told by people who have experienced meaningful life events such as living with a disability or chronic illness, witnessing the death of a loved one, or parenting a teenager with a substance abuse problem. Many narrative approaches exist in qualitative research. Some of these approaches are closely related to phenomenology, whereas others are more grounded in the arts and humanities, such as literary analysis. In other narrative designs the researcher produces a piece of literature, such as a novel, poetry, or a play, based on the lived experience of health or illness, healing, or dying. Stories are powerful ways to describe the lived experience. Narrative themes can illustrate important lessons of life and health useful for understanding or explicating appropriate health care interventions or policies.

11. When is a life history approach useful in nursing research?

A life history approach may be the most suitable design when a researcher finds that describing a significant life event or series of events from the perspective of the experiencing person may facilitate understanding a cultural, personal, or societal theme or pattern of life experience. Similar methods are used in life history and other qualitative designs, with the interview being the primary mode of data generation. However, the idea of life history implies a more longitudinal approach to data gathering, with multiple interviews over time with a small sample or even a single participant. Often the episodes of life are recounted around specific marker events that are identified jointly by participant and researcher; each event is discussed and reflected upon during the interviews. Collecting other data, such as letters or inter-views with friends or family members of the participant, often assists life history data generation.

Examples of nursing research questions associated with life history approach include:

- Childbearing experiences of women from varying cultural or ethnic groups
- Development of leadership roles and experiences as told by contemporary nursing leaders
- Illness trajectory of a person living with multiple sclerosis or other chronic illness

Nurse researchers use biographical studies, autobiographies, oral history, and interpretive biography in this type of design.[3]

12. Is qualitative research as easy as it seems?

Qualitative research is deceptively difficult and time-consuming but quite satis-fying. The researcher is the instrument of research and uses her or his best skills of interviewing, observing, photographing, and sometimes participating in the events or phenomena of interest. The work of data generation/collection can be tiring as the researcher tries to take in and make sense of the many activities or ideas presented by the participants and research environment. Sometimes a rest break is needed during data generation activities to permit the researcher to reflect and refocus on the topics at hand. Tape-recorded interviews and researcher field notes or journal en-tries must be transcribed into computer files, and the activities of the research, such as photographs, artifacts, and text data must be catalogued carefully. Data manage-ment is often problematic because of the volume of data gathered from interviews and observations. Such activities often produce researcher fatigue.

The process of analysis and interpretation of data can add additional burden but also generate a sense of excitement and discovery. Engagement in data analysis is often referred to as "dwelling with the data" because of the numerous times that the researcher reads, hears, examines, considers, interprets, and reflects on the meaning of the data. All of these processes take considerable time and effort, but by knowing the data so intimately, the qualitative researcher can create a rich description of the lived experiences of participants. The writing of qualitative research is part of the analysis, just as the analysis process is part of data generation. Telling the story and providing rich description are important parts of the research. The outcomes of quali-tative research are the satisfaction that a story has been well told or an experience or phenomenon well described or interpreted so that the participants or others who have experienced the phenomenon will recognize them as credible and authentic. From the findings of qualitative research in nursing, nurse clinicians and scientists can develop appropriate interventions based on evidence grounded in nursing practice.

13. How does the research question lead to selection of the most appropriate qualitative design?

Just as in any research project, the purposes of the study and the research prob-lem or question are the best indicators of the design. For example, an ethnographic design may be preferred if the research problem or question asks, "How is a nursing intervention or health care delivery approach practiced in a cultural context?" or "How do people in a culture experience a certain health or illness condition (e.g., chronic illness in Hispanic older persons or terminal illness and hospice services in a rural population)?" On the other hand, if the research question is related to the meaning of a lived experience, such as the death of a life partner or military battlefield nursing care, phenomenology is a good choice. Life experiences that involve the remembering or telling of stories at one point in time, such as an experience with temporary disability, may indicate a narrative inquiry design; however, the telling of stories over a lifetime, such as child-bearing and rearing experiences of immigrant women, may indicate a life history approach. If the purpose of the study involves developing a theory grounded in nursing practice, such as describing the process of rehabilitation or preparing for hospital discharge by people with head injuries and their families, a grounded theory approach is appropriate. Researchers who enjoy a critical theory philosophic approach often ask a question that indicates a critical research approach, such as critical ethnography, feminist inquiry, or action research. Rather than selecting the design and making the question fit, the qualitative nurse researcher is much better served by letting the question determine the design.

14. What researcher characteristics facilitate use of different qualitative designs?

Of interest, certain designs also choose their researchers. People who are comfortable with ambiguity and research that unfolds during the investigation make good qualitative researchers, as do people who enjoy surprise, discovery, and listening and learning about lived experiences directly from the experiencing persons. The researcher who enjoys a more structured approach to data generation and especially analysis may prefer the grounded theory approach. Researchers who enjoy anthropology, transcultural nursing, or learning about life in different cultures also enjoy ethnographic research. Such researchers must have the ability to see the big picture and to handle complex data on many levels of analysis. On the other hand, researchers interested in the meaning of a lived experience as told by the participating person and researchers with skills in interpretation and philosophical analysis may enjoy phenomenology. Narrative inquiry intrigues researchers who are curious about story or enjoy literary analysis; likewise, interest in historical research leads to an interest in life history, oral history, or historiography designs. Most qualitative researchers enjoy the discovery that unfolds as their research question and preferred design become congruent. Personal characteristics play an important role in this process.

REFERENCES

1. Munhall PL: Nursing Research: A Qualitative Perspective, 3rd ed. Sudbury, MA, Jones & Bartlett, 2001.
2. Denzin NK, Lincoln Y: Handbook of Qualitative Research, 2nd ed. Thousand Oaks, CA, Sage, 2000.
3. Creswell JW: Qualitative Inquiry and Research Design: Choosing among Five Traditions. Thousand Oaks, CA, Sage, 1998.
4. Oiler C: Philosophic foundations of qualitative research. In Munhall PL (ed): Nursing Research: A Qualitative Perspective, 3rd ed. Sudbury, MA, Jones & Bartlett, 2001.
5. Sandelowski M: Focus on research methods: Whatever happened to qualitative description? Res Nurs Health 23:334–340, 2000.
6. Lincoln YS, Guba EG: Naturalistic Inquiry. Beverly Hills, CA, Sage, 1985.
7. van Manen M: Researching the Lived Experience. Albany, NY, SUNY Press, 1990.
8. Reeder F: The phenomenological movement. Image J Nurs Scholar 19:150–152, 1987.
9. Magilvy JK, Congdon JG: The crisis nature of health care transitions for rural older adults. Public Health Nurs 17:336–345, 2000.
10. Fetterman DM: Ethnography: Step by Step, 2nd ed. Thousand Oaks, CA, Sage, 1998.
11. Charmaz K: Discovering chronic illness: Using grounded theory. Soc Sci Med 30:1161–1172, 1990.
12. Witherell C, Noddings N (eds): Stories Lives Tell: Narrative and Dialogue in Education. New York, Teachers College Press, 1991.

15. MEASUREMENT AND VARIABLES

Martha H. *Stoner,* RN, PhD

1. What is measurement?

Measurement is the process of systematically assigning numbers or other symbols to observations of phenomena of interest, such as behaviors, traits, or a program's characteristics. Numbers are assigned to indicate the amount of some variable. Measurement requires the assignment of numerical scores to descriptors of severity, such as 0 = no pain to 10 = the worst pain possible, and frequency, such as 1 = rarely to 5 = every day.

2. Why is measurement important in nursing research?

Human responses to health and illness are complex and the interaction among multiple variables add to the challenge of nursing research. A critical concern is the measurement of variables. A research study's quality is only as good as the appropriateness of the research design and the quality of measurement procedures. Nurse researchers must understand measurement, the attributes of a good measure, and how to identify or develop a psychometrically sound measure.

3. What are measurement frameworks?

Measurement frameworks provide direction for the development of instruments and for interpretation of findings. See Chapter 16 for a discussion of norm-referenced and criterion-referenced frameworks of measurement.

4. What do research instruments measure?

Research instruments measure variables. A variable represents a behavior or characteristic that can change on some dimension. A variable can be observed and measured and sometimes controlled and manipulated. Height is an example of a variable that can be measured. A variable that can be controlled or manipulated for research purposes may be a patient education program. The content, format of delivery, and timing of delivery are aspects of the educational program that can be modified by the researcher.

5. What are conceptual definitions of research variables?

Conceptual definitions of research variables are an important and early step in measurement. The variable of interest to the nurse researcher may be an unspecified abstract phenomenon that must be defined by identifying all of the possible elements of what the variable is as well as what it is not. A comprehensive review of the literature from all relevant disciplines is essential to place the phenomenon within a conceptually meaningful context. For example, there are two distinctly different conceptual definitions of pain: (1) pain is whatever the experiencing person says it is and (2) pain is a set of physiologic measures. Measurement of pain would be quite different for each definition.

6. What are operational definitions of research variables?

Operational definitions specify the way in which the phenomenon of interest will be measured. Operational definitions narrow the focus for measurement by eliminating nonrelevant aspects and by specifying what you want to study and what methods you will use to study the variable. Content experts are often asked to evaluate the conceptual and operational definitions for accuracy and completeness. Operational definitions of pain based on the conceptual definitions above may include a response to a single-item indicator rating pain on a 0–10 scale or measurement of blood pressure and pulse.

7. How are numbers assigned to variables in research instruments?

Number assignment is easy to understand in the measurement of height and weight. Numbers can also be assigned arbitrarily; for example, when 1 = male and 2 = female. To minimize the risk of meaningless or questionable findings, measurement theory is used to guide the selection of numbers so that they are a more accurate reflection of reality. Formal scaling methods from both psychometrics and econometrics are used in the development of instruments for health research instead of simply assigning numbers as responses to instrument items.

8. Discuss other important features of variables.

Measurement of each variable must include an exhaustive list of optional responses. All possible responses or the most common attributes must be listed, including an "other" response with a request that respondents write in their specific answer. Such responses must also be mutually exclusive so that only one answer for each item is selected on the instrument. In measuring income, categories of responses may range from $1–4999, $5000–9999, and so on, to greater than $100,000. Categories do not overlap, and respondents select only one response.

9. What is important to know about the research types and the terms applied to variables?

Although the terms applied to variables are sometimes used interchangeably across types of research, many people distinguish between terms used in experimental studies and terms used in correlation studies. In experimental research the researcher investigates a cause-effect relationship between two or more variables: the hypothesized cause or independent variable, which can be manipulated, and the anticipated effect or dependent variable, which is not manipulated.

The independent vs. dependent distinction is less critical in correlation research because the goal is to discover or explore relationships among sets of variables without specifying a cause-and-effect relationship. Variables are measured, not manipulated, in correlation research. A cause-and-effect relationship is not the goal and cannot be verified. Based on findings from a correlation study in which a strong relationship is found, a researcher may design an experimental study to test for causality. Correlation research may be used in prediction studies in which the researcher seeks to determine whether the scores on one variable can be forecast by the scores on one or more other variables. A question for a prediction study may be whether scores on the Graduate Record Exam predict success in graduate school.

10. Define discrete variables.

Discrete variables are those with no possible intermediate value. They are measured using a nominal scale and are sometimes called categorical or dichotomous.

Employment status may be a two-value (dichotomous) variable, as indicated by 1 = employed or 2 = unemployed. Marital status is often a four-value variable, as measured by selection of one of four categories: 1 = single, 2 = married, 3 = divorced, and 4 = widowed.

11. Define continuous variables.

Continuous variables have values between points and are measured using an ordinal, interval, or ratio level of measurement. Continuous data are generated by variables for which the response set is a request for an actual number (e.g., weight in pounds). Continuous data are preferable to categorical data because they represent more precise measurement and allow more options for statistical analysis. If the researcher sees a need to do so, a continuous measure can always be converted into categories, whereas data gathered as discrete variables cannot be changed to continuous variables.

12. Define independent variables.

Independent variables (IV) are factors under the control of the researcher that are thought to have some impact on or potential to change a dependent variable. IVs may also be thought of as the cause and are sometimes called treatment variables. In a study comparing types of diabetic education for patients newly diagnosed with diabetes, the educational program is the independent variable. The researcher manipulates and controls the IV by using different methods of instructing patients—for example, group vs. one-to-one teaching. The research question may be, "Which teaching method produces greater learning and increased diabetic control?" Independent variables may also be classified as predictor variables.

13. Define dependent variables.

Dependent variables (DVs) are behaviors or responses expected to be affected by the IV. They are the response or result and depend or rely on something that precedes them. DVs are measured but not manipulated and may be classified as criterion variables. In the experiment with diabetic patients, more than one DV may be included because increased knowledge, skill in self-care, and good diabetic control, as evidenced by a desirable hemoglobin A1c laboratory report, are all appropriate outcome measures to evaluate the impact of the patient education program.

14. Define antecedent variables.

Antecedent variables come before the measurement of the variable of interest. They may be preexisting factors, such as a confirmed diagnosis or height and weight, or demographic characteristics, such as gender, ethnicity, socioeconomic status, and educational level.

15. Define a predictor variable.

A predictor variable in correlation research is an antecedent variable that, unlike an independent variable in experimental research, is not under the control of the researcher and cannot be manipulated. It is simply measured. Data about the variable are gathered because the researcher has theoretical rationale to predict the existence of a relationship between the predictor variable and the outcome or criterion variable of interest. For example, smoking history cannot be manipulated, but it can be measured as the number of packs per day for the number of years that the person smoked and can serve as a predictor variable in a study of the incidence of lung disease later in life. Predictor variables are sometimes called explanatory variables.

16. Define a criterion variable.

A criterion variable is a term used in correlation research that is most like the dependent variable in an experimental study. Like the dependent variable, a criterion variable is measured but not manipulated. The researcher is interested in the relationship between the antecedent, predictor variable and the criterion variable. Outcome variable and response variable are other terms for the same concept.

17. Define extraneous variables.

Extraneous or nuisance variables are all variables other than the independent variable that may have an influence on the dependent variable. They are undesirable and, if not controlled, may affect the outcome variable and threaten the validity of findings. Extraneous variables may limit the researcher's ability to attribute a change in the dependent variable solely to the independent variable. Efforts to control extraneous variables include holding the variable constant and allowing random variation. Random assignment to group does not eliminate the influence of extraneous variables, but it distributes the error equally between groups. A particular type of extraneous variable is a confounding variable, which introduces systematic error associated with the independent variable when random assignment is not used.

18. Define intervening variables.

Intervening variables, specific extraneous variables, come between the independent and dependent variables and directly affect the action of the independent variable on the dependent variable. For example, the personality and teaching style of the nurse implementing the patient education program may influence how well patients learn, regardless of the content or format of the program.

19. Define demographic variables.

Demographic variables are characteristics such as age, gender, ethnicity, and health used most often to describe a sample. A continuous demographic variable such as age describes a person in terms of a single value on some underlying scale (e.g., actual age elicited by asking subjects to give their age at their last birthday). Age as a categorical demographic variable describes a person in terms of discrete categories by asking subjects to place themselves in an age category such as 20–29, or over 65

20. What are the levels of measurement? Why are they important?

The four measurement levels are nominal, ordinal, interval, and ratio. The level of measurement influences how much information can be obtained about a variable and is critical to determining the appropriate statistical analysis to apply to answer the research question. Level of data is important because it is associated with the types of statistics (i.e., parametric and nonparametric) that can be used for analysis. In most circumstances, parametric statistics are reserved for interval and ratio data. The table below provides examples of the four levels of measurements.

Four Levels of Measurement

SCALE	DEFINING CHARACTERISTICS	EXAMPLES
Nominal	Mutually exclusive categories	Race, gender, blood type, marital status, diagnosis
Ordinal	Rank or ordered levels	Socioeconomic status (e.g., low, middle, high) Level of anxiety (e.g., high, moderate, low) Level of agreement (e.g., always, some-times, disagree)
Interval	Numerical scale with equivalent interval size	Fahrenheit, Celsius temperatures; IQ scores
Ratio	Numerical scale with an absolute zero point	Weight, age, measures of force and time

21. What is nominal level of measurement?

Nominal scales/variables are those for which only qualitative classification (naming) can be done. Values are assigned arbitrarily to a variable, and measurement of nominal variables is limited to placement of items into categories indicating that they are different from one another. Nominal measures classify by using numbers as labels for categories. Differences are qualitative rather than quantitative because one category is not more or better than another. For example, subjects can be categorized as having A-positive blood type, which makes them different from but not better than other subjects whose blood type is O-positive.

22. Describe the ordinal level of measurement.

Like nominal measures, ordinal measures assign arbitrary numbers to response categories, but the numbers reflect an increasing order of the measured characteristic. Ordinal scales/variables have a calculable value in that one value is greater than another, but it is not possible to specify how much greater. The distance between measuring points may not be the same. For example, on a patient satisfaction instrument with a scale from 1 = not satisfied to 4 = very satisfied, we know that 4 is both more than and better than 3, but we do not know how much better. We do not know if the difference between 3 and 4 means that 4 is 25% better than 3. We also do not know that the difference between 1 and 2 is the same as the difference between 3 and 4.

23. Describe the interval level of measurement.

Interval scales/variables give information about the size of the difference between scores in addition to ranking them in order. We know what score is higher and can specify how much higher because the distance between each value is equal. A temperature of 100° is higher than a temperature of 90°, and the difference between 38° and 48° is the same as the difference between 90° and 100°. We also know that an increase from 80° to 100° is twice as much as an increase from 90° to 100°.

24. Describe the ratio level of measurement.

Ratio scales/variables have all of the properties of interval measures but are unique in that they have an identifiable absolute zero point. When we weigh a person, we know that 180 pounds is greater than 170 pounds and that the difference between 170 and 180 is the same as the difference between 6 and 16 pounds. We also know that 16 pounds is twice 8 pounds and that the scale can be balanced to a measurable and meaningful zero. Counts are often considered a ratio level of measurement. For example, the number of nurses or patients could conceivably be zero; thus, a count of either nurses or patients allows construction of a fraction or ratio. You can identify that twice as many patients were admitted this week compared with last week. Similarly, you can note that twice as many nurses were on duty today as yesterday.

25. What are reliability and validity issues in measurement?

Reliability and validity are critical in the development and evaluation of instruments. An instrument that is both valid and reliable measures what it is supposed to measure (valid) and does so accurately and consistently (reliable). Measurement error is a threat to reliability and validity (see Chapter 16 for more details). The fact that it is nearly impossible to construct an instrument that is completely reliable and valid makes it imperative that instrument developers provide evidence of methods to address measurement error. The goal of reliability and validity assessments is to minimize the portion of the observed score that is due to error and to increase the portion that is true score.

26. What is measurement error?

Measurement error is the difference between the measurement (actual score) and the hypothetical true value (score) of whatever is measured. An observed score is a combination of a true score (the score obtained if the instrument is perfect) plus random and systematic error. No instrument is perfect. All instruments are beset with errors of measurement, making it impossible to measure variables with complete accuracy. Sources of measurement error include:
- Situational contaminants
- Response set biases
- Transitory personal factors
- Administration variations
- Instrument clarity
- Response sampling
- Instrument format

27. What is constant (systematic) measurement error?

Systematic or constant errors of measurement occur when a measuring device consistently provides an incorrect measure of the variable each time that it is measured. Thus, the error is the same for all subjects. For example, an incorrectly calibrated blood pressure gauge yields consistently elevated (or lowered) readings for all subjects. The error becomes a consistent part of the obtained score and makes the true score unclear. Because the measure is affected in the same way each time, the mean of a set of scores is biased in a specific direction. Validity is directly threatened because, as error increases, validity decreases. Acquiescence, the consistent agreement or disagreement with response set choices, and social desirability, the selection of choices based on what is believed to be the socially correct answer whether the respondent agrees with it or not, are common sources of constant error.

28. What is random measurement error?

Random error of measurement is sometimes considered noise because the error adds variability to the data but does not affect average performance for the group. Random errors vary from one measurement to the next because they are produced by chance, temporary factors that confound the measurement of a variable and yield inconsistent data. Random error raises or lowers observed scores randomly, resulting in inconsistent data and often raising questions about what exactly is being measured. Mean scores are not affected because scores vary randomly around the true score and affect the variability around the mean score. Examples include such factors as respondent fatigue and pain. The data collector may introduce random error just by being present during data collection or by being bored or distracted and making errors in collecting data. Environmental factors (noise or poor lighting), inconsistent data collection procedures (changes in the test instructions or poor directions), or problems with the instrument (ambiguous items) may also produce random error.

29. How can measurement error be reduced?

Instrument pilot testing can reduce measurement error by providing the researcher with an opportunity for practice and learning as the instrument is administered to a small number of subjects similar to the target population. In the process, the researcher follows planned procedures and makes improvements to maximize the quality of the research study. Additionally, preliminary reliability and validity assessments can be made. Pilot study subjects can provide helpful suggestions to make data collection more efficient and of the desired quality. Thorough training of data collectors is another way to reduce errors. Reduction of errors can be enhanced by double-checking data as it is collected and as it is entered into a computer. Using multiple measures of the major variable is another way to limit error by allowing triangulation. Statistical procedures, based on the advice of a statistical expert, can also be useful strategies to reduce error.

30. What is sensitivity of a measure?

Sensitivity refers to the ability of a measure to detect a difference, primarily in isolating hypothesized changes in an outcome variable (improved health status) that can be attributed to the independent variable (nursing educational intervention). Sensitivity may be reflected in the degree of discreteness included in the response set. Pain can be measured using a categorical scale of yes and no or a visual analog scale with infinite points. The visual analog scale has a higher degree of sensitivity than a dichotomous yes-or-no format. Another important issue to consider regarding the sensitivity of an instrument is the ability of the respondent to use the scale appropriately. For example, a 0–4 scale to measure pain is likely to be more appropriate for a young child, whereas an adult may be able to handle a greater number of points, such as a ten point scale or a visual analog. Hence, the degree of scale sensitivity should be tailored for the intended user.

31. What is a psychometrically sound measure?

A psychometrically sound measure is developed within and remains consistent with an appropriate and adequate conceptual framework. A detailed description of the ways in which items were identified and refined is essential information in evaluating an instrument's quality. The intended subjects should be specified to ensure that the instrument is used with appropriate people, based on socio-demographic characteristics. Guidance for administering and scoring the instrument is an important inclusion in reports about the instrument. Psychometrically sound measures are used over time and in settings with samples large enough to obtain meaningful estimates of reliability and validity. Evidence of sensitivity of the instrument should also be provided.

32. How are data about variables gathered?

Questionnaires, self-administered paper-and-pencil forms, or researcher-completed structured interview guides are used to gather demographic, health, and illness data. Data collection for other variables may use single-item indicators (e.g., pain). Other instruments are composed of multiple indicator items with response sets that yield quantitative data for analysis (e.g., a quality-of-life scale for people with multiple sclerosis). Some scales use discrete responses with categories such as excellent, good, fair, or poor. Likert or Likert-like scales ask subjects to rate agreement or disagreement with a series of statements or opinions. For visual analog scales subjects mark on a line of fixed length where they would place themselves in relation to defining anchor words located only at the extreme ends of the line. Data from instruments may be analyzed as individual items, as subscales or factors, and as total scale scores.

33. What is item analysis?

Item analysis refers to item-total correlation that compares the correlation of each item in an instrument with the total instrument score to determine how much an individual item contributes to the overall concept being measured. When items with low item-total correlations are eliminated, the accuracy and utility of the instrument are increased and an internal consistency or homogeneity of the scale is indicated.

34. What is factor analysis?

Factor analysis is a mathematical technique used in instrument development to reduce and organize a large number of items into smaller groupings that fit together. The smaller group is called a factor. All of the items in a factor are highly correlated with each other but less correlated with items in other factors and with the overall items. As an example, a factor analysis of an 18-item instrument to assess health may distinguish groups of items about physical (8 items) and emotional health (6 items). The remaining 4 items may have an identifiable conceptual link that justifies being named a factor, or they may be deleted from the instrument because of a lack of fit. Thus, factor analysis provides evidence of validity instrument structure.

35. Are all published instruments considered reliable and valid?

No. Researchers who develop instruments must make a thorough evaluation of the psychometric properties of the instrument (as described in Chapter 16) and publish those findings to provide sufficient information to enable readers to judge the quality of the instrument and the resultant research findings. The fact that an instrument is published does not ensure that its development and evaluation were rigorous. The burden of responsibility for selection of an instrument for use in research lies with potential users, who must evaluate both the quality of its development and its appropriateness for the proposed research.

BIBLIOGRAPHY

1. Aday LU: Designing and Conducting Health Surveys: A Comprehensive Guide, 2nd ed. San Francisco, Jossey-Bass, 1996.
2. Brink PJ, Wood MJ: Basic Steps in Planning Nursing Research: From Question to Proposal, 5th ed. Boston, Jones & Bartlett, 2001.
3. Fry ST, Duffy ME: The development and psychometric evaluation of the ethical issues scale. J Nurs Scholar 33:273–277, 2001.
4. Jacobson SF: Evaluating instruments for use in clinical nursing research. In Frank-Stromborg M, Olsen SJ (eds): Instruments for Clinical Health-Care Research, 2nd ed. Boston, Jones & Bartlett, 1997.
5. Lewis RJ: Reliability and validity: Meaning and measurement. Presented at the 1999 Annual Meeting of the Society for Academic Emergency Medicine (SAEM) in Boston, MA. Available at <http://www.ambpeds.org/ReliabilityandValidity.pdf>.
6. McDowell I, Newell C: Measuring Health: A Guide to Rating Scales and Questionnaires. New York, Oxford University Press, 1996.
7. Norwood SL: Research Strategies for Advanced Practice Nurses. Upper Saddle River, NJ, Prentice Hall Health, 2000.
8. Saile WS: Measurement theory: Frequently asked questions. 1996. Available at <http://www.creative.net.au/mirrors/neural/measurement.html>.
9. Trochim WMK: Research Methods Knowledge Base. 2002. Available at <http://trochim.human.cornell.edu/kb/measure.htm>.
10. Yen M, Lo LH: Examining test-retest reliability: An intra-class correlation approach. Nurs Res 51:59–62, 2002. Available at <http://www.nursingcenter.com>.

16. INSTRUMENTATION

Richard W. Redman, RN, PhD

1. What is a research instrument?

An instrument can be defined as a tool or an implement for performing a task. It also can be thought of as a device for measuring or controlling conditions, such as those in cars or airplanes.

These aspects of an instrument have meaning in research. Research instruments are used as tools for performing different facets of research. They help us to measure phenomena, such as attitudes, blood pressure, or particular behaviors, that are directly related to our research questions. They are also used to produce data that represent potential answers to the research questions.

2. What are instruments supposed to measure?

In any research study, the phenomena that we want to observe and measure can have different values. If only one value were possible, we would not have to measure it. These values are referred to as variables (i.e., changeable values). Instrumentation is the process of determining how to measure a variable as well as what processes and devices to use for measuring the characteristic or quality of interest in research.[1]

Instruments are used to measure nearly all study variables of interest. Although some variables may be quite straightforward, such as sex or age, we still need some way to capture the information using a variety of guidelines and a method for collecting the data. In this sense, a questionnaire can be viewed as an instrument in the same way that a thermometer is an instrument. Both measure a specific characteristic or value with a set of rules to help us interpret the obtained data. The more directly we can measure something, the more accurate the measurement is. For example, measures of physiologic characteristics, such as serum cholesterol levels, are performed using laboratory instruments and agreed-upon rules and standards. If we are measuring something that is less easily quantified, such as attitudes about health or assessment of the quality of nursing care, the task and the measurement become more challenging. All, however, require instrumentation for gathering data about the variables of interest.

3. Give examples of biophysiologic instruments.

We use instruments continuously in clinical practice to measure various biophysiologic phenomena. A variety of quantitative instruments are used to measure height, weight, and related characteristics. In this sense, a tape ruler and a scale are instruments to measure something that we can see or estimate with our eyes. Other biophysiologic characteristics are not easily or directly visualized, but they, too, require instruments to help us measure and assess patient characteristics. Again, many instruments are available in clinical practice: a sphygmomanometer to measure systolic and diastolic blood pressure, a thermometer to measure body temperature, a glucometer to estimate blood glucose levels, and an electrocardiogram to measure various aspects of the electrophysiology of the heart. A wide array of laboratory results used in clinical practice are produced by technologic instruments.

These same instruments can be used to measure phenomena or gather data that will provide answers to research questions. The resultant measures are often considered objective because the laboratory or diagnostic report of findings is the indicator. Often, if the measurement is complex or requires sophisticated analysis with biochemical techniques, the researcher collaborates with a scientist from another discipline.

4. Give examples of psychosocial and behavioral instruments.

Instruments that measure attitudes and psychological variables are likely to be the most familiar to nurses. Intelligence tests are instruments designed to measure "intelligence quotient" as an indicator of cognitive ability. Counselors also use various types of personality measures to assess aptitudes for characteristics such as creativity or ability to manage anger. All of these instruments are designed to measure some psychosocial or behavioral variable.

In nursing research, phenomena of interest often require instrumentation to measure some psychosocial variable directly related to practice. For example, an instrument to measure parenting ability is likely to be of interest to a researcher working with young or first-time parents. We may be interested in assessing attitudes toward healthy lifestyles. Such instruments are designed to measure behavioral or psychological variables much in the same way that laboratory instruments are designed to measure physiologic characteristics. Laboratory or diagnostic tests are often considered "objective" because of greater agreement on the criteria used to establish them, whereas psychosocial measures often are considered to be "subjective" because they are indirect. The researcher has to make a judgment about the indicator.

5. What psychometric properties are used to describe a research instrument?

Psychometric properties describe how well the instrument performs. The standards against which any instrument is judged are validity and reliability. The various techniques used to measure validity and reliability have come primarily from statistical measurement experts in the behavioral and social sciences, especially psychology. Specifically, the term *psychometrics* refers to the validity and reliability of an instrument. Various recognized techniques are used as indicators or "properties" of the validity and reliability of an instrument. These agreed-upon indicators often are used by researchers to evaluate whether an existing instrument performs satisfactorily. Statistical indicators of test-retest reliability, internal consistency reliability, and construct validity are examples of performance indicators that describe the psychometric properties of an instrument.

6. Discuss reliability of a research instrument.

Reliability is a major criterion for assessing quality and performance of an instrument. Reliability refers to the consistency of performance or dependability that an instrument provides. An instrument that measures weight or length can be compared with a standard measure to ensure that it is measuring accurately and that we can depend on the results. Such a scale or measure is said to be reliable. This same dependability, or reliability, is expected of any instrument we use. If an instrument designed to measure the concept of interest produces results that are highly variable or inconsistent, it is said to have low reliability. The less variability an instrument produces, the higher the reliability. Reliability can be equated with the following characteristics[2]:

- **Stability over time** refers to the extent that repeated uses of the instrument produce the same results. Sometimes this is called test-retest reliability or stability. If the instrument is administered to the same subjects on two different occasions and the results are compared, stability over time is being addressed. If the instrument has high reliability, the results at the two different times should be identical or very similar.
- **Dependability** is sometimes referred to as equivalence. If an instrument requires observation and rating by two different observers or researches, the results should be the same. Intrarater reliability is another form of stability assessment—one rater's consistency in assigning scores at two points in time. This type of reliability evaluates the equivalence of an instrument.
- **Internal consistency** refers to how well all items of an instrument measure the same underlying construct or phenomenon of interest and do it better than any one item.

Reliability continues to be measured whenever an instrument is used. Just like support for validity, evidence for the reliability of an instrument is an ongoing activity. Reliability and validity must be evaluated every time that the instrument is used and with every sample. Reliability and validity always have potential for change as research subjects change.

7. Discuss validity of a research instrument.

Validity, one of the criteria used to evaluate the quality of a research instrument, refers to the extent to which an instrument measures what it purports to measure. Validity addresses the meaning or interpretation of the data produced by the instrument.[2] For example, if the instrument has been designed to measure depression, do the data obtained by the instrument actually identify depression and, perhaps, distinguish it from other affective states? Measures of validity indicate the level of confidence that the instrument actually measures depression. The precision with which an instrument measures the concepts or phenomena refers to its validity. Several types of validity are important to know and understand: content validity, criterion-related validity, and construct validity.[2]

Because validity assessments are less data-based than reliability assessments, validity is difficult to establish and is generally an ongoing endeavor. Perfect validity is probably unobtainable, but a researcher always strives for a validity index as high as possible. Often a researcher continues to seek evidence for an instrument's validity even if initial support is solid.

Types of Validity

TYPES OF VALIDITY	DEFINITION
Content validity	The degree to which the contents of the instrument accurately examine the dimension/characteristics that it purports to measure
Criterion-related validity	The degree to which the instrument or measurement agrees with other approaches for measuring the same characteristic
Construct validity	The extent to which an instrument measures the concept or construct it was designed to measure

8. Explain content validity.

Content validity refers to how well or thoroughly the instrument measures the underlying concept or theoretical trait. That is, how adequate is the instrument in measuring all aspects of the concept of interest? If a concept has three critical dimensions, an instrument must measure all three critical dimensions with an adequate number of items from the dimensions before it can be stated to have content validity. Judgment of content experts and consistency with the literature are methods used to assess content validity.

9. Explain criterion-rated validity.

Criterion-related validity refers to how well the instrument compares with another indicator or concept of interest (e.g. test score with skill performance). The interest is not in how well the instrument measures some underlying concept (i.e., content validity); rather, the aim is to establish that the instrument distinguishes between different concepts, such as satisfaction and dissatisfaction. Criterion-related validity can be predictive or concurrent. Predictive validity describes how well the instrument actually predicts that something will occur in the future. This measure requires that the instrument meets the "criteria" for a concept and can actually predict that the concept will be measurable in the future. Concurrent validity provides an assessment of how well the instrument compares with another recognized measure or gold standard of the concept of interest.[3]

10. Explain construct validity.

Construct validity is the most challenging type of validity to establish, because it requires evidence that the instrument measures what it claims to measure. The more abstract the phenomenon of interest, the more difficult it is to provide evidence for construct validity.[4] The most direct way to demonstrate construct validity is comparison with another instrument that measures the concept of interest and has established construct validity. Both instruments are administrated to the same individuals and the scores or results compared. If both measure the same construct, scores should be similar.

11. What is the difference between a norm-referenced and a criterion-referenced instrument?

A **norm-referenced** instrument measures or evaluates the performance of a subject relative to the performance of other subjects in a defined norm or comparison group.[1] A wide variety of concepts or phenomena in clinical practice are norm-referenced. Examples include physiologic measures, such as blood pressure, blood glucose, height, and weight. Many attitudes are viewed as norms as well. Test scores are another example of norm-referenced values. The challenge in developing a norm-referenced instrument is to capture variance. Because a norm-referenced concept can hold a range of values, the key is to ensure that it measures the differing amounts of the concept across the full range of possible scores.

Criterion-referenced measures are used to determine whether a subject can perform a particular task or has acquired a particular characteristic.[4] The subject is measured against a standard, such as ability to perform a certain behavior or procedure. The important point to measure is whether a subject has a particular characteristic or behavior, not how well the subject performs on that measure in relation to all other subjects. In clinical practice, competency-based measures provide a good example of criterion-referenced measurement. In competency-based measurement, we are interested in whether a clinician can perform a certain clinical task, not how their performance compares with all other people who also perform that task.

Determining whether a measurement framework will be norm- or criterion-referenced is important. The design, scoring, methods of reliability and validity measurement, and the statistics that may be used vary, depending on the underlying framework for instrument development.[1]

12. How are validity and reliability of instruments assessed?

Techniques range from use of expert opinion to highly sophisticated statistical techniques and vary with the type of data that are gathered, the availability of other measures, the design of the instrument, and whether the instrument is norm- or criterion-referenced. Generally, if one is designing an instrument, collaboration with an expert researcher and/or statistician is prudent. It is essential to use the right techniques for measuring validity and reliability. In general, an instrument is no better than its validity or reliability.

Reliability is often assessed in different ways. One approach is to examine the internal consistency, or homogeneity, of an instrument. This type of reliability measures how well each item in the instrument agrees with the overall score produced by the instrument. One common approach is to examine the item-total agreement of an instrument by correlating each item in the instrument with the total score. Items that do not agree or correlate highly with the total score may be deleted from the instrument. Another method examines the average correlation among all items in a scale and the total number of items in that scale. Values range from 0 to 1, and the closer the value to 1, the stronger the reliability or internal consistency on the instrument. Values of 0.70 and higher are generally desired.[2,3] When clinical decisions are based on a measure, a value of 0.90 is generally used.

Nursing research texts provide general information about how to assess and interpret different types of validity and reliability. A classic text in this area is *Measurement in Nursing Research*.[1] Additionally, research methods resources from any scientific discipline are helpful in learning more about different approaches to measuring validity and reliability. Many statistical analysis packages have features to perform analyses for certain types of reliability and validity testing.

13. Where do I find research instruments for possible use in a research project?

Generally, instruments used by other researchers are identified through a literature review, including published studies of instruments that have been newly developed or revised as well as research reports that describe the use of particular instruments. If you read the research regularly in a particular clinical area or have conducted an extensive literature review as part of the development of a research project, you will begin to have an understanding of the research instruments in your area of interest. If you are interested in investigating an area where little research has been conducted, you may find that no instruments are available and that your first step is to develop an instrument that you can use in your research.

The majority of nursing and health services research reported in the literature uses some type of instrumentation. If you do a literature search on a topic of interest, you generally will have to search through the results to separate the research articles from conceptual or review articles. Most research articles describe some type of instrumentation used to gather data and measure the variables of interest. A section of the research article describes the instruments used. Occasionally, a research study uses existing data from another study (called a secondary analysis) and does not directly report on the instrument. Reviewing articles that have used various instruments is one way to begin to identify instruments used in your area of interest.

Various compendiums and directories contain standardized instruments in particular content areas. These directories are particularly helpful because they often contain well-developed instruments with evidence of reliability and validity in the specific sample. In addition, they generally provide all of the available information about the psychometric properties of the instrument or at least references to the literature where such information may be found.

14. Which references provide instruments that can be used in clinical research projects?

An excellent source of instruments for clinical nursing research is Frank-Stromberg and Olsen's *Instruments for Clinical Health-Care Research.*[5] The literature occasionally contains review articles of standardized research instruments in a particular clinical area.[6] Instruments and rating scales to measure various aspects of health status, quality of life, and psychological indicators are also available in multiple sources.[7,8,9] Increasingly, resources of this type are available on the worldwide web (WWW) or CD ROM and can be accessed in most university and health science libraries. The Health and Psychosocial Instruments (HAPI) database includes over 15,000 instruments in the health and psychosocial areas. It is available as part of standard health sciences literature databases, such as Medline and Ovid, using keywords as outlined in the National Library of Medicine's Medical Subject Headings (MeSH). These are the same keywords used for conducting a Medline search of the literature. Many directories to instruments can be identified and accessed on the web. An excellent example, the *Guide to Tests and Measurement Instruments*, can be found at the website for the Taubman Medical Library at the University of Michigan[10] <http://www.lib.umich.edu/taubman/info/testsandmeasurement.htm>.

Some online sources may have restricted use if you are not a member of the sponsoring organization. Many directories and compendiums are available at health science and medical libraries, often in the reference section. A librarian can help identify useful resources.

15. How do I evaluate an existing instrument for possible use in my research project?

Because an instrument is designed to measure an underlying concept, the first step is to evaluate conceptual fit with the topic and concepts central to your study. The instrument must fit the variables and their operational definitions. One way to assess fit is to examine the instrument to make sure that the items address the variables that you wish to measure.

One also wants to review the psychometric properties of the instrument to determine whether its reliability and validity have been tested. It is important to make sure that these characteristics are acceptable for your purposes and that the instrument actually measures the concept of interest in your study and provides high-quality data to answer your research questions. It is also helpful to review whether the instrument has been used by other researchers and, if so, how well it performed with other samples. Typically at the end of a research article authors discuss limitations of the study, some of which may be related to the instruments.

In the end, the results of your study will be no better than the instruments used in gathering the data. Adequate time must be devoted to reviewing the available instruments. As the investigator, you need to defend your instruments as the best measures available for the key variables in your study and their underlying concepts or theoretical constructs.

16. What do I do if a credentialed or standardized instrument does not exist?

If a thorough search does not produce a standardized instrument for use in your research project, you are faced with the task of developing your own measurement tool. This task is always challenging and adds time to your research project. In fact, developing the research instrumentation may become a research project in itself. Sometimes a standardized instrument can be used to address part of your research question. In this case, you may have to develop additional questions or an additional scale to answer your research question completely. (*Caution:* Any additions or modifications to an existing instrument alter the psychometric properties.) Another possibility is that the research project originally intended may have to be simplified in some way.

All of these approaches have differing advantages and disadvantages. The critical point to keep in mind is that the quality of the data obtained by an instrument is directly related to the quality (i.e., validity and reliability) of the instrument. A revised research question or redesigned project is preferable to one in which inadequate or inappropriate instrumentation is used to gather data that do not answer the research question of interest.

17. How do I go about developing and testing my own instrument? Where can I find help?

Several resources are available to help with this challenging task. Many health care agencies have staff members who may be of some assistance. Typically, people with a doctoral degree have had some course work in research methods and statistics that address many of the approaches for developing instruments. Sometimes this knowledge and skill is available from people with master's preparation. In academic health settings, an office of nursing research or clinical research with doctorally prepared researchers is often available. Sitting down and talking with them is a necessary first step in identifying what actually needs to be done. In turn, this step helps to identify whether they have the resources to assist you.

If your organization does not have a specific research office, think of people with graduate-level preparation who may serve as resources. Examples include master's prepared nurses who are working in specialized clinical roles, such as a clinical nurse specialist. If they do not have the expertise to assist you in instrument design, they often can provide some assistance and direct you to other resources. If help is not available within nursing, check the organization for other people who have some clinical responsibilities related to your area of research interest and who may be able to help. Examples include clinical psychologists, social workers, physical therapists, and pharmacists.

Another good source of assistance is the local college or university. If a school of nursing is nearby, a faculty member who teaches and/or does research in your interest area would be ideal. If the school of nursing has a master's and/or doctoral program, faculty members may connect you with students who have degree requirements for some type of research. Such connections can be invaluable in finding technical expertise and provide students or faculty with opportunities that benefit them as well. If nursing is not available in the college or university, other disciplines can be approached. Social and behavioral scientists often have the expertise to assist with instrument design and development. (*Caution:* If you lack expertise or resources, you should not try to develop an instrument on your own.)

18. If I develop and test an instrument, how do I describe it and make it available to other researchers?

As you review the literature, you become aware of a number of new instruments that have been developed. In fact, many articles in the literature describe new instruments, their psychometric properties, how they were developed and tested, and how they should be used. These articles can serve as a guide for describing an instrument that you have developed and want to make available to other researchers or clinicians.

Proposed standards[11] for a publishable report of instrument development include:
* Description of the conceptual basis for the tool
* Methods used for item generation and refinement of those items
* Sociodemographic characteristics for the intended respondents
* Guidelines and requirements for administration of the instrument
* Method of scoring
* Description of the type of data obtained with the instrument
* Range of scores and values for the scales for comparative purposes
* Sample items or a copy of the instrument.
* Minimal standards for psychometric properties: test-retest reliability, internal consistency reliability; at least one measure of validity such as content or construct validity or criterion-related validity

Publishing in a recognized journal is the key way to disseminate information about an instrument that you have developed. If an article describing the instrument is published in a journal, it will be indexed by key words in standard literature databases such as Medline or CINAHL and can be identified by other researchers looking for instruments to use in their studies.

19. Do I have to get permission to use an instrument developed by someone else?

It depends. If the instrument has been copyrighted, you must request permission to use it. If the instrument is reported in a journal article, with a complete copy of the instrument and all information about its use, administration, and scoring, the instrument is considered to be in the public domain and is available for use without permission.

Under all circumstances, proper citation of the source of the instrument is mandatory. In addition, if an instrument in the public domain is altered or adapted in any way, permission to do so should be sought from the author.

20. If I use a researcher's or testing firm's instrument, do I have to pay for it?

It depends on the nature of the instrument. If the instrument was developed by a researcher in a college or university as part of their research program, it is unlikely that you will have to pay to use it. The instrument was developed by a scientist who is making a contribution to knowledge or some aspect of science. Instruments developed by public funds, such as research grants, are usually considered to be in the public domain and available for use by all.

If the instrument was expensive to develop and required years of testing or was developed by a firm in the business of selling instruments, you may have to pay for its use. This type of proprietary orientation is becoming increasingly common in the biologic arena. The recent developments and special measurement techniques in genomic science offer examples of how scientists, research firms, and universities are trying to recapture some the investment that they have made in developing highly specialized instruments.

21. If I use a standardized instrument, do I still need to assess its validity and reliability in my study?

Yes. Every time an instrument is used, the reliability and the validity should be tested to the extent possible. Reliability is easier to test than validity. A researcher always needs to monitor how well instruments perform. Special characteristics in a population may alter how an instrument functions and thus affect the reliability or validity of the instrument and the data it produces. For example, cultural values and beliefs influence health behaviors. If an instrument was developed and tested to measure beliefs and values of African Americans, it may not perform in the same way if used to measure the same beliefs and values in Hispanics. Assessing the reliability and validity of the instrument with Hispanic clients helps evaluate the performance of the instrument. Whenever an instrument does not perform as intended (i.e., the psychometric indicators are different from previous uses), further examination is required.

22. Why are some instruments copyrighted?

Copyright is a form of legal protection available to authors of original works. The owner of the copyright has the exclusive right to control use of the copyrighted materials. Copyright protection exists as soon as something is created and fixed in a tangible form; it does not require official registration. Sometimes, however, researchers may register instruments with the Copyright Office at the U.S. Library of Congress. This step may be taken to control how the instruments are used, to ensure that they are used and scored correctly, or to ensure that royalties or fees associated with the use of the instrument accrue to the owner. Typically, when an author publishes a research report, the copyright is transferred to the publisher. Whenever the report is referenced by others, the full citation to the copyrighted material must be given. If a researcher gives a copy of the complete instrument along with scoring instructions in the published report, others can use it as long as the original source and author are cited. If the full instrument and related information are not provided in the research report, the author must be contacted for permission to use the instrument.

Information about copyright law and how to go about registering an instrument that you have created can be found at <http://www.loc.gov/copyright/circs/cir1.html>. If you develop an instrument, you are faced with deciding whether you want to have it copyrighted. Typically, in the interest of science and the advancement of knowledge, researchers readily share their instruments with others. However, if a measurement device has been developed with a considerable investment of money and time, you may want to receive fees in an attempt to repay your investment. Sometimes these fees are paid for analysis because of the complexity of the measure and the fact that few of the instruments exist. This scenario is most common with instrumentation in the biophysiologic realm.

REFERENCES

1. Waltz CF, Strickland OL, Lenz ER: Measurement in Nursing Research, 2nd ed. Philadelphia, F.A. Davis, 1991.
2. Polit DF, Beck CT, Hungler BP: Essentials of Nursing Research: Methods, Appraisal, and Utilization, 5th ed. Philadelphia, Lippincott, 2001.
3. McDowell I, Newell C: Measuring Health: A Guide to Rating Scales and Questionnaires, 2nd ed. New York, Oxford University Press, 1996.
4. Jacobson SF: Evaluating instruments for use in clinical nursing research. In Frank-Stromberg M, Olsen SJ (eds): Instruments for Clinical Health-care Research, 2nd ed. Boston, Jones & Bartlett, 1997, pp 3–19.
5. Frank-Stromberg M, Olsen SJ (eds): Instruments for Clinical Health-Care Research, 2nd ed. Boston, Jones & Bartlett, 1997.
6. Beck CT: A review of research instruments for use during the postpartum period. Am J Matern Child Nurs 23:254–261, 1998.
7. Mental Measurements Yearbook. Lincoln, NE, Buros Institute of Mental Measurements of the University of Nebraska at Lincoln, 1992.
8. Bowling A: Measuring Health: A Review of Quality of Life Measure Scales, 2nd ed. Philadelphia, Open University Press, 1997.
9. Bowling A: Measuring Disease: A Review of Disease-specific Quality of Life Measurement Scales, 2nd ed. Philadelphia, Open University Press, 2001.
10. University of Michigan, Taubman Medical Library: Guide to Tests and Measurement Instruments. Available at <http://www.lib.umich.edu/taubman/info/testsandmeasurement.htm>.
11. Norbeck JS: What constitutes a publishable report of instrument development? Nurs Res 34:380–382, 1985.

17. SAMPLING, POWER, AND DATA ANALYSIS PLAN

Souraya Sidani, RN, PhD

1. What is a sample? Why is it needed?

Research is undertaken to investigate phenomena of interest within a target population, which is characterized by certain attributes. Populations targeted in nursing research include patients with chronic obstructive pulmonary disease, pregnant women, registered nurses, and family caregivers of patients with Alzheimer's disease. Because the target population is large in number and spread throughout a country or the world a researcher does not have the resources, time, and money to study all possible members. It is, therefore, more economical and efficient to gather data from a sample. A sample refers to a subset of persons that make up the target population.

2. What characteristics should a sample have?

A sample has to be representative of the target population, of a large size, and nonbiased to help the researcher obtain pertinent data and make appropriate generalizations of the results to the target population.

3. What is a representative sample?

A representative sample is like the target population, with similar attributes (e.g., sociodemographic profile) and similar range of values on the variables under study (e.g., varying levels of anxiety). For instance, if the study is set to examine the satisfaction of general medical and surgical patients with nursing care, the sample should include patients with varying degrees of satisfaction, of different age groups and gender, and with various diagnoses. A representative sample provides information about the study variables that reflect the information in the target population. In other words, the statistical scores on the variables obtained in a sample (such as mean values) are precise estimates of the scores of the target population (called parameters). Over the years, researchers have realized that a sample is not identical to the target population; it may differ from the population to some extent on some variable(s).

The difference between the sample and the population scores on the study variables is called **sampling error**. Sampling error, which is due to chance, results from the sample selection process. Large sampling error indicates that the sample does not adequately represent the target population, which limits the generalizability of the results to all persons in the target population.

4. Explain the role of sample size.

Sample size is critical to interpreting data because sampling error is associated with sample size. The larger the sample size, the smaller the sampling error. Therefore, large samples tend to be more representative of the target population than small ones.

5. What is a biased sample?

We can think of a biased sample as the opposite of a representative sample. A biased sample under- or overrepresents certain subgroups of the target population. For example, a sample containing only patients who are highly satisfied with nursing care overestimates the level of satisfaction. A biased sample may result from selecting, consciously or unconsciously, participants with particular characteristics or with a certain level on a study variable to the exclusion of the others. Results of biased samples are of limited validity, because the participants' characteristics may confound the scores on the study variables. For instance, a sample containing a large proportion of older persons may have, on average, a low level of anxiety. Biased samples also have limited generalizability, because the results are applicable only to a subgroup of the target population with similar characteristics.

6. On what basis is a sample selected?

A sample is carefully selected on the basis of well-defined inclusion and exclusion criteria, which consist of characteristics that delimit the target population. As such, they inform the researcher when making a decision about whether a particular person is considered a member of the population and, therefore, is eligible to participate in the study.

7. Define inclusion and exclusion criteria.

The **inclusion criteria** are characteristics that participants must possess to identify them as members of the target population. These characteristics include qualities that define the population (such as medical diagnosis or experience of a symptom) as well as demographic features that enable the persons to participate in the study (such as ability to read and write the language used in the study and ability to provide written informed consent).

The **exclusion criteria** are characteristics that some members of the population may have but may influence the study variables. They are often considered as extraneous factors that confound the results and present threats to the validity of the study conclusions. Participants with these characteristics are excluded from the study sample. The exclusion criteria control for extraneous, confounding factors and make the sample homogeneous. Sample homogeneity is essential in studies evaluating the effectiveness of nursing interventions. It reduces variability among participants in outcome variables that is not attributable to the intervention, which in turn, increases the statistical power to detect significant intervention effects (for more details, refer to Lipsey,[1] Sidani and Braden[2]).

8. Why is it important to specify inclusion and exclusion criteria?

Inclusion and exclusion criteria should be specified carefully because they may affect the ability to find eligible participants and to obtain the required sample size, the results of the study, and the validity of conclusions.

In some studies, researchers specify a set of restrictive inclusion and exclusion criteria to control for as many extraneous factors as possible. Restrictive criteria, however, have some limitations. First, they make it difficult to find enough participants who meet all of the specified criteria; thus, the researcher may not obtain the required sample size within the study period. Second, the accrued sample is homogeneous. The results, therefore, are applicable to a subgroup—not the full range—of elements in the target population. Close and colleagues[3] recognized the limitations of setting restrictive criteria. They reported that they were able to recruit 20% of the potential participants within the 5-year study period and that those excluded represented a large proportion of the target population frequently seen in the practice setting.

In other studies, researchers predetermine a set of loosely defined or less restrictive criteria. The advantages of this set of criteria are twofold: it increases the representativeness of the sample in that the sample reflects all subgroups of the population of interest, and it makes easier the selection of participants and less time-consuming the accrual of the required sample size. A less restrictive set renders the sample heterogeneous. Heterogeneity is associated with increased variability in the study variables, which may confound the results. A researcher setting less restrictive criteria has to account for this variability when analyzing the data by doing subgroup analysis. The question of which set of criteria (restrictive vs. less restrictive) to use can be best addressed, at the moment, by encouraging researchers to maintain a balance when formulating the sample selection criteria to avoid the limitations of each set.

9. How are the sample selection criteria specified?

Careful specification of the sample selection (i.e., inclusion and exclusion) criteria depends on the following factors:

- The **nature of the research problem** points to the population to be targeted, which is defined, at least, by the experience of the phenomena under investigation. For example, if the problem is about women's coping with sexual assault, the sample consists of women who had experienced such an event.
- The researchers' **knowledge of the target population** contributes further to elucidating the selection criteria. To continue with the previous example, the researchers' awareness of when exactly after the event the women feel comfortable to discuss the experience informs them of which women to approach, based on the length of time since the event (e.g., within 1 or 3 months).
- The **variable definition and measurement** are other factors to consider in specifying the selection criteria. For instance, the American Sleep Disorders Association defines insomnia as difficulty in initiating or maintaining sleep. This definition implies that persons who experience either type of sleep difficulty are to be sampled. Insomnia is a symptom; its subjective nature is best captured through self-report and keeping a daily diary. This measurement requires the selection of persons with insomnia who are cognitively able to complete the daily diary.
- The **purpose and design** of a study guide the specification of selection criteria. Studies aimed at exploring new phenomena or at describing a phenomenon in the population (e.g., epidemiologic studies) benefit from sampling participants on the basis of less restrictive criteria to ensure adequate representation of all subgroups. Studies aimed at testing hypothesized relationships among study variables demand somewhat restrictive selection criteria for the purpose of controlling extraneous factors that may confound the hypothesized relationships.

10. How does the specification of the sample selection criteria vary across types of research and designs?

In **quantitative designs**, the criteria are predetermined and precisely defined before recruiting participants. They form the basis on which participants are selected or excluded. In *descriptive, correlational, survey-type designs*, the selection criteria tend to be less restrictive because the sample needs to be representative of all sub-groups of the target population; hence, some heterogeneity in the study variables is necessary. Furthermore, in large-scale surveys, it may not be possible to screen potential participants for eligibility. Screening for eligibility requires that the researchers (1) have adequate information about the characteristics of all elements of the population, which is not available most of the time on lists enumerating them and used to mail out questionnaires; or (2) begin the questionnaire with items to determine whether the respondents meet the eligibility criteria and explaining to the respondent to return the questionnaire unanswered if she or he identifies her- or himself as not eligible. This strategy is a waste of time, energy and resources and may be cumbersome to respondents. In *comparative* (e.g., case-control or cohort), and *true* or *quasi-experimental designs*, the selection criteria tend to be restrictive to control for extraneous factors that may confound the results. The researcher plans to screen potential participants by conducting a short interview or laboratory tests to determine eligibility before enrolling them in the study. This strategy has some resource implications.

The specification of sample selection criteria differs in **qualitative designs**. Researchers usually start with general, loosely defined criteria that lead to the inclusion of persons who experienced the phenomenon of interest and who have the potential for providing "rich" information. They revisit the selection criteria based on the early findings, the quality of informants, and the purpose of the inquiry. That is, the preliminary emerging themes guide the selection of additional participants, who are purposefully sought to represent persons with similar characteristics as those who already participated, with characteristics that differ from those of early participants, or with "typical" reflection of the average case.

11. What is a sampling plan?

Once the target population is defined and the selection criteria are delineated, a sampling plan should be devised. The plan consists of identifying the accessible population and choosing the sampling approach and strategy.

12. Define accessible population.

Accessible population refers to the part of the target population that is available to the researcher. To access potential participants, the researcher needs to identify a location within the community where they can be found, obtain approval to recruit them, and gain assistance of staff to recruit eligible participants.

The nature of the population points to the location where potential participants can be found. For example, if the interest is inpatients scheduled for surgery, surgical inpatient units or presurgical clinics are suitable sites to recruit participants. In some cases, the identified sites have a small number of participants, and the researcher plans to include multiple sites to increase the pool of participants and the opportunity to obtain the required sample size.

Researchers must obtain approval to access participants from the appropriate site authority. This process involves obtaining approval from the institutional review board (IRB) as well as support from managers and staff to facilitate recruitment. Staff support requires clear communication of the study purpose and discussion of procedures and staff contribution. The less demanding the study in terms of staff involvement, the more likely they are to support it. Gaining the staff's assistance in recruiting eligible participants is essential. Lack of staff cooperation interferes with the ability to access, approach, and enroll participants, thereby reducing the pool of available cases.

13. What approaches are used to select a sample?

Two general approaches are available for sampling participants: probability and nonprobability. The corner stone of probability sampling is random selection of participants. Random selection is a process in which each participant in the accessible population has an equal chance of being selected. Random selection is not used in nonprobability sampling. Within each approach, there are specific strategies to choose from.

14. What strategies can be used to achieve a probability sample?

Four strategies can be used to achieve probability sampling: simple random, stratified random, cluster, and systematic sampling.

15. How is a simple random sample obtained?

Simple random sampling consists of randomly selecting a sample from a sampling frame. A sampling frame is a complete list or enumeration of all participants in the accessible population, such as a list of registered nurses or a cancer registry. Randomly selecting the required number of participants is done by

- Drawing names of participants written on a piece of paper. The pieces of paper are placed in a container and mixed well before they are drawn one at a time. The pieces of paper are replaced in the container before the next draw to ensure that participants have an equal chance of being selected.
- Assigning a code number to each participant and using a table of random numbers (available in most research books), wheel, or computer program to select participants.

16. Explain stratified random sample.

Stratified random sampling involves dividing the accessible population into strata and taking a random sample of participants within each stratum. Strata are mutually exclusive subgroups of the population based on known characteristics, such as gender, ethnicity, or socioeconomic status. Stratification ensures that all subgroups of the target population are represented in the sample. The researcher classifies participants into their respective strata, then randomly selects participants belonging to each subgroup. The number of participants selected within the subgroups may be either proportional or disproportionate to their occurrence in the population. For instance, a proportional stratified random sample includes numbers of Caucasians and African Americans that are consistent with the proportions of these subgroups in the target population. Proportional selection is preferable, because it enhances the representativeness of the sample.

17. How is a cluster sample obtained?

Cluster sampling, also called multistage sampling, is often used in large-scale surveys targeting persons in various geographic locations for whom a sampling frame is not available. The persons are located within clusters such as state, city, and institution. The researchers develop a list of the clusters, moving from the larger or inclusive cluster (e.g., state) to smaller ones (e.g., hospitals). Then they randomly select larger clusters, followed by smaller ones that are nested within the larger ones; within the smaller cluster, they randomly select the participants. For example, if researchers are interested in conducting a nationwide survey of registered nurses (RNs), they randomly select RNs working in randomly selected hospitals within randomly selected cities located in randomly chosen states.

18. How can a systematic sample be obtained?

Systematic sampling involves selecting every k^{th} participant enumerated on a list. K is the sampling interval or the size of the gap between participants to be selected from the list. K is computed by dividing the accessible population size by the required sample size. For example, if the population size is 3,000 and the sample size is 300, then $k = 3,000/300 = 10$. The researchers then select every tenth participant listed, starting with a randomly selected participant, until the required sample size is achieved. The researchers consider the list as circular; they can run through the list as many times as needed to select the sample.

19. How are nonprobability samples derived?

Three strategies can be used for nonprobability sampling: convenience, quota, and purposive. Selection of the sampling approach and strategy is guided by the researchers' knowledge of the advantages, disadvantages, and feasibility of each strategy.

20. Explain convenience sampling.

Convenience, also called accidental, sampling entails selecting available persons; that is, those who happen to be present at the place and time of recruitment. Eligibility of participants is determined before they are included in the study. Snowball or network sampling is a special type of convenience sampling that is used when it is difficult to find eligible participants by usual means (e.g., persons with substance use). It involves asking colleagues or early participants to identify and refer other persons who meet the selection criteria.

21. What is quota sampling?

Quota sampling is similar to stratified random sampling. Participants are classified into strata and are selected by nonrandom means. The number of participants selected within strata may be either proportional or disproportional.

22. How is a purposive sample obtained?

Purposive, also called theoretical or judgmental, sampling refers to situations in which the researchers "handpick" participants. The selected participants are thought to be typical cases representative of the target population, which is often not precisely defined. This strategy is commonly used in qualitative research and some quantitative studies, such as those involving experts in a field (e.g., the Delphi technique).

23. What are the advantages and disadvantages of the different sampling strategies?

Advantages of **probability sampling** include:

- Random selection eliminates researchers' biases in including or excluding participants for reasons not related to the selection criteria, such as excluding uncooperative participants.
- The obtained sample is considered a "random" subset of the target population; as such, any difference in the value of sample variables from those of the population is a function of chance. Sampling error is minimal, which improves the precision of the parameter estimates.
- A random sample is more representative of the target population than a non-random sample, which allows more accurate generalizations of the results to the population.

Probability samples are difficult, expensive, and tedious to obtain, which makes them inconvenient, particularly for small-scale studies.

Nonprobability sampling is more convenient, less complicated, easier to implement, and less expensive. However, it yields samples that may not be representative of the target population, which limits the generalizability of the findings.

The advantages and disadvantages of the specific sampling strategies are presented in the table below. A word of caution: random selection does not guarantee that the sample is representative of the target population and/or unbiased. Bias can result from pure chance.

Advantages and Disadvantages of Sampling Strategies

SAMPLING STRATEGY	ADVANTAGES	DISADVANTAGES
Simple random	• Eliminates researcher bias • Requires limited a priori knowledge of the target population • Provides a means for estimating sampling error	• Does not guarantee that the sample is representative of the population • Time-consuming, laborious process
Stratified random	• Provides a means of including participants representative of all subgroups of the population	• Difficult to implement if the stratifying information is not available • Requires a priori knowledge of the target population • Requires more labor and effort
Systematic	• Fast, easy, and an inexpensive strategy for drawing a random sample	• May lead to biased sample if participants are listed in a particular order and this order is not taken into account (as forming subgroups)
Cluster	• Economical, time-saving, and practical when the population is very large	• Introduces sampling error at each stage, which adversely affects the sample representativeness
Convenience	• Easy to implement • Saves time and resources	• Includes atypical participants, which results in biased sample • Yields results that are of limited generalizability to the full range of the target population
Quota	• Ensures that diverse segments of the target population are represented	• Includes atypical participants, which results in biased sample • Yields results of limited generalizability to the full range of the target population

(*Table continued on next page.*)

Advantages and Disadvantages of Sampling Strategies

SAMPLING STRATEGY	ADVANTAGES	DISADVANTAGES
Purposive	• Yields selection of typical cases	• Is highly subjective since selection criteria are not explicitly stated or objective • Results in biased, unrepresentative sample

24. How feasible are the various sampling strategies?

Probability sampling strategies are not always feasible in nursing research. They require the availability of a comprehensive and up-to-date list of all participants in the accessible population. Such lists may not be kept for populations of interest to nurses. When available, the lists may not be comprehensive and up-to-date, they may not present information needed to classify participants into strata, or they may not be given to researchers for ethical reasons. For instance, a cancer registry may not be released to researchers in some settings for fear of breaching patients' privacy and confidentiality. The random selection process is time-consuming; if done with replacement, the selection of random numbers is nonproductive because an already selected number may be randomly selected again. Random selection with computer programs is resource-intensive, expensive, and complicated.

Nonprobability strategies are simple, easier to carry out, and convenient. They are used most frequently and are familiar to researchers and participants.

25. How does ethical conduct of research affect selection of random samples?

The ethical conduct of research requires respecting the participants' right for self-determination. Voluntary participation results in self-selection, which increases the likelihood of having a biased sample. Empirical evidence suggests that some subgroups of the population tend to volunteer, whereas others refuse to participate. For instance, clients who volunteer for psychosocial intervention studies tend to be women, Caucasian, unemployed, old, and of low socioeconomic status; they also have an internal orientation to locus of control. This point raises the question of whether it is possible to obtain truly random samples.

26. To what extent is selecting participants from multiple settings efficient and beneficial?

Researchers often resort to selecting participants from multiple sites to increase sample size and representativeness. This practice is efficient and beneficial because it ensures the accrual of the required sample size within the constraint of the study period and increases the opportunity of including participants reflecting all subgroups of the target population. Although advantageous, selecting participants from multiple sites has some limitations. It increases the heterogeneity of the sample in terms of extraneous factors that confound the results; this diversity, if not controlled for, can lead to erroneous results. Clinical and empirical evidence indicates that persons in different sites vary in some characteristics, even though they are members of the same population. For example, older adults with dementia admitted to long-term care units in a VA medical center tend to be men of a younger age than those admitted to a nursing home, who tend to be older women. Researchers should recognize, test, and account for differences in characteristics of participants selected from multiple sites.

27. Which strategies can be used to recruit participants?

- Advertising the study by putting advertisements in local newspapers, newsletters, or radio and TV stations; by posting flyers or leaving brochures in settings visited by potential participants; or by adding information about the study on relevant websites (such as those for support groups).
- Contacting potential participants by mailing a letter or calling them by phone to introduce the study.
- Approaching participants in a particular setting and explaining the study to them.
- Having staff or colleagues introduce the study to and refer eligible participants.

Some of these recruitment strategies will be more tightly regulated when HIPAA standards are in place. Local IRBs will provide more direction and oversight to subject recruitment plans. Researchers can come up with other innovative strategies to recruit participants. Information about the study should cover:

- The affiliation of the investigators (which gives credibility to the study)
- The purpose of the study (which introduces the general research topic and the importance of the study)
- Who is being recruited (which identifies the sample selection criteria and may serve as an initial screening)
- The research activities in which participants will be involved and the time needed to accomplish them (which provides an idea of the nature and amount of effort the participants will invest)
- Compensation that the participants may receive (which serves as an incentive for participation)
- Benefits and risks associated with participation
- Information about who to contact if interested in taking part in the study.

28. Which of these recruitment strategies are most effective?

No study has investigated the effectiveness of different recruitment strategies. Experience suggests that the usefulness of the strategies varies with the type of population targeted and the study design. Community-wide advertisement can reach various subgroups of a target population defined with less restrictive criteria and difficult to identify by other means. Contacting potential participants by mail is useful in large-scale surveys of the general population. Approaching participants in a particular setting is effective in recruiting a rather captive population (e.g., those attending a clinic). Referrals by staff can be used to recruit participants into a study addressing a sensitive topic or "hard-to-get" participants. Combining strategies that are feasible and appropriate for the target population is most useful.

The manner in which the study is introduced to potential participants is very important. The information needs to be comprehensive and convincing, yet to-the-point. The presentation has to be neutral, clear, not rushed, and not coercive. Participants should not feel pressured to make a decision about volunteering in the study. Their questions need to be answered; they should be given time to think about participating before deciding.

29. What tips can a researcher use to enhance recruitment?

- **Advertisement.** The content of the ads has to be informative, brief, and written in simple terms (usually sixth-grade level) that raise interest. For instance, an ad to recruit persons with insomnia may begin with the question, "Do you have trouble sleeping?" The layout is equally important: a large, simple font is easier to read. Crowding of words on a page makes reading difficult. Interspersing figures with words and using high-quality, colored print are appealing strategies.

• **Contacting participants**. The letter needs to be carefully composed so that it is persuasive, pointing to the importance of the study and appreciating the participants' time and decision. It also should be formal and neutral in presentation, respective of the participants' rights as research subjects, and clear but concise. The letter is printed on institution letterhead, using large font and high-quality print. The same points are followed when contacting potential participants by phone. Courtesy and politeness are also critical, as well as ensuring that the time of the call is convenient to the participant.

• **Approaching participants**. The researcher approaching participants in a face-to-face encounter, whether in group or individually, must consider the following points: (1) showing respect, courtesy, and politeness; (2) presenting the information in a clear, nonrushed, and neutral way; (3) being formal yet understanding of individuals; (4) dressing appropriately (e.g., wearing casual clothes when recruiting participants in a poor neighborhood); and (5) adapting the information to the learning needs of individual participants.

• **Referral**. The researcher has to discuss the study with staff to gain their support and to devise strategies that make their involvement in recruitment simple, easy, not time-consuming, and least disturbing to their practice. For example, physicians can be given a pad of small advertising papers that they can keep in their pocket and from which they can tear a paper and hand it to eligible participants. Maintaining regular contact with the staff to discuss their referral pattern serves as a reminder and as an opportunity to address any difficulty encountered.

30. How can a researcher determine whether a study sample is biased?

Researchers can develop a form to keep track of all persons recruited and to document their status at each stage of the research project. The information to be recorded includes:

• The person's assigned code number
• Decision about participation
• Reasons for refusals
• Demographic characteristics of refusers (researchers can request refusers to provide such data, if they do not mind)
• Decision to drop out of the study
• Reasons and time of attrition

The researchers can analyze such information to examine sample bias. Content analysis of the reasons for refusal to participate and for attrition identifies themes underlying the person's decision and sheds light on the profile of refusers and dropouts. For example, patients who are "too sick" tend to refuse to take part in the study. Patients assigned to the control or experimental group, who do not experience improvement in their condition, tend to drop out of the study.

Refusers and participants are compared in terms of demographic profile, using appropriate statistical tests. The results indicating significant differences in some characteristics suggest that the obtained sample is biased, over- or underrepresenting certain subgroups of the target population. Similar comparisons are made between those who dropped out and those who completed the study on demographic characteristics, pretest outcome measures, and group assignment (e.g., experimental and control). Significant differences imply that drop-outs and completers do not come from the same target population, and the final sample, composed of completers, is biased.

Another strategy involves comparing the sample mean values to normative values available for the target population. For example, the sample mean values of blood pressure or on the Medical Outcome Study SF-36 are compared with available norms for the target population. The sample gender distribution is compared with census data maintained by the hospital or clinic. Significant differences indicate sample bias. Biased samples limit the generalizability of the findings to the target population.

31. How many participants are needed?

Researchers are strongly encouraged to consider participant refusal and/or attrition rates when determining sample size. They should plan to recruit more participants than required on the basis of power analysis. Researchers have to recruit an additional 20% of cases to account for refusals and an additional 10–15% cases to account for attrition. For instance, if power analysis indicates that the researchers need 100 cases in a survey study, they mail out at least 120 questionnaires to achieve the required sample size. If 50 cases are required for an experimental study with repeated measures, they enroll 5 (i.e., 10%) or 8 (i.e., 15%) additional cases. In qualitative research, the sample size is determined by reaching data saturation. If researchers do not account for refusal or attrition rates before obtaining approval from an IRB, they must resubmit the protocol to the IRB to gain approval to recruit additional participants.

32. Define statistical power in a research study.

Statistical power refers to the capacity of the study to detect differences or relationships that actually exist in the population.[4] It is the probability that a statistical test will yield sample results that accurately reflect those of the target population.

33. How does sample size affect statistical power?

Sample size is one criterion for determining the statistical power of the study and consequently for reaching correct conclusions or avoiding error of inference from the sample to the target population values. Two types of error are of concern:
- **Type I error**. The sample results fail to reject the null hypothesis at a time when the null hypothesis is true in the population. That is, the results indicate that two variables are correlated, or an intervention is effective, when in fact they are not.
- **Type II error**. The sample results accept the null hypothesis at a time when the null hypothesis is not true in the population. That is, the results indicate that two variables are not correlated, or an intervention is not effective, when in fact they are.

A large sample size is associated with increased power.

34. How is the adequacy of a sample size determined?

Power analysis is the most accurate method for determining the adequacy of the sample size. The analysis is based on four elements considered essential for determining the power of a study:

- The level of significance preset for the study (i.e., the alpha or p-level, conventionally set at 0.05 or 0.01)
- The sample size
- The effect size, defined as the magnitude of the relationship between variables or treatment effect investigated in the study
- Power, referring to the probability that a statistical test will detect a significant relationship between variables or difference between groups; usually, a power of 80% is considered acceptable.

A formula representing the functional relationship among these four elements forms the basis of a power analysis.

35. When should a power analysis be done?

The power analysis can be done during the planning of the study and/or during analysis of data. At the planning stage, the researchers set the desired level of significance and power and estimate the effect size based on theoretical predictions or previous findings. The analysis is then performed to identify how many cases are required for the study. In some situations, the required sample size may not be obtained because of limited resources and time constraints. The power analysis is then conducted during analysis of data. At this stage, the researchers use the level of significance set for the study, the estimated effect size based on the sample data, and the obtained sample size to determine the power of the study. This analysis informs the researcher about the adequacy of the sample size and validity of conclusions.

36. How is a power analysis done?

Researchers have three options for doing a power analysis. They can refer to a table published by Cohen,[5] which assists in identifying the required sample size for small, medium, or large effect sizes, at 0.05 or 0.01 alpha-level, and a fixed power of 80%. The table is simple and easy to use but may not provide an accurate estimate of the required sample size. Researchers also can use computer programs to run a power analysis. Programs are available with some statistical packages (e.g., SPSS) or on-line. Finally, researchers can consult statisticians, particularly when the research design is complex and power analysis demands complicated formulas.

37. Does the power analysis differ across types of research design?

Yes. For correlational studies examining relationships among study variables, the analysis takes into account the number of variables included in the model to be tested in addition to the four elements discussed above. For comparative, experimental studies, the effect size is computed as the standardized mean difference in the primary outcome variable at post-test; the number of study groups is also taken into consideration. In studies involving comparison between groups, measured on repeated occasions, power analysis requires an estimate of the within-group variance in the primary outcome.

38. Which aspects of a study influence power? How?

- **Level of significance**. A larger level of significance (e.g., alpha between 0.05 and 0.10) makes it easier to attain statistical significance but increases the likelihood of type I error.

- **Effect size**. Large effect sizes increase the probability of statistical significance and, therefore, the statistical power.
- **Sample size**. Large sample sizes reduce sampling error and increase statistical power.
- **Statistical test**. The test should be appropriate for the data and the data should meet the assumptions underlying the statistical test. Researchers should be aware that nonparametric and nondirectional tests have generally less power than parametric and directional tests.
- **Reliability and sensitivity of measures**. Unreliable measures introduce error, which decreases the power to detect significant correlation/regression effects or intervention effects. Measures that are not sensitive to change cannot detect significant differences in the variable expected over time.
- **Integrity of treatment**. Variability in implementing an intervention across participants assigned to the experimental group results in increased within-group variance in the outcomes, which decreases the statistical power to detect significant intervention effects.
- **Extraneous factors** not controlling for extraneous sources of variation in the study variables, either experimentally (by carefully selecting participants) or statistically (by residualizing their effects), decreases the statistical power.

Astute researchers take these factors into consideration when planning a study or analyzing the data and interpreting the results. Prevention is better than cure. At the planning stage, researchers can devise appropriate strategies to prevent or minimize the potential influence of these factors, such as carefully selecting reliable and sensitive measures. Attending to these factors is critical for reaching valid conclusions. They are more important than sample size in determining power in a study. For instance, unreliable measures and inconsistent implementation of the intervention definitely yield incorrect results, even if the sample size is quite large.

39. What does a plan for data analysis include?

A plan for data analysis is prepared at the proposal writing stage. It describes the steps to be followed and the statistical tests to be performed for analyzing the data.

40. What are the steps for data analysis?

Three general steps are usually followed for analyzing the data. They are done in the following sequence: preliminary steps, descriptive analysis, and statistical analyses to address the research questions or objectives or to test the study hypotheses.

41. What are the preliminary steps in data analysis?

The preliminary steps involve data cleaning and assessing the reliability of measures. Data cleaning consists of the following:

- Ensuring that data entered into the data files are accurate, reflecting the actual responses provided by participants and having no erroneous values that are out of range. This step can be accomplished in two ways. The person who entered the data compares the values in the data file with the responses recorded by participants on the hard copy of the questionnaires, either for all cases or for a randomly selected portion of the cases (e.g., 10%). Alternatively, the person enters the data into two separate files and the values in the two files are compared, using special programs (available with some statistical packages).

- Identifying the extent of missing data and selecting appropriate techniques for managing this problem.
- Identifying outliers (i.e., cases with extreme values) and deciding how best to handle them (i.e., either exclude them from the analysis or lump them into a subgroup of the sample and analyze their data separately).
- Examining the distribution of scores on the variables and applying appropriate transformation for skewed distributions to normalize them before running parametric statistics. Empirical evidence indicates that most parametric statistics are robust when the data violate the assumption of normal distribution, thus minimizing the need for transformation.
- Computing total scale or subscale scores on each study variable measured with multi-item instruments. The formula for computing total scores is available in the instrument manual; it usually consists of taking the sum or the mean of the individual items' scores.
- Assessing the reliability of measures informs the researchers of the extent of measurement error. The internal consistency reliability is most commonly examined, using the Cronbach's alpha coefficient. The test-retest or interrater reliability is also assessed, as appropriate.

42. What is descriptive analysis?

Descriptive analysis is conducted on sociodemographic variables to characterize the total sample or subgroups. It is also done for each study variable, measured at each point in time, for the total sample or relevant subgroups. The purpose is to have an idea of how participants performed on the variables of interest. Descriptive analysis includes frequency count and measures of central tendency (i.e., mean, median, or mode) and dispersion (i.e., standard deviation and range of scores). The descriptive analysis also assists in determining the success of the measures taken to clean the data (e.g., the transformation normalized the data, all outliers were excluded).

43. What is statistical analysis?

Statistical tests that address each research question or objective or test each study hypothesis are identified. Some of these tests are discussed in Chapter 22. In general, correlation and/or regression analyses are used to examine relationships between one or more independent variables, and one dependent variable. Path or structural equation analysis tests a complex model of relationships among multiple independent and dependent variables, measured with multiple indicators. Comparisons among groups on one outcome variable are made with t-test or analysis of variance, whereas comparisons on several interrelated outcomes are done with multivariate analysis of variance. Repeated measures analysis of variance and hierarchical linear models analyze changes in outcomes over time and/or between groups.

REFERENCES

1. Lipsey MW: Design Sensitivity. Statistical Power for Experimental Research. Thousand Oaks, CA, Sage, 1990.
2. Sidani S, Braden CJ: Evaluating Nursing Interventions. A Theory-driven Approach. Thousand Oaks, CA, Sage, 1998.
3. Close P, Burkey E, Kazak A, et al: A prospective, controlled evaluation of the home chemotherapy for children with cancer. Pediatrics 95(6):896–900, 1995.

4. Burns N, Grove SK: The Practice of Nursing Research. Conduct, Critique, and Utilization, 4th ed. Philadelphia, W. B. Saunders, 2001.
5. Cohen J: A power primer. Psychol Bull 112:155–159, 1992.

BIBLIOGRAPHY

1. Cohen J: Statistical Power Analysis for the Behavioral Sciences, 2nd ed. New York, Academic Press, 1988.
2. Kalton G: Introduction to Survey Sampling. Newbury Park, CA, Sage, 1983.
3. Munro BH: Statistical Methods for Health Care Research, 3rd ed. Philadelphia, J.B. Lippincott, 1997.
4. Patton MQ: Qualitative Evaluation and Research Methods, 2nd ed. Newbury Park, CA, Sage, 1990.
5. Polit DF, Hungler BP: Essentials of Nursing Research. Methods, Appraisal, and Utilization, 5th ed. Philadelphia, Lippincott, 2001.

18. LEVELS OF ANALYSIS

Mary A. Blegen, RN, P*h*D, FAAN

1. What is meant by level of analysis?

Level of analysis refers to the focus of an investigation. The analysis can be focused on small details of a certain component of the research or on large data-sets. For example, the analysis can focus on micro-events such as psychological phenomena within the individual or groups of people. The term *level* is appropriate because it indicates the place on a continuum of events from micro to macro phenomena. Many levels of analyses are of interest to nurse researchers. Most nursing research asks questions about characteristics, behaviors, attitudes, patient interventions and outcomes or about individual nurse actions, behaviors, attitudes, and characteristics. Researchers may want to know the effect of a particular nursing intervention on one or more patient outcomes or whether a particular patient characteristic affects the patient's outcome.

Researchers may also want to know the effect of a care delivery model on patient outcomes. For example, if a primary care model is used on a patient care unit, are patients on that unit more satisfied? Do they have better outcomes than patients on other units? The nursing care model (e.g., primary care, team nursing) is not a behavior or characteristic of an individual nurse but a characteristic of the patient care unit as a whole or the hospital. A typical research question currently of interest to nurse administrators is, "Does the safety climate on a patient care unit affect the occurrence of accidents and errors in patient care on the unit?" Safety climate is clearly a characteristic of the unit; the occurrence of accidents and errors is less clear and may be conceptualized at the level of the patient or group of patients during a particular time frame.

Another level of analysis may be systems or events within patients. An individual patient has many different heart rates, serum glucose values, or pain episodes over the time that they receive care. Such patient events can be studied at the level of the episode. The interventions may be different for each episode, and the effect of an intervention may be questioned at the level of the episode. The levels of analyses are episode of pain, glucose level, or heart rate. The unit of analysis is each measure of pain, glucose, or heart rate.

2. How does unit of analysis differ from level of analysis?

The **unit of analysis** may be an individual patient or nurse, patient care unit, pain episode, or whole communities of potential patients. Each of these units is relevant to a specific research question and requires appropriate measurement, sampling, and analysis. For example, a researcher may ask whether a public health intervention such as public education has any effect on exercise and the development of type I diabetes. Or the researcher may ask whether opening a nurse-managed clinic has an effect on prenatal care and the birth of low-birth-weight infants. In such cases, the researcher may compare the rate of type II diabetes or the rate of low-birth-weight infants in the community with rates in other communities without public education or nurse-managed clinics. The analysis of communities uses resident data, probably collected and compiled by governmental surveys from individuals, that are aggregated to produce rates. The unit of analysis in these examples is communities, and the number (N) of communities is likely to be small.

The **level of analysis** follows the unit of analysis. In comparing the pain episodes, multiple repeated measures of pain within a small group of patients are appropriate. The statistical analysis is based on the number of episodes measured. However, as discussed below, the analysis also has to account for the dependence of those episodes within each patient.

3. How does level of analysis differ from level of measurement?

Unfortunately, research terminology often contains multiple overlapping terms. In this instance the level of measurement is quite different from level of analysis and refers to a characteristic of the concept itself and its measurement. Levels of measurement may be nominal, ordinal, interval, or ratio (see Chapter 15).

4. Why would a nurse researcher consider any unit other than a patient or a nurse as the main unit of level of analysis?

Many phenomena that influence a patient's health and nurses' actions are external to the patient or nurse. For example, current issues in health care, such as the nursing shortage and how the health care institution responds to this crisis, exist on a larger scale than individuals yet have a major impact on individual nurses and patients. Health maintenance is affected by entities beyond the individual. The most pertinent entity that affects humans' health status is the family, followed by community and immediate environment. At a larger level, public policy also has a major impact. The knowledge that nursing builds through research must address these levels beyond the individual patient and nurse to be useful in directing health care delivery.

5. Is the unit of analysis the same as the sampling unit?

The answer to this complex question is maybe and maybe not. Some units of analysis can be selected directly through a sampling procedure; other units of analysis must be accessed after the sampling has been done. For example, if episodes of pain are being studied, the first sampling unit is the patient. Next, a procedure is created for selecting episodes of pain (perhaps all, perhaps one each 4 hours). If the unit of analysis is communities, you would most likely select them directly using either a random procedure or a procedure designed for the researcher's convenience.

6. Do we measure at the unit of analysis level?

When possible, all data should be collected and measured at the same level at which the analyses will be conducted. For some levels or units of analyses this approach is obvious and easy to do; for others, it can be quite challenging. Measurement of pain at any level other than the episode of pain requires that we first collect data about pain episodes and then combine these data to produce an aggregated measure, such as a mean pain measure for each patient. Measurement of a patient care unit characteristic such as primary care nursing is straightforward. The researcher most likely asks the nurse administrator or nurse manager to report the nursing care model. To validate the nurse administrator or manager's report, the researcher may observe how nursing care is organized. Measuring a patient care characteristic such as safety climate is more difficult. This concept indicates a set of social norms (informal rules) that are not documented and may not be part of the consciousness of persons working on the unit. Safety climate involves capturing perceptions at the individual level and calculating a group statistic (i.e., average for the group of individuals). In such cases, a survey questionnaire may be developed and administered to nurses working on the unit. This questionnaire may contain an item set that tapped the nurse's perceptions of group norms about patient safety on the unit. Research studies often examine rates. If the researcher wants to know and calculate the rate of health care accidents and errors, the usual measurement route is to count the number of reported or observed incidents and divide by the total number of patients or observations. Disease rate at a community level should be obtained by dividing the number of persons with the disease by the total number of people. Disease rates may be reported as percentages or proportions but more often are presented as the number of persons with a disease for each 10,000 (or 100,000) people.

7. Can most variables be measured at more than one level or unit of analysis?

Many variables can and are measured at more than one level. If measured first at the individual level, group statistics such as rates or averages are calculated. If measured first at the group level (e.g., individuals on a unit with primary care nursing), the characteristic can be assigned to the individual patients. In assigning group characteristics to individuals within the group, caution must be used. This approach makes sense with some but not all variables. For example, a particular nurse on a unit with a low safety climate does not necessarily ignore safety precautions.

8. How can more aggregated units of analysis be measured?

Guidelines for aggregation of data have been developed over the past 20 years. Verran, Gerber, and Milton[1] describe and apply these guidelines to data about nursing practice collected by survey questionnaires. They discuss four criteria: content validity, representativeness, reliability, and validity. Overall, the criteria allow the researcher to show that the aggregated variable has construct validity; i.e., that the variables at the aggregated level function similarly to the variables at the lower level. This step requires specifying theoretically the relationships among variables at both levels and showing the similarities.

- To establish **content validity**, the survey tool should contain items that refer to the phenomena at the level used for aggregation and analysis. For example, for a safety climate measure, the items should refer to "the nurses on this unit" rather than to the individual respondent "I".
- **Representativeness** means that the persons who responded to the survey (provided the data that will be aggregated to produce the group score) are representative of the group as a whole. That is, the response rate was adequate and the number of responses was sufficient to analyze. Rules of thumb suggest that the response rate should be at least 50% and that 6–10 responses should be received from each group.
- For **reliability and validity**, techniques used for other psychometric analyses can be used with some modification. For example, inter-item consistency measures can be calculated (i.e., Cronbach's alpha) with the item scores calculated

at the group level rather than the individual respondent level. Glick[2] suggests that the intraclass correlation coefficient provides useful information. This coefficient compares within-group variation to between-group variation with the assumption that a valid aggregated measure shows more between-group than within-group variation.

9. Why not just reduce all variables to the lowest level?

As the complexities of multiple levels become clear, it is tempting to use the lowest common denominator (unit of analysis at lowest level), assign group characteristics to the lowest level of analysis, and conduct the research at that level. Problems can be encountered when such reductionistic methods are used. For example, individuals in communities with high rates of type II diabetes may or may not have the condition. Patients on units with high rates of accidents and errors may or may not have experienced an accident themselves. Fortunately, accidents and errors are relatively rare events, and even on units with high rates of adverse incidents most of the patients do not experience them. Although it makes sense to study the group rates of errors on the patient care units in relation to the safety climate on the unit, one cannot conclude that individual patients on that unit experienced an adverse incident.

Another problem with reducing group-level information to the individual level is that the statistical assumption of independence maybe violated. This assumption states that each unit's values are independent of the other units. That is, whether patient A experiences or does not experience an accident or error is independent of whether patient B experiences or does not experience errors. Whereas the experience of an error is independent for each patient, the variable to which we relate the error experience (unit safety climate) is not. All patients on a given unit must have the same safety climate value; that variable is dependent across the unit of analysis (individual patients). Special multilevel analysis techniques are needed for these situations.

10. What about aggregating all variables to the highest level?

The most obvious problem with aggregating all variables to a higher level is that the richness of variation for the individual units of analysis is lost. This variation often contains important information. With some phenomena this approach can be done with useful results, whereas with other phenomena the results are not clear. Social scientists discuss such problems as ecologic and reductionistic fallacies as defined by Babbie.[3]

11. What are the ecologic and reductionistic fallacies?

Ecologic fallacy (also called aggregation fallacy) refers to the danger of making assertions about individuals as the unit of analysis based on the examination of groups or other aggregates. A well-known example of ecologic fallacy in sociology (conducted in the 1930s) was the conclusion that people born in other countries had higher levels of English language literacy than people born in the U.S. This conclusion came from an analysis of regions that showed the northeastern U.S. had both higher levels of foreign-born residents and higher literacy rates compared with the southeastern U.S., which had lower levels of foreign-born residents and lower levels of literacy. In this case the relationships discovered for regions did not hold when individuals were examined.

Reductionistic fallacy (also called individualistic fallacy) refers to the opposite tendency to draw conclusions about groups from individuals. A common social science example may be concluding that Democrats are richer than Republicans because a particular study of wealthy persons showed that the majority were Democrats.

12. Can the relationship between two variables be studied when one variable is at one level and the other variable is at a different level?

It is possible to do studies with variables at different levels. We often want to know the effects of group or structural variables on individuals. Examples of research questions include (a) which characteristics of patients who have had hip fractures and (b) which characteristics of their health care best explain patient outcomes. Among the characteristics of interest are the patient's age and other physical conditions, the hospital unit's staffing model and average hours of nursing care provided on the unit, and the presence of a rehabilitation service in the hospital. There are variables at three possible levels: patient level characteristics, nursing unit level staffing, and hospital level services. An advanced statistical procedure that can take into account these variables across the three levels of analysis is needed to answer this research question.

13. What are cross-level analyses?

The most basic cross-level analysis is analysis of variance (ANOVA), which, in the previous example, could examine the variation within patient care units (differences among the outcomes of patients in each unit) and the differences between patient care units with low vs. high staffing. If patient characteristics were included in the model, an analysis of covariance (ANCOVA) would be used. However, the number and types of variables that can be included in each analysis are limited. In recent years, more advanced statistical techniques have been introduced to handle multiple levels of variables. Although known by several names, collectively they are referred to as multilevel analyses. Large data sets are needed to conduct such analyses.

14. What types of data are needed to conduct a multilevel analysis?

If the researcher asked about the effect of rehabilitation facilities in the hospital, staffing levels on the unit, and patient characteristics on patient outcomes, it would be necessary to have multiple observations at all three levels. That is, you would need multiple hospitals, some with and some without rehabilitation facilities; then, within each of these hospitals, you would need multiple units with different staffing levels, and within each unit you would need multiple patients with different values on the characteristics of interest. For example, you may have 50 patients on each of 5 units in each of 10 hospitals, or 2500 patients on 50 units in 10 hospitals. Special considerations for measurement and analysis are needed to conduct research at more aggregate levels of analysis. However, research at these levels of analysis provides knowledge that is important to healthcare and to nursing. Consulting additional references[5] may assist in further understanding the complexities of research at multiple levels of analysis.

REFERENCES

1. Verran JA, Gerber RM, Milton DA: Data aggregation: Criteria for psychometric evaluation. Res Nurs Health 18:77–80, 1995.

2. Pedhazur E: Multiple Regression in Behavioral Research: Explanation and Prediction, 3rd ed. Fort Worth, TX, Harcourt Brace College Publishers, 1997.
3. Glick WH: Conceptualizing and measuring organizational and psychological climate: Pitfalls in multi-level research. Acad Manage Rev 10:601–616, 1985.
4. Babbie E: The Practice of Social Research, 6th ed. Belmont, CA, Wadsworth, 1992.
5. Bryk A, Raudenbush S: Hierarchical Linear Models: Applications and Data Analysis Methods. Newbury Park, CA, Sage, 1992.

IV. Collecting and Interpreting Data

19. DATA COLLECTION

Dana R. Epstein, RN, PhD

1. What is data collection? How does it fit in the research process?

Data collection is the step-by-step process of gathering information from a specified sample of subjects about the variables of interest in your research study. The data are used in the statistical analysis to address the purpose and aims of the study, answer the research questions, and support or refute the hypothesis(es). The work of the study begins with data collection. Until this point, the the primary focus was the development and planning stages. You developed the problem statement, reviewed the literature, constructed the purpose of the study, and formulated research questions, aims, and/or hypotheses. Based on the questions, aims, or hypotheses, you know the variables that you need to measure and the instruments needed to measure them. Now you are ready to begin the process of data collection.

2. What does the researcher need to begin data collection?

The most critical issue is to know and understand the data requirements of your study. The steps of the research process should provide a clear guide to what type of data needs to be collected. More than the major research variables is involved. Data must also be collected to describe the characteristics of the subjects in the study. Without this information, the major variables of interest may not make sense. The characteristics of the sample provide the context in which to understand the major variables of the study. In addition, be sure to include instruments that measure extraneous variables if the study design does not control for them. Therefore, give careful consideration to all variables that need to be measured during the data collection process.

Subjects, patient records, or an existing data set may be needed, depending on the purpose of the study. You must specify where you will find your data and how to gain access to it. The process of gaining human subjects approval or permission to review patient records helps clarify the issue of access to subjects, records, or data sets.

3. How does the researcher develop the data collection plan?

A plan needs to be developed before data collection begins. Before you pick up your instruments and head out the door, sit down and lay out a step-by-step plan for gathering the necessary data. This plan should be made in the most efficient manner possible and requires careful forethought. The start of data collection assumes that all preliminary steps in the research process have been described to provide the direction needed to proceed with data collection. In the development of the study, a review of the literature pertinent to the research problem was completed. Take careful note of the data collection processes used in the studies reviewed:

• Are the populations similar to your population of interest?
• Do the data collection protocols seem appropriate for your purpose?
• What can you use from the studies?
• What problems did the researchers encounter during their data collection?

The problems provide guidance as to what to avoid. The researchers may have suggestions about how the process can be improved. Pay attention to these helpful recommendations and incorporate them into your data collection plan.

4. Why is a consistent data collection plan needed?

A data collection plan must be implemented in the same way by all data collectors. Data collectors can influence subjects' responses. As the number of data collectors increases, this point becomes more salient. However, even if you are the sole data collector, the data need to be collected in the same way from subject to subject to avoid bias. Although it is often assumed that bias is introduced when more than one person collects the data, a single data collector can introduce bias if he or she does not follow a structured protocol. Bias can be introduced when data collection methods other than self-report are used, such as behavioral observation. More complex studies with multiple data collectors demand more precise protocols. The training process for data collectors is important; thus, developing and writing a protocol to ensure consistent data collection are essential. Aside from the immediate concerns of a consistent data collection plan, when personnel in the study change the researcher needs a protocol to train others. Additionally, a clear data collection protocol allows other researchers to replicate your study in the future.

5. How does the researcher ensure consistency in the data collection plan?

A written protocol helps to ensure consistency. Consider the following components in developing a protocol for the study:
• Start with an overview of the project to familiarize the personnel with the study and its aims.
• Identify the type of subjects that you are looking for through an explanation of inclusion and exclusion criteria. Explain where subjects are found and how they are approached. If data collection sites are used, include a list in the protocol. Note information about the contact person at each site and any idiosyncrasies of the sites.
• List any advertising sources used for the study.
• Include a way to keep track of the participants. Your protocol should include a procedure to maintain an accurate count of persons who were interested and eligible, refused to participate, participated, and remained or dropped out of the study, including the reasons for refusal or dropping out. An understanding of the reasons why people refuse to participate or drop out is useful for interpreting the results of the study as well as for future research projects. Describe how to maintain a master list of subjects and their contact information. This list is necessary during the immediate research phase and critical for any follow-up measurement.
• Describe the screening and measurement phases of the study, including all of the instruments and tasks that need to be completed during each phase. For each phase of the study, include an example of the instruments and an explanation of any physiologic measures.

- The protocol should detail the steps of data collection once the data collector meets with the subject. If the design entails assigning subjects to groups for descriptive or experimental purposes, this procedure should be clarified. If the study includes an intervention, refer to the treatment manual in the protocol or place the treatment manual in the protocol.
- When raw data are returned to the study site after collection, describe how the data are securely stored while awaiting entry, keeping in mind the policy of your institution. Indicate who is responsible for and the process for data transformation, entry, and analysis.

A study protocol facilitates the often complex process of data collection. Everyone involved in the study, including new study personnel, will have a consistent reference to consult when questions arise about the data collection process. When study personnel change, you will have a reference for orienting the new study staff.

6. What are the sources of data for a study?

To answer the research question(s), you need to know where your data will come from. Who or what will provide the data? Will the data be primary or secondary? These questions are answered during the review of the literature and the development of the design of the study. Primary data come from sources such as persons or observations of behavior; examples of secondary data include patient records or previously collected data sets.

7. Discuss the importance of accurate and reliable data.

The quality of the data collected influences the outcomes of the study. Therefore, plan to use instruments that effectively operationalize the concepts proposed in the framework of the study. Adequate operationalization of the concepts results in accurate measurement of the variables. The reliability and validity of the instruments used for data collection affect the stability and accuracy of the data. Data collector(s) must be trained to follow the protocol to ensure consistency. When more than one person is collecting data (i.e., the data collector completes the instruments rather than the subject), the issue of interrater reliability arises. Supervision of data collectors and the collection process, including random checks of collected data, helps maintain consistency and accuracy in data collection. The concepts of reliability and validity of instruments are addressed in Chapter 16.

8. Who collects the data?

Depending on the research budget, it may be only you! If you have sufficient money to hire research personnel, determine all of the tasks associated with the research study and decide who will do which tasks. At some point in the development of the study, make a list of the tasks and the type of person(s) best suited to carry them out. In making the list, consider the phases of the study and the type of data that need to be collected in each phase. The staff at the study site may also collect data. You need to consider how much training is needed and what can be reasonably asked of data collectors who are not employees of the study. You must also determine how the quality of the data will be affected if collected by clinical staff. For health care providers, you may need to emphasize the research vs. clinical aspects of the problem under investigation.

9. How do you select persons to collect data?

It depends on the type of data needed for the study. Think about what you want the data collector to do. The researcher must consider data collectors and their characteristics in such terms as educational background, skills, and age. You need to know what type of people can serve as data collectors in your study. They may be nurses, students, or other types of people. When selecting data collectors, think about the type of data and the subjects from whom the data are collected. Subject characteristics may influence the type of data collector. You may need to match personal characteristics to the population of the study. For example, to build rapport quickly with subjects, you might want someone of similar age. You must also ascertain the potential data collector's experience. Are resources, including time, available to train the person in data collection tasks, or must the person bring such skills to the study? For instance, if the data collector must draw blood samples, will this skill be taught or will the person come with phlebotomy competency already certified? Are there any certifications or licensing requirements within the site where the blood will be drawn? Your belief that the person is capable of drawing blood does not mean that the site where the data collection occurs will allow it.

10. How does the researcher train data collectors?

Very carefully! Some researchers develop training manuals for the staff of their projects in addition to a data collection procedure. A training manual may not be necessary, depending on the complexity of the study. The data collection protocol may suffice. Determine the amount of time needed to train the data collectors by reviewing all required tasks and the skills that they bring to the project. If they must be taught certain skills, you will need more time. You may need to hire someone to teach data collection skills. Company representatives may be needed to train the data collectors to use specialized equipment. Before the data collectors begin, they need to practice the protocol in a training session. Ideally, the practice precedes a pretest of the protocol or pilot test of the study. Practice gives the data collectors a chance to become comfortable with the instruments and the procedure.

Data collectors may be staff employed by the site where data are collected. Using staff from the site as data collectors may affect the way you develop the training protocol, the data collection procedure, the study budget, and the quality of the data. It may be advisable to avoid using study site staff to collect data, because they may be a source of bias.

As discussed in question 4, if more than one data collector is involved, interrater reliability becomes an issue and may be part of the psychometric evaluation of the instruments during a pretest or pilot study. As the data collection procedure is tested, the collectors and the investigator should keep notes about the process. Ideally, feedback from the subjects will also be collected. After the data collection procedure has been tested, the protocol is modified as needed. The data collectors must then be retrained according to the latest version of the protocol, with special attention to how and why the process has changed from the initial trial run.

The investigator or a designee should provide ongoing supervision from the initial training through the completion of the full-scale version of the study. The data collectors and the investigator should continue to keep notes on the data collection process. The notes can inform the outcomes of the study and are useful for future studies. Keep in mind the possibility of personnel turnover, particularly in a lengthy study. You will be grateful for a modified and updated data collection protocol when a new data collector is hired, when you are writing the results of your current study, or when a future study is being developed.

11. Where are the data collected?

The place where you collect your data depends on the clinical problem, study variables, required instruments, and the subjects in your study. If advertising is used to find subjects, you want to keep track of the response elicited by each advertisement. This step helps you make the best use of your advertising budget. When a data collection site is used, the persons at the site must have the subject characteristics necessary for inclusion in the study. The sites should also be able to provide enough subjects for the study. A site may seem ideal, but the researcher must determine how many subjects can reasonably be accrued at the site and over what period. The determination may steer the researcher to evaluate additional sites in order to complete data collection within the proposed time frame. Alternatively, subjects may come to your research office or laboratory for data collection or may be asked to take home the data collection instruments, such as self-report measures, and return them later to the study office in person or by mail. Additionally, certain physiologic instruments may be used by subjects in the home at different times of day and for varying lengths of time.

12. What issues must be considered in choosing data collection sites?

Before data can be collected, access to the site must be granted and permission obtained. Identify the key person to contact at the site. If available, start with a personal contact who may work at the site to direct you to the appropriate person. You may also contact the nurse executive of the facility for direction. A research department may be available, hopefully with a research nurse coordinator or nurse scientist.

Once contact has been made with the appropriate person, you can determine whether the site can provide the type and number of subjects required. Then the process of gaining permission to collect data from the subjects can begin. If human subjects approval from the institutional review board has been obtained, bring it with you to any preliminary meetings. It is a good idea to have human subjects approval from the institutional review board of your own institution beforehand. However, this may not be possible without an established data collection site agreement.

When you meet with the representatives of the data collection site, be prepared to explain succinctly the study and what will be required from the site. Depending on the site's preference, take the research proposal to the meeting or send it in advance. Also prepare a summary of the proposal that highlights the important points, particularly what is expected from the staff, how the study will fit into their routine without disrupting the flow of patient care, and how human subjects are protected. Be prepared to undergo institutional review board procedures at the site and/or a review of the study by a site research committee.

13. How do you build a rapport with the clinical site personnel to accomplish your research goals?

Establish meetings with all persons who will be involved in any way in the data collection process. Bring your research personnel—and bring food! Depending on the structure and staffing of the site, more than one meeting may be required to make contact with all persons involved. Before attending any meetings, think about what you need from the site to formulate any special study-related requests. Listen carefully to what personnel at the site say that they can do to help supply data collection needs. Tell them what you will do to avoid impeding the flow of patient care. Be prepared to be flexible to the extent that the scientific integrity of the study is not compromised. Ask for the staff's ideas and feedback about the process. They may be able to warn you in advance of what will and will not work at their site. As the data collection process proceeds, be sure to keep the staff informed of your progress. If you are not involved in data collection at the site, get feedback from your research personnel about how the process is working at the site and address any problems immediately, since you want the site to welcome you back for future studies. Inform the staff of the final study results, perhaps presenting the findings in a meeting with site staff. Give the staff some kind of recognition for their participation and, if possible, acknowledge them in the manuscript at the time of publication.

14. When are the data collected?

Once you have developed your data collection protocol, hired and trained the staff, obtained human subjects approval, gained access to the data collection site(s), pretested the instruments and/or pilot-tested the study, you are ready to collect data.

15. How much time should be allocated to data collection?

The pretest of the instruments or pilot test of the study provides a good estimate of how long it takes to complete data collection. However, it is often difficult to determine how long it will take to recruit subjects. Examining similar studies (i.e., a similar research problem, subjects, and setting) may help to estimate the time frame. The study site can identify how many patients who meet the study criteria are seen in a certain period. This information may help to estimate the time frame. The time necessary to complete the instruments should also be considered. A pretest of instruments or pilot test of the study provides feedback about the burden of instrumentation. The data collection method also affects your time frame. Data from mailings to subjects, face-to-face meetings, telephone administration, laboratory tests, or home monitoring entail different collection methods and require differing amounts of time.

16. When planning for data collection, how do you match your study aims to the resources of the study?

The sources of funding for a study may vary from none to a federal or private foundation. Keep in mind that data collection is usually the most expensive part of the study because it is a time-consuming process. In the planning stages, determine the volume of data to be collected and the time required to collect it. If you have conducted a preliminary study or have an opportunity to pretest the instruments before requesting research funds, you are ahead of the game; you already have an idea of the resources needed to accomplish the data collection. Otherwise careful planning is required. Become familiar with the instruments, and consider the type of personnel needed to collect the data. Talk with experienced researchers, especially those who have conducted similar studies. Their input will help you formulate a budget for data collection. Keep in mind the recommendations made in question 15.

17. How do you track the completion of data collection, especially in studies with more than one time point for measurement?

You need to develop a system for tracking data completion. Some investigators track data management using computer-based methods, whereas others use hand-written logs. The more complex the data collection, such as studies involving many subjects, several instruments, and many time points, the more sophisticated the tracking method will need to be. For example, in our insomnia intervention studies, in addition to electronic methods and paper logs, we keep a table posted on our study office bulletin board. The table includes the phases of the study (e.g., baseline, treatment), a space for subject identification numbers, and a place to mark the dates of each phase. We also use a large wall calendar to help keep track of dates, particularly follow-up measurement phases. Data tracking needs to be assigned to someone as a special responsibility and monitored regularly, depending on the time frame of the data collection process.

18. Discuss the fit between data collection and other components of the study.

Thoughts about data collection begin as soon as the ideas for the study are formulated. Look at the sections of this book. As you get started, you begin to develop your research question and review the literature. You formulate hypotheses. You take note of how other researchers have operationalized the concepts of interest. As you plan the study design, the concepts transform into study variables as your ideas about how to measure them become clearer. You may start to contact researchers to gain permission to use their instruments. The conduct of the study includes the data collection process. In evaluating the results of the study, the data are managed and interpreted to reach conclusions that answer your research questions and either support or refute your hypotheses. The data are then communicated in a variety of ways to inform health care providers of your findings.

19. What are the implications of the data collection procedure for the timeline of the study?

Data collection is lengthy and always takes longer than planned. The advantage of a pretest of instruments or a pilot study is the ability to estimate the time required to complete the instruments. A pilot study has the added advantage of determining how long it takes to recruit a certain number of subjects. Input from experienced researchers, especially those who have conducted similar studies, also contributes vital information for planning the timeline. During the planning phase of the study, you developed a timeline for all phases of the project. Because data collection will take the most time, develop a fairly accurate estimate of how long it will require. If you have a funded study and the data collection takes longer than estimated, arrangements must be made with the funding source to extend the study timeline. If you are a student conducting research, prolonged data collection may delay the completion of your course or degree. Because changes in the study timeline hold major implications for the progress of the study, potential obstacles need to be fully examined.

20. What are the implications of the data collection procedure for the budget of the study?

Data collection not only takes the most time, it also eats up most of your budget. When you have a consistent protocol, capable and trained personnel, and an estimate of the time to complete the protocol, you are likely to remain within the financial resources of the study. Problems can occur during any study. Research personnel may leave the project. The data collection site may no longer have the type of subjects needed. Talk to researchers who have conducted similar studies, and determine the kind of problems that affected their budget. Solicit recommendations about strategies to avoid the problems.

21. How do you ensure that researchers who follow your data collection procedure in another study will be able to obtain the same results?

A detailed, consistent protocol is the key to ensuring replication. Another researcher needs the details of your study to conduct a similar study. This is a reminder of the importance of writing and modifying the study protocol.

22. What do you do with the data after they are collected?

Do *not* wait until you have collected all of your data to begin the process of data management. You must get the data ready for management and analysis. Part of the data collection process includes a plan for how to move data in their raw form into the data management system. When the data collectors return to the study office with the completed instruments, secure a place to store the instruments while they await entry into the data management system. Be sure to follow institutional regulations for storage. You need to determine the turnaround time between the arrival of the instruments and the entry of data into the management system. Data from physiologic instruments may need to be downloaded by a software program associated with the equipment and imported into the study's data management and analysis systems. This process may need to be done quickly to make the equipment available for new subjects. Self-report instruments may be able to wait for entry—but do not wait too long! Data pile up quickly. You may also need to transform some data before its entry. No matter what type of data you have, develop a plan for handling it after collection.

ACKNOWLEDGMENT

The preparation of this chapter was supported by National Institutes of Health/National Institute of Nursing Research grants NR04951 and NR05075.

BIBLIOGRAPHY

1. Brink PJ, Wood MJ: Basic Steps in Planning Nursing Research, from Question to Proposal, 5th ed. Monterey, CA, Wadsworth, 2001.
2. Burns N, Grove SK: The Practice of Nursing Research: Conduct, Critique and Utilization, 4th ed. Philadelphia, W.B. Saunders, 2001.
3. Gillis A, Jackson W: Research Methods for Nurses: Methods and Interpretation. Philadelphia, F.A. Davis, 2002.
4. Granger BB, Chulay M: Research Strategies for Clinicians. Stamford, CT, Appleton & Lange, 1999.
5. Hedrick TE, Bickman L, Rog DJ: Applied Research Design: A Practical Guide. Thousand Oaks, CA, Sage, 1993.
6. LoBiondo-Wood G, Haber J: Nursing Research: Methods, Critical Appraisal, and Utilization. St. Louis, Mosby, 2002.
7. Norwood SL: Research Strategies for Advanced Practice Nurses. Upper Saddle River, NJ, Prentice Hall Health, 2000.
8. Polit DF, Hungler BP: Nursing Research: Principles & Methods, 6th ed. Philadelphia, J.B. Lippincott, 1999.

20. QUALITATIVE DATA GENERATION

JoAnn G. Congdon, PhD, RN, CNS

1. Is *data collection* or *data generation* the preferred term? Why?

Qualitative researchers prefer data generation. Data, however, are not simply collected or compiled; they are instead produced, constructed, created, or developed through the interview. The interview is not a neutral, passive tool but rather an interactive, negotiated, cooperative text between at least two people and is influenced by the personalities of the participants.

2. What is the setting for data generation in qualitative research? Where are the data generated?

The setting for qualitative research data is the field. The field is the unchanged natural setting where the participants live, work, and experience life. Data are generated in the natural setting or the field. The field may be a cultural group, deaf community, inner-city community, rural area, ethnic neighborhood, hospital, school, daycare center, or prison.

3. How does one gain entry into the field? What problems are commonly encountered?

Gaining access or entry into the field may be one of the most difficult parts of the study. Researchers are not usually part of the group, culture, or social situation being studied. Gaining entry requires building trust and drawing on interpersonal resources and strategies to gain permission to enter the field. Developing a trustful relationship with a key informant or someone who is well established in the field can be a successful strategy for access. Common problems include:

- Choosing a site
- Overcoming personal discomfort with gaining entry to an unfamiliar site
- Identifying and obtaining support of gatekeepers who control the setting
- Unanticipated length of prefield work time needed to gain access
- Ethical considerations, such as honesty and confidentiality with the participants

4. Once a researcher is in the field, how is access maintained?

Maintaining access to the field can be problematic for the researcher. Data generation takes time, and the researcher must keep in mind that the participant's time is valuable. The researcher must respect the use of time and exercise flexibility in the data generation process. Scheduling interviews or participant observations at a time that fits with the participant's schedule is critical. Maintaining community or institutional support, nurturing participants, taking time for social amenities, and maintaining a pleasant climate facilitate data generation and participant cooperation. Participants who believe in the significance of the study are most likely to continue, and this commitment can be strengthened through active nurturing and sincere interactions with the researcher. Reciprocal contributions by the researcher, such as offering an education class, workshop, or volunteer session, can facilitate participant interest and commitment.

5. Is there a difference among the terms *subjects*, *informants*, and *participants*?

Most qualitative researchers use the terms *participants* or *informants* for individuals who inform or participate in their studies. These terms connotate a position of active involvement or a partnership between participants and researchers. The term *subjects* is generally not used because it implies being acted on or detachment, which is contrary to the philosophical underpinnings of qualitative research.

6. How is the sample selected for qualitative data generation?

Participants are recruited or selected for qualitative research based on their personal knowledge or experience with the culture or phenomenon of study. The goal of sampling is to develop a rich, thick description of the phenomenon of inquiry. The sampling principles are not based on numbers of interviews, participant observations, or ability to generalize data, but rather on how accurately the data represent the full context of the phenomenon under study. The sample is selected based on familiarity and understanding of the study's focus.

7. What is purposive sampling?

Purposive sampling refers to sampling that is purposefully selected by the researcher. The researcher selects participants or situations that fit with the phenomenon under study and meet the criteria for selection. For example, a researcher who is studying the phenomenon of postpartum depression will recruit women who have experienced postpartum depression.

8. Define theoretical sampling.

Theoretical sampling is a form of purposive sampling that is used primarily in the qualitative design of grounded theory. Theoretical sampling is based on the need to generate more data to examine, further analyze, and elaborate on an emerging theory. Further sampling is purposefully sought to refine, validate, or test the accuracy of the initial conceptualizations of the findings and/or theory.[1]

9. Who is the insider and who is the outsider in qualitative research? Are these terms important?

These terms are frequently used in qualitative ethnographic research and are important for the understanding and interpretation of culture. The insider's (emic) view is the native participant's view of the culture or phenomenon being studied. It is the view of the person experiencing the phenomenon of interest. The qualitative researcher's goal is to describe and understand the culture or phenomenon of interest from the insider's or native's perceptions or point of view. The outsider's (etic) view is the researcher's or interpreter's view. The etic point of view is based on the researcher's perceptions of what is occurring in the culture or with the phenomenon under study. The researcher generates data and analyzes and interprets the culture according to his or her perceptions. The aim of ethnography is to obtain an in-depth emic perspective.

10. Define reflexivity. Why is it important in qualitative data generation?

Reflexivity, also referred to as reflective thought or reflective critique, is an interactive process that the researcher goes through to uncover underlying factors that may influence the study's findings. Researcher reflexivity is important because in qualitative research the researcher becomes part of the research and may influence the study during data generation and analysis. The researcher explores the dynamic interaction between the self and the data and integrates this added insight and understanding into the study.[2] This introspective process requires critical thinking and self-awareness. Researchers are encouraged to keep a record of their feelings, thoughts, reactions, and biases to determine how their personal views may have influenced their interpretation of findings.

11. What are the most common methods for generating data in qualitative research?

Interview, participant observation, record or document review, focus groups, photography, or combinations of these approaches are the most commonly used methods to generate data in qualitative research. Face-to-face interviews, the most frequently used data generation method, may extend from minutes to hours and may take place on one occasion or be repeated over a prolonged period.

Interviews can be unstructured or open-ended, semistructured, or structured. **Unstructured interviews** are appropriate when little is known about a phenomenon. This type of interview usually begins with open-ended questions and allows the participant unlimited opportunity to elaborate on the phenomenon of interest. The interviewer asks few specific questions. In **semistructured interviews** the researcher exerts more control over the interview and commonly has a set of questions prepared to guide the interview. The questions may not be strictly followed to allow latitude in the participant's responses. The interviewer may also guide the discussion by asking specific questions. The **structured interview** is used more often in quantitative research than qualitative research. In a structured interview, the researcher asks each participant a series of preestablished questions with little or no latitude for expansion by the participant.

12. What makes an interview successful?

Qualitative interviewing builds on one's skills as a conversationalist and listener. The successful interviewer understands that the interview is an intentional way of learning about the other person's experiences, perceptions, thoughts, and feelings. The interviewer conveys respect, interest, and importance to what is shared. Listening is key; questions and answers must flow logically as the interviewee speaks. Cues for forming the next question are taken from what is said rather than from a prescribed format. Listening intently helps to frame questions and comments to fit with the conversation. Encouraging the participant to elaborate facilitates meeting the goal of obtaining a rich, thick description of the phenomenon of interest. No two interviews will be the same—be prepared for the unexpected, and be flexible. At the end of the interview, make an attempt to keep the door open for continuing discussion.

13. List common pitfalls of interviewing.
- Asking more than one question at once, thus confusing the participant
- Asking closed questions or those than can be answered by a yes or no, thus closing off the conversation
- Correcting participant information or counseling the participant, thus taking over the interview

- Allowing interruptions, such as telephones, children, or visitors, that distract the participant from fully engaging in the conversation
- Competing distractions, such as a noisy room, a tape recorder that does not work properly, or time commitments of participant or researcher that create the feeling of being rushed
- Asking embarrassing questions, thus discouraging further conversation
- Using an interpreter who does not accurately translate the question or the response, resulting in frustration to both researcher and participant[3]

14. What is a focus group? When is it an appropriate strategy for data generation?

A focus group is a type of group interview in which specific people assemble to give their opinions or impressions about the phenomenon of interest. The groups can be convened for various reasons, such as evaluating a new product, sharing feelings about an upcoming policy or discussing experiences with a particular form of treatment. Focus groups generally range in size from 5 to 10 people who have been selected because they share qualities that can inform the study's questions. Focus groups can be used as the sole means of data generation or as a supplement to other qualitative methods. An advantage of the focus group is that the researcher can benefit from the interaction among group participants. The group discussion can generate data that may not be elicited from a single guided interview. Creative thinking and collective responses stimulated by a focus group can lead to improvement of whatever is evaluated, marketed, or discussed.

15. Discuss advantages and disadvantages of focus groups.

Focus groups can be especially effective for discussing a sensitive topic because no one person is put on the spot. The conversation is shared by the group, creating an environment that encourages, supports, or stimulates others to elaborate on the topic. People often reflect on and evaluate their own opinions as they listen to others. Data from individual interviews may not be as rich as data from focus group participants because individual interviewees may not have had the opportunity to reflect on the topic or hear the reflection of others. Focus groups are less intimidating than meeting alone with an interviewer. The use of focus groups increases sample size quickly and provides immediate results.

A major disadvantage of focus groups is the phenomenon known as **group think**, a process that occurs when certain members of the group control, take over, or strongly influence the responses of other group members. The researcher has less control in such a group than in an individual interview, and the process can take more time to generate meaningful data. Additional disadvantages are that it can be difficult to find a meeting time and setting convenient for several people, the groups may be highly diversified, and the researcher or moderator may need additional training or skills to conduct focus groups.[4]

16. Explain participant observation.

Participant observation is a data generation method in which the researcher becomes immersed in the field and observes the activities of the participant. The researcher uses all of his or her senses to generate data about the observations. Involvement in the natural setting of the participants allows the researcher to experience firsthand the phenomenon under study. It is the second most common approach to qualitative data generation after the interview. Detailed, descriptive, and systematic recordings of the observations are kept as field notes.

17. What are the different approaches to participant observation? Are there specific requirements for using a particular approach?

There are four basic types of participant observation. The first is **complete observer**, in which the researcher fully observes but has no direct social interactions with the participant or the setting. In the second type, called **observer as participant**, the researcher may minimally participate in activities or do some interviewing, but the majority of the time is spent observing. In the **participant as observer** approach, the researcher becomes part of the group; that is, he or she can be a worker in the setting as well as the researcher. Role discord and conflict with primary responsibilities may occur in this type of observation role. In the fourth type, called **complete participant**, the researcher participates in the setting as a member of the group and the researcher's identity and purpose are concealed. This approach, sometimes referred to as "going native," is difficult to justify and is considered unethical by current standards.

There are no specific requirements for any of the approaches of participant observation, nor are there any rules for adopting only one type. Researchers are encouraged to choose the approach (or approaches) that best fits with the purposes of the study and is comfortable for both observer and participants.

18. How does the researcher record the generated data? What strategies are commonly used?

Most researchers record or document their data through the use of field notes and/or tape recorders. Field notes document the researcher's observations and interviews; they may be handwritten or dictated into a tape recorder and transcribed later. Data from interviews or focus groups can be recorded as handwritten field notes or tape-recorded; the researcher also can use a combination of these methods. Field notes can supplement audiotaped interviews by documenting facial expressions, gestures, interactions, and general responses. At the end of a tape-recorded interview, the researcher may choose to dictate field notes into the tape recorder so that the tape includes both the interview and the field notes. Eventually all tape-recorded data are transcribed for analysis. To minimize interference with data generation, researchers should become familiar with and practice using their equipment, carry extra batteries, and develop good habits for immediately labeling and organizing data.

19. How can data be generated with visual methods such as photography, films, and videos?

Photographs, films and videos provide visual records of daily and life events of the phenomenon under study. Visual methods can document cultural and life events, ceremonies, and behaviors in the natural setting. Their use has been recognized for added communicative and descriptive effects in presenting research results.

Photography is the least expensive and most commonly used of the three visual methods. The addition of photography can complement qualitative strategies of data generation, such as interviewing, participant observation, and examination of records and cultural artifacts. Photographs can capture nonverbal data, provide visual records, create permanent artifacts, stimulate meaning of the lived experience, help researchers gain insight into the phenomenon under study, and elicit emic (insider) descriptions and perceptions from participants.[5] Photographs can generate data from participants during interviews by stimulating further recall and details of an experience, thus enriching the depth of the interview. Because photographs are a part of family life, cameras can easily be given to participants to use as tools to capture life events, to symbolize human conditions and lived experiences, and to generate rich, thick descriptions of the phenomenon under study.

20. How do artifacts and written records or documents contribute to the data?

Artifacts, archival data, and written records and documents can contain rich data that are useful in creating and enriching an understanding of the phenomenon or culture of interest. Such data may be the primary source or supplement other methods of qualitative data generation. The data can be in the form of any communication materials, such as newspapers, books, letters, e-mails, speeches, music, photographs, works of art, or household goods.

21. When is written narrative an appropriate strategy for data generation?

Written narratives are created by participants. Instead of audiotaping an interview, the researcher requests that the participants respond to questions related to the phenomenon of interest by writing them by hand or word processing. The narratives may be a one-time written response, or they may be serial responses over time as the participant experiences the phenomenon. Because the researcher is not usually in attendance when the narratives are written, clear and explicit instructions need to be given to the participant. Advantages of this type of data collection are that the participant can think about what he or she wants to say beforehand and refine the narrative. In addition, transcription costs are eliminated. The disadvantages include the potential loss of spontaneity or naturalness by the participant and the risk of not understanding the directions.

22. Can more than one researcher generate data in qualitative research? Is interrater reliability important?

More than one researcher can generate data in a single qualitative study. Team research is commonly used in qualitative research, especially if the study is complex. Conducting large field studies takes an immense amount of time and can be done more efficiently and effectively by a team of persons than by an individual researcher. The interviews or participant observations can be made together or individually. Another observer or interviewer can also reinforce and validate the data. Interrater reliability can add to the credibility of the data but is not necessary in qualitative research. The researcher is the instrument or tool in qualitative research, and qualitative researchers acknowledge the reflexive nature of data generation.

23. What about collecting data using computers? Can one collect data on line?

The massive proliferation of communication technology invites new ways of conceptualizing data generation and research methods. Computerized data generation techniques are in the process of being developed and are a promising method of data generation for the near future. Opportunities to collect online data are growing rapidly with the increased use of computer-mediated communications, along with rising public comfort and satisfaction with the technology. Web-based chat rooms and conference centers allow participants to interact in real and delayed time, allowing flexibility in data collection time. However, accompanying this growth in technology are challenging methodologic and ethical implications, such as appropriate or compatible software for all participants and the ease of data manipulation and alteration.

REFERENCES

1. Chenitz WC, Swanson J: From Practice to Grounded Theory. Menlo Park, NJ, Addison-Wesley, 1986.
2. Burns N, Grove S: The Practice of Nursing Research: Conduct, Critique, and Utilization, 4th ed. Philadelphia, W.B. Saunders, 2001.
3. Morse J, Field P: Qualitative Research Methods for Health Professionals, 2nd ed. Thousand Oaks, CA, Sage, 1995.
4. Marshall C, Rossman G: Designing Qualitative Research, 3rd ed. Thousand Oaks, CA, Sage, 1999.
5. Magilvy JK, et al: Visions of rural aging: Use of photographic method in gerontological research. Gerontologist 32:253–257, 1992.

21. DATA MANAGEMENT: QUANTITATIVE AND QUALITATIVE

Lauren Clark, RN, PhD, and Anne Marie Kotzer, RN, PhD

1. Why should I bother with data management for my study? It sounds like extra work.

Although managing data may seem like an unnecessary burden to the researcher, it is in fact the secret to being organized, effective, and rigorous. In the process of managing data, you also protect yourself, your data, and your subjects from a variety of risks, including breaches in confidentiality and research errors. Data management gets done one way or another, even by people who do not want to do it. If you fail to construct a data management strategy, you will end up with piles of papers, loose notes, and scores or documents that you cannot track to subjects. Ultimately, nonmanagement of data requires far more work to sort through and fix than formulating a thoughtful data management plan early in your research.

2. How can literature and resources related to my research area be managed in a database?

In the precomputer era, researchers kept bibliographic cards for each reference that they collected. Although a good method at the time, carrying around and shuffling cards can be cumbersome and inefficient. Now computer programs can do the same job, only faster and more efficiently. Special programs designed for managing references include ProCite, Bibliolinks, and Reference Manager. Databases using software such as Microsoft Access can also be created to track references.

3. How does data management help protect the human subjects in my research?

Human subjects who participate in research are generally provided **confidentiality** (you do not reveal their identities) or **anonymity** (even you do not know their identity). If your data are confidential, you are likely to keep a master list linking subject name, hospital record number, or social security number to your subject identification number or other identifying variables. This master list is a key part of data management that you may need to use on several occasions. For example, you may refer to your master list to be sure that follow-up data are collected for particular individuals at subsequent data collection points. Or you may need to check to be sure that the same individual is not enrolled twice in the study. Sometimes master lists are helpful if suspicious data require you to go back and double-check actual numbers in a medical record or retrieve data missing from the study records of a particular subject. Keeping this master list secure (in a locked filing cabinet or a password-protected computer file) is critically important to the protection of study subjects. Only individuals with prior approval and a need to know the information on this sensitive master list should have access to it. As a researcher, your job is not only to manage data about human subjects but also to arrange for a data management system that safeguards the confidentiality of subjects' identities and the anonymity of subjects' research results.

4. How are subject code numbers assigned?

Coding subjects can be as easy as numbering returned surveys in order—1, 2, 3, and so on. For other studies, you may want to number subjects with embedded codes so that all subjects from research site A have a prefix or suffix indicating that site and all those from research site B have a different prefix or suffix. Similarly, subject codes can indicate a particular month or year of data collection if the same subject participates in repeated measures or interviews. Codes can even specify whether a particular subject is in a control or experimental group for quick reference.

Subject Codes

EMBEDDED SUBJECT CODE INFORMATION	EXAMPLE
Research site as a prefix	Site A: 101, 102, 103, 104... Site B: 201, 202, 203, 204...
Child's age at data collection as a suffix	1-month visit: 101-1, 102-1, 103-1... 6-month visit: 101-6, 102-6, 103-6...
Control or experimental group membership as a prefix	Control group: C101, C102, C103, C104... Experimental group: E201, E202, E203, E204...

The most important point to keep in mind when assigning subject code numbers is that they cannot reveal the subject's identity. For example, one researcher was recently disciplined by an internal review board for assigning a subject's initials to a tissue sample. Birthdates and social security numbers are inappropriate subject identifiers for the same reason—they do not maintain confidentiality. Someone who knows the subject well could identify him or her from the birthdate, thus compromising confidentiality.

5. How does data management help me keep track of recruitment and attrition statistics in my study?

You will encounter people who refuse to participate in your study or agree to participate but later drop out. It is a good idea to keep a record of the number of people approached for study participation, those who formally consented to participate, and then the stage at which dropouts left the study. For some studies you may also want to record the reason given by people who chose not to participate. Information about recruitment success, attrition, and retention are important for describing the sample of a study and also for estimating sample sizes and the effort needed to enroll subjects in similar studies in the future. A simple table can be used to record recruitment statistics, with subject identifiers listed for those who chose to participate, chose not to participate, and dropped out. No names or other identifiable subject information should be recorded on the forms, because those who refused to participate also refused to allow you to record their name. Often statistics about the percentage of those who agreed to participate, the return rate of surveys, or the rate of attrition are important to include when you write about your study. Lack of planning in the early phases of your research may prevent you from having such data when you need them.

6. How are data coded?

- **Numeric data** are the simplest kind of data to code, because the result of the measure is the number that you enter. Examples are weight, height, and age.
- **Fixed, nonnumeric responses**. Often subjects are asked to provide a rating in response to a question. This response must be changed into a number. For

example, we may ask subjects to rate their health as excellent (4), good (3), fair (2), or poor (1). The number corresponding to the response is assigned by the research team as a code that refers to the descriptor. When subjects complete the question, it is a simple matter of entering the code previously assigned to the response as the coded data. This format for coding also applies to categorical data such as gender [male (1), female (2)] and yes (1)/no (2) responses.

- **Short answers**. Some open-ended questions can be coded through a content analysis process, in which the researcher assigns codes to the responses after the data are collected. Instead of asking subjects to rate their health, the researcher may simply ask, "How would you describe the idea of health,?" and then see what kinds of answers subjects offer. From reading their responses, the researcher may conclude that a specific number of typical responses can be summarized, such as:

(1) Health is not having any aches or pains.

(2) Health is being able to function and do the things I want to do.

(3) Health is being in top form spiritually, mentally, and physically.

Thus, word data are reduced to categories. Data coding of short-answer responses into numerically indexed categories has to be done after a significant portion of the data are collected so that a comprehensive and nonoverlapping set of response codes can be developed.

- **Discourse or narrative**. In coding discourse or narrative for meaning, subjects are asked to discuss an experience, such as what it is like to have a miscarriage or undergo a heart transplant. The coding that the researcher does with whole interviews and narratives involves reading the transcript of the interview, thinking about the meaning of the subject's response, and then identifying "chunks" (sentences or paragraphs) that can be tagged with a code word. Later these data can be grouped with other similarly coded chunks of data to form categories. Many different qualitative researchers have written about the process of coding data in this manner. The reference list gives several examples.

For quantitative data, coding sometimes means simply entering numeric data into a specified place on a spreadsheet. For nonnumeric data, coding involves transforming word data into numbers or beginning the process of data analysis by coding word data (sentences or paragraphs) with a shorter code word for later retrieval.

7. Do I need a code book or data dictionary?

Whether your research is qualitative or quantitative, you definitely need a code book or data dictionary. For quantitative research, the code book consists of the variable name and label, value labels, and any other notes that help you remember all of the details of that particular variable. Do *not* rely on memory to help you when you reexamine your data years from now! Some statistical packages create a code book or data dictionary as you set up your database within the system.

Quantitative Code Book

VARIABLE NAME	VARIABLE LABEL	VALUE LABEL
DIAG	Primary diagnosis	1 = appendicitis
		2 = hernia
		3 = fractured leg
CHRONILL	Chronic illness	1 = yes
		2 = no

In qualitative research, the code book lists the codes used to index parts of discourse or narrative and also offers definitions of each code word that you choose. For example, if the mothers and grandmothers in a particular study talked about different ways to predict the sex of a baby while a woman is pregnant, the researcher may want to assign a code for each method. "Twirling wedding ring" and "heartbeat" are likely codes.

Qualitative Code Book

CODE WORD	DEFINITION
Twirling ring	Using the mother's wedding ring, hold it suspended by string over the mother's pregnant abdomen. The direction the ring twirls will indicate if the baby is a boy or girl.
Heartbeat	Either a slow baby heart rate or a fast heart rate will indicate whether the baby is a boy or girl.

A definition of each code is useful to ensure that codes are not too similar and to define the limits of a particular code.

8. How do I handle multiple sources of data for each subject?

If your study results in a demographic questionnaire, survey, measure of blood pressure, and interview, you need a way to keep track of each kind of data. In some studies, all data about an individual subject are stored in the subject's file. In the file drawer subjects are arranged in chronological order by identification code. Sometimes it is easier for the researcher to separate each different kind of data and file it with other subjects' data on the same measure. In this case, the file drawer contains one file for demographic questionnaires, one for blood pressure measures, and one for interviews. Generally, a master list, table, or chart is helpful to keep track of which kinds of data are on record for each subject, because some subjects may provide only the demographic questionnaire and blood pressure reading but not be available for the survey or interview. Whichever method you choose, it is critical that each piece of paper containing subject data is labeled with the subject's code. Do not rely on paper clips or staples to keep multiple sheets together. One loose piece of paper with no identifier indicates that you have lost data that otherwise could enrich and inform your results.

9. When should I begin to enter data into the computer?

Ideally, you should set up the database as part of the study design and start entering data as soon as the first pieces are collected. More likely than not, however, there is enough to keep you busy during the early phases of the study, and data entry may be postponed until it becomes critically important. With large studies, you may want to hire a person to enter data as it is collected so that preliminary or interim analyses can be done or to avoid scurrying at the last minute to enter and analyze data when abstract submissions are due. Some data collection is amenable to immediate entry into a laptop or hand-held computer on the spot. Teleform is a computerized solution that allows data collected in the field to be scanned directly into a digitized data management file. By choosing to enter data at the earliest possible time, you can find glitches in your coding scheme or even in your data collection instruments. Even better, you may find that you are collecting interesting results and are well on your way to completing your project.

10. Some data for some subjects are missing. Is this a data management problem?

Missing data are not so much a management problem as they are a problem when you begin to analyze your data. Be sure that missing data are coded as such so that they are not confused with a refusal to answer, a not-applicable response, or an actual value of zero as a valid answer. Each computer program has its own process for interpreting blanks or missing data. Know what it is, and code your data accordingly.

11. Can computer programs help with data management?

Computer packages are available for both quantitative and qualitative data management and analysis. An Internet search is a good starting point to find a program that meets your study needs. Comparisons of different analysis packages are published in books and periodically in journal review articles. More critical than finding software is setting up some kind of system or mechanism by which you log in, check off, file, or otherwise track your subjects and their data throughout the course of your study. The following qualitative and quantitative software programs are excellent resources.

- **ATLAS.ti** is a computer program for qualitative analysis of textual, graphical, audio, and video data. It offers a variety of tools for accomplishing the tasks associated with any systematic approach to qualitative data.
- **Ethnograph** is a computer program for the analysis of interview transcripts, field notes, open-ended survey responses, or other text-based documents. It offers a variety of tools for coding and managing text.
- **HyperRESEARCH** is a computer program for the analysis of qualitative data. It enables the researcher to code and retrieve, build theories, and conduct analyses with text, graphics, audio, and video sources.
- **SPSS** (Statistical Package for the Social Sciences) is a quantitative data management and analysis product produced by SPSS, Inc. in Chicago. Among its features are modules for statistical data analysis, including descriptive statistics such as plots, frequencies, charts, and lists, as well as sophisticated inferential and multivariate statistical procedures such as analysis of variance (ANOVA), factor analysis, cluster analysis, and categorical data analysis.
- **TeleForm** is a high-volume, network-based program that enables researchers to capture information and convert existing paper forms into digital data, thereby decreasing the need for manual entry.

12. Can I store my data electronically, or do I need to keep paper files with raw data?

You want to save data electronically and more than once to ensure that back-up files are available. Even so, do not throw away your paper data too soon. If your data are saved on a computer hard drive, be sure to have at least one back-up copy on a floppy disk. A word of caution: some people make several back-ups on floppy disks for fear that they may lose one. This can create a problem when you start editing your data files because you must remember to change all versions on each floppy disk. Additionally, be sure that the disks are not kept in the same place. Be prudent! You can save subject data for as long as you need, but you must destroy the data when you told subjects that you would. If your subjects were told that their tape-recorded interviews will be held in your research office for 5 years, you must destroy their data after that period. In the future, direct data entry strategies will completely eliminate the need for paper. Voice recognition software can help researchers transfer audiotapes into transcripts. TeleForm and other scannable software forms can help researchers scan or even key data directly into a computerized database to bypass the need for paper copies.

13. Will I need to start over with new data management processes each time I do a new study?

A well-conceived study design and rigorous methods will serve you well in future studies. We all learn from our experiences, both the good and the disappointing. Although no two databases are identical, the structures and formats used in your past research project may be transferable to your future study. New technology will change what you do. Stay current, but do not throw out strategies that worked well for you in the past. Good data management should boost the rigor and parsimony of your research. You will be clearer, more organized, and more accurate in conducting and reporting your research if your data are managed appropriately from the start. Your data are all you have—protect them!

BIBLIOGRAPHY

1. Miles MB, Huberman AM: Qualitative Data Analysis. Thousand Oaks, CA, Sage Publications, 1994.
2. Riessman CK: Narrative Analysis. Thousand Oaks, CA, Sage Publications, 1993.
3. Weitzman EA, Miles MB: Computer Programs for Qualitative Data Analysis: A Software Sourcebook. Thousand Oaks, CA, Sage Publications, 1995.
4. Woods NF, Catanzaro M: Nursing Research, Theory, and Practice. St. Louis, Mosby, 1988.

22. QUANTITATIVE DATA ANALYSIS

Carol P. Vojir, PhD

1. What are statistics?

Statistics consist of procedures that help you (1) summarize the information collected from your research (descriptive statistics) and (2) to test any hypotheses that you may have developed (inferential statistics).

2. How can I understand the thought process underlying statistics?

Evaluation or analysis of information to answer data-related questions is something that we do every day. For example, if you look outside in the morning and see that it looks like rain, based on your past experiences you may decide to take an umbrella when you go out. It may not rain, but your experience (your database) tells you that it looks threatening enough to carry an umbrella. Statistics as a part of research is a formalized thinking process, whereas the example of the weather is an informal thinking process. The approach is the same.

3. What must I do before beginning data analysis?

- Your data must be in an automated file that has been verified for accuracy and that uses a format compatible with your chosen data analysis program (e.g., SPSS, SAS, or Excel).
- You must have access to a computer with a data analysis program such as SPSS, SAS, or Excel.
- You need a data dictionary or code book that relates the short and often cryptic names used in the automated data file to your variables (see question 5).

4. Once I have completed these preparations, how do I analyze data?

Whether you are conducting an exploratory (descriptive) or hypothesis-driven (inferential) study, you should begin the data analysis process with frequency distributions and summary statistics for your variables.

5. What are frequency distributions and summary statistics?

The tables below show portions of the data matrix and data dictionary from a 32,374-subject, 1,275-variable file of survey data (National Health Interview Survey, 2000). This data matrix, although potentially interesting, is too large to draw conclusions about the data without the use of frequency distributions and summary statistics. **Frequency distributions** inform the researcher about the values of a variable and the number of subjects with each of the values. **Summary statistics** are single numbers used to characterize the variables in a data matrix.

The First Ten Subjects and Nine Variables in an Example Dataset

SEX	AGE	ETHNIC	EDUC	SMKEV	LCANCER	BMI	SAD	EFFORT
1	53	2	5	2	2	2233	5	5
1	50	2	6	2		2510	5	5

(Table continued on next page.)

The First Ten Subjects and Nine Variables in an Example Dataset (cont.)

SEX	AGE	ETHNIC	EDUC	SMKEV	LCANCER	BMI	SAD	EFFORT
2	74	2	5	2		2048	5	5
2	33	2	4	2		2489	4	4
1	36	2	2	2		2233	4	4
2	62	2	2	1		2232	5	5
1	34	1	1	2		2833	4	5
2	25	2	3	2		2145	5	4
2	25	1	3	2		3719	5	5
1	35	2	2	1		2951	5	5

For key to abbreviations, see table below.

A Portion of the Data Dictionary from the Example Dataset

NAME	LABEL	VALUES
SEX	Gender	1 = M; 2 = F
AGE	Age	Continuous
ETHNIC	Ethnicity	1 = Hispanic; 2 = White; 3 = Black; 4 = Asian; 5 = American Indian; 6 = Multiracial
EDUC	Education	Continuous
SMKEV	Ever smoked?	1 = Yes; 2 = No
LCANCER	Had lung cancer?	1 = Yes; 2 = No
BMI	Body mass index	Continuous
SAD	How often sad?	1 = All of the time; 2 = Most of the time; 3 = Some of the time; 4 = A little of the time; 5 = None of the time
EFFORT	How often is everything an effort?	1 = All of the time; 2 = Most of the time; 3 = Some of the time; 4 = A little of the time; 5 = None of the time

6. Give a specific example of a frequency distribution.

A frequency distribution is a table of the values included in a variable as well as the counts of subjects (frequencies) associated with those values. The table below shows a portion of a frequency distribution table obtained from the SPSS program for the variable AGE (example dataset). Note that unlike the data matrix in question 5, the values for AGE are displayed in increasing order. This strategy provides a useful summary for the AGE variable.

The First Six Values of the Frequency Distribution Table for the Variable AGE

VALUE	FREQUENCY	PERCENT	CUMULATIVE PERCENT
18	403	1.2	1.2
19	462	1.4	2.7
20	452	1.4	4.1
21	546	1.7	5.8
22	523	1.6	7.4
23	566	1.7	9.1

Frequency distributions also can be displayed graphically. Below is a histogram plot of the categorized frequency distribution for the variable AGE with a line representing an ideal "normal" distribution superimposed. (This histogram plot was obtained directly from the statistical program, SPSS.) Note that the age values have been categorized into 5-year groups, such as 17.5 to 22.5, against which the frequency of occurrence of these values is plotted. From this histogram we know something that was not obvious from the matrix of raw data about the ages of the 32,374 subjects (for instance, that ages ranged between approximately 18 and 88). We also can see that the four largest 5-year age categories in terms of frequencies (counts)—32.5–37.5 years, 37.5–42.5 years, 42.5–47.5 years, and 47.5–52.5 years—are in the middle of the horizontal axis.

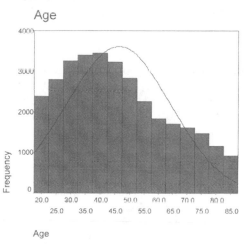

A histogram plot of the variable AGE.

7. Explain summary statistics.

Summary statistics are single numbers that help to characterize attributes of a variable's frequency distribution. The most common summary statistics describe the center and spread of the distribution. Measures of a distribution's "height" along the vertical axis are called measures of central tendency. Measures of a distribution's "spread" along the horizontal axis are called measures of variability.

8. What is the difference between mean, median, and mode (all well-known measures of central tendency)?

The **mean** is the arithmetic average. The **median** is the data value dividing the 50% of the subjects with lower values from the 50 percent of the subjects with higher values. The **mode** is the value or values with the largest frequency. The AGE frequency distribution has a mean of 46.4 years, a median of 44.0 years, and a single mode of 38 years. All of these summary statistics, obtained from a statistical program such as SPSS, describe the middle or center of the AGE distribution where most of the subjects' ages are clustered.

9. What are measures of variability? How are these obtained?

Useful measures of variability, such as range and standard deviation, can be calculated or obtained from a statistical analysis program (e.g., SPSS or SAS). For our example data, the age **range** was approximately 67 years, increasing from a low of 18 years to a high of over 85 years. The **standard deviation**, which is essentially the average of the differences between the individual subject values and the mean, was 17.9 years for the example dataset. You often see the standard deviation reported in conjunction with the mean to summarize the center and variability of a distribution.

$$\bar{X} \text{ (mean)} \quad \pm \quad s \text{ (standard deviation)}$$

For our example data, $\bar{X} \pm s$ would be 46.4 ± 17.9. These two numbers tell us that the center of the age distribution is approximately 46 years (a middle-aged person) and that much of the data is contained within a 36-year band around the mean (17.9 years above the mean and 17.9 years below the mean). The 36-year band is the contribution of the standard deviation; it shows that quite a spread of ages is represented in the sample. About two-thirds of the subjects were aged between 28.5 years (46.4 − 17.9) and 64.3 years (46.4 + 17.9).

10. Can I use frequency distributions and summary statistics for variables at all levels of measurement?

We can obtain and use frequency distribution tables for all variables. However, summary statistics that are computed (e.g., mean, median, or standard deviation) can be applied only to variables whose levels of measurement are at least interval. If the differences between sequential numbers on the scale are not equal, the premises on which mathematical operations are based do not hold. Thus we cannot use computed summary statistics to characterize nominal or ordinal level variables.

Nominal- and ordinal-level variables usually do not have many values; therefore, data can be summarized through use of the values that represent the majority of subjects. For example, a frequency distribution table obtained from the SPSS program of the counts for males and females in the example data file showed that 18,388 (57%) were female. This is a perfectly valid way to summerize nominal- and ordinal-level variables. SPSS charts like the bar chart shown below also work well.

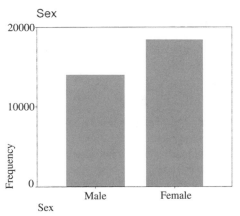

A bar chart for the variable SEX.

11. What is the purpose of superimposing a line representing an ideal normal distribution on the frequency distribution of the variable AGE?

The bell-shaped and symmetric form called the normal distribution has important properties that enable a researcher to make the correct inference from the sample to the population when certain statistical procedures with requirements for approximate normality are used. Therefore, assessing whether the distribution of an interval- or ratio-level variable such as AGE is approximately normal in shape is important for the beginning researcher. A line superimposed on a frequency distribution allows one to judge the approximate normality of the variable. This is one of several methods to assess normality.

12. Is the distribution of the variable AGE approximately normal?

Inspection (the "eyeball" test) of the histogram in question 6 shows that the variable AGE is roughly normally distributed. Can we say that it is "normal enough" that statistical procedures using the variable AGE will yield accurate results? Not without information from other indicators of approximate normality.

13. What other tests can be used to judge approximate normality?

The summary statistics called **skewness**, which is a measure of asymmetry, and **kurtosis**, which is a measure of deviation up or down at the center from the bell shape of a normal curve, provide additional clues about approximate normality for an interval- or ratio-level variable. **Fisher's coefficient of skewness** and **Fisher's coefficient of kurtosis** can be computed by dividing the skewness index or the kurtosis index, which are obtained from a statistical analysis program such as SPSS, by their standard errors (the names given to the standard deviation of a statistic). For our example dataset, the skewness index for the variable AGE was reported from the SPSS program as 0.42 and its standard error as 0.014. Fisher's coefficient of skewness, therefore, is 0.42/0.014 or 30. Fisher's coefficient of kurtosis for the variable AGE is –0.78 divided by 0.027, which equals –28.9. (The kurtosis index of –0.78 and the standard error of –0.27 were obtained from SPSS.) Values for these coefficients between 2 and +2 are consistent with approximate normality.

By these criteria, AGE is *not* approximately normally distributed. The distribution is positively skewed, that is, pulled to the right, shown by the positive sign on the skewness coefficient. The distribution is also flatter than a normal distribution, as shown by the negative sign on the kurtosis coefficient. We must do something about this non-normal distribution to ensure that analyses involving AGE do not yield inaccurate inferences about the population.

14. Are there any other components of descriptive analysis?

The next important process is to look for **patterns of relationships** among the variables in the dataset. This concept is a component of the descriptive characterization of the dataset, not an hypothesis-driven activity. To examine patterns, the researcher uses the statistical analysis program to obtain a matrix of correlation coefficients among important variables. A count of the number of statistically significant results showing that a given variable has relationships with at least half of the other variables constitutes a pattern for that variable. Patterns are useful to uncover unsuspected interactions among variables. Below is an example from the dataset.

Correlation Matrix

	SEX	AGE	EDUC	SAD	EFFORT
SEX		0.049	–0.022	–0.100	–0.053
AGE			–0.16	–0.023	0.021
EDUC				0.149	0.081
SAD					0.554

This example is a matrix of statistically significant correlations among five variables (SEX, AGE, EDUC, SAD, AND EFFORT) in the example dataset. Because our example dataset is so large (32,374 subjects), all correlation coefficients are statistically significant; our criterion for determining patterns is not helpful. However, inspection of the significant correlations shows that only the AGE and EDUC, AGE and SAD, and SAD and EFFORT correlations exceeded ±0.1. As no single variable is part of more than two of these three correlations, we will consider that we have no particular patterns. If patterns are deemed to be present, their interpretation requires knowledge about correlation, to be discussed in a subsequent question, as well as knowledge of the involved variables.

15. What information do I need to choose a statistical procedure to test my hypothesis?

The figure on the following page shows a systematic scheme that is based on the type of hypothesis, the level of measurement of the variables, and the nature of the independent variable (the "cause," or the variable considered to affect the dependent variable, the "effect"). The level of measurement of the dependent variable puts you on the correct entry branch of the figure. Then you must decide whether your hypothesis is one of difference or one of relationship. Often but not always, the wording of the hypothesis gives you this answer. However, the word "relationship" frequently is used when the word "difference" is meant; thus you need to think about whether in fact you are looking at associations/relationships or at differences. For some procedures, no more information beyond the above is needed. For others, there are third and even fourth steps to the process.

If appropriate, the third step on the pathway is based on the independent variable(s), either the number of these or the number of values in a single independent variable. We often refer to the values contained by a nominal-level variable as "groups." For example, the variable of gender has two values or groups, male and female.

The final step, if required, refers to the nature of the data. In unrelated groups, such as male and female, we expect that the males and females in the sample are not closely related; they are independent of one another. If subjects were related and we thought otherwise, our results from a statistical test requiring that the groups be unrelated may be biased because one person may have influenced another's response to the dependent variable. We then could draw an incorrect inference from the sample results to the population of interest.

16. What procedure can I use to test the hypothesis, "There is a relationship between age and sadness"?

AGE is a ratio-level variable, and SAD is strictly an ordinal-level variable but can be treated as an interval-level variable because the measurement literature confirms that such an action has minor impact on the analysis. AGE is the independent variable as it occurs before SAD. According to the table in question 14, we start on the topmost entry branch because we consider SAD to be an interval-level variable:

Interval/ratio-level DV

This is a relationship hypothesis; we truly are interested in the relationship or association between the two variables:

Interval/ratio-level DV → Relationship hypothesis

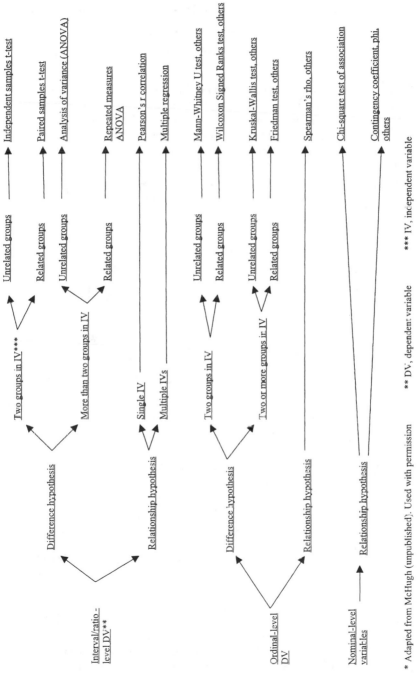

Simplified process for choosing basic statistical techniques.

* Adapted from McHugh (unpublished). Used with permission   ** DV, dependent variable   *** IV, independent variable

As we have but a single independent variable (AGE), we take the single IV path and follow it until we arrive at Pearson's r correlation on the right side of the table:

Interval/ratio-level DV→Relationship hypothesis→Single IV→Pearson's r correlation

This type of correlation is appropriate, given the hypothesis and variables.

17. What is the result when we test the above hypothesis with Pearson's r correlation?

Pearson's r correlation is a parametric procedure, which means that to produce accurate results, certain assumptions about the data must be met. These assumptions are that (1) the variables are approximately normally distributed and (2) there is a linear relationship between the two variables. Before we can interpret the result for the Pearson's r correlation, we first must test whether these assumptions are valid for our data.

We have determined that AGE is not approximately normally distributed. Using a similar process, we can see that the variable SAD also is not approximately normally distributed (see figure below).

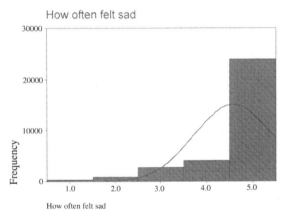

A histogram plot of the variable SAD.

Because neither variable is approximately normally distributed, we will use two types of correlation coefficients, Pearson's r correlation coefficient and Spearman's rho correlation coefficient, which has no distributional assumptions and is typically used for ordinal-level measures or when there is a violation of the assumption of normality for Pearson's r correlation. When the assumptions are violated for the Pearson's r coefficient, the Spearman's rho coefficient is the more accurate and powerful correlation coefficient.

The other assumption (for Pearson's r) of a linear relationship is determined through a scatterplot, which is a plot of the values held for the two variables (see figure, next page).

The scatterplot obtained from the program SPSS and displayed below resembles a rectangle more than any other figure. Linearity appears as an oval- or cigar-shaped figure. What is displayed is more consistent with a circle. A circle is one of the figures that we can accept as evidence of a linear but not a strong relationship. A circle is at one end of the shape continuum; a straight line is at the other end of this same continuum. Between are oval and cigar-shaped figures. We do not want to see horseshoes or sine waves; nonlinear shapes are not consistent with this type of correlation.

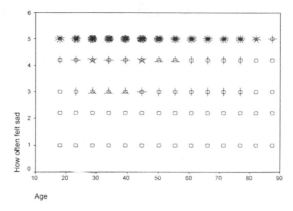

Weighted scatterplot of the variables AGE and SAD.

We conclude that the variables are non-normally distributed but linearly related. Because violations produce inaccurate results, we apply both Pearson's r correlation and Spearman's rho correlation to get an idea of how much of an impact non-normality had on the statistical procedure. The table below shows the output from the program SPSS.

The Correlation between AGE and SAD

		SAD		SAD
AGE	Pearson Correlation	−0.023	Spearman's rho	−0.016
	Sig. (2-tailed)	< 0.001	Sig. (2-tailed)	0.004
	N	31,905	N	31,905

First, examine the row with Pearson's r correlation and Spearman's rho correlation. Pearson's r correlation is −0.023; Spearman's rho is −0.016. Because these results are close, we know that the violations did not have much impact. The correlations are similar in value and identical in sign so we can be more confident that we have obtained results from this sample that are the same as those we would find if we tested the entire population.

There are two parts to a correlation: the sign and the value of the number. The sign, in this case a negative one, tells us that the relationship is inverse. As age increased, sadness increased (lower numbers for sadness mean more frequent sadness). Although weak, this is the outcome that we might expect.

The second component to correlation is the number. Correlation ranges between −1, a perfect inverse relationship, and +1, a perfect direct relationship. Zero means no relationship. The obtained Spearman's rho coefficient, −0.016, is small and close to zero. This is consistent with the scatterplot showing a more circular figure. We have a weak relationship between the variables AGE and SAD. The next step is to determine whether that relationship is statistically significant and thereby inferable to the population.

We find statistical significance in the sig. (two-tailed) row in the table above. A significance, called a p-value, that is less than or equal to 0.05 (the typical cut-off value referred to as alpha) is considered to be statistically significant. In our case, the p-value for the Spearman's rho coefficient is 0.004, which is much smaller than

0.05. Therefore, the answer to our hypothesis is that there is a relationship between AGE and SAD.

18. Is it possible that we made a mistake in our conclusion about the correlation hypothesis?

This practice of using a probability (the p-value) to infer that something is or is not statistically significant in the population because we have or have not gotten statistically significant results with our sample leaves us open to errors, called **conclusion errors**. In the correlation example, we decided that because we got statistical significance in our sample, a relationship between AGE and SAD exists in the population of U.S. adults. If that decision were incorrect, we would make what is called a **type I** conclusion error—that is, finding significance in the sample when it is not present in the population. Researchers actively design their studies, test assumptions, and engage in similar safety procedures to avoid conclusion errors. An example is the cut-off value, alpha, which can be manipulated as a part of research design to change the probability of a type I error. Another indicator is the actual p-value obtained from the statistical procedure. The smaller the value, the less the chance of a type I error.

19. What is the practical significance of a small statistically significant correlation?

First of all, statistical significance is required before practical significance can be evaluated because if we play by the rules of statistics, results that are not statistically significant are considered to be indicative of no relationship in the population. There is no practical significance to "no relationship."

When appropriate, practical significance in correlation is estimated by squaring the obtained correlation coefficient. Such a squared correlation estimates how much information is shared between the two variables—if there is quite a bit of shared information (perhaps 20% or higher), the variable pair may be useful for further work in building models or as evidence for evidence-based practice changes. In our test example, the correlation was –0.016, which, when squared, is not even 1%. We obtained a statistically but not practically significant result from the test of our hypothesis.

20. What procedure do I use to test the hypothesis, "There is a positive association between having ever smoked and lung cancer"?

You certainly could use an appropriate correlation coefficient because this is a relationship hypothesis, but we can use another helpful procedure to answer the question. In our example datasets SMKEV and LCANCER (see table in question 5) are dichotomous (two values), nominal-level variables.

We start on the bottommost entry branch of the figure on page 199: nominal-level variables. There are two analysis choices, one for correlation (contingency coefficient, phi, others) and one for the chi-square test of association, which we will use for this analysis. The chi-square procedure compares the counts of the various combinations of the two variables: smokers with lung cancer; smokers without lung cancer; nonsmokers with lung cancer; and nonsmokers without lung cancer. If our research hypothesis is correct, we expect to find higher counts of people in the smokers with lung cancer and nonsmokers without lung cancer categories than in the other two categories.

21. What are the results if we test our hypothesis with the chi-square test of association?

Again we start with the assumptions underlying the technique. Although the chi-square test of association is a nonparametric technique, it also has assumptions:

- Each observation is classified into only one combination of the two variables (called a cell).
- The variables are categorical, ordinal at highest.
- The cells contain counts (frequencies).
- No more than 20% of the cells have counts of less than 5; no cell is empty (zero count).

We use a cross-tabulation (two-variable frequency distribution) table to examine these assumptions:

Cross-tabulation of the Variables LCANCER and SMKEV

			SMKEV 1 YES	SMKEV 2 NO	TOTAL
LCANCER	1 Yes	Count	38	12	50
		% within LCANCER	76.0%	24.0%	100.0%
		% within SMKEV	3.2%	1.2%	2.3%
	2 No	Count	1136	950	2086
		% within LCANCER	54.5%	45.5%	100.0%
		% within SMKEV	96.8%	98.8%	97.7%
Total		Count	1174	962	2136
		% within LCANCER	55.0%	45.0%	100.0%
		% within SMKEV	100.0%	100.0%	100.0%

This table shows counts for the four combinations of the variables LCANCER and SMKEV as well as totals for each variable. (Each total column or row is a frequency distribution table for one variable.) Data were obtained from the SPSS program.

The variables are categorical; that assumption is satisfied. Because each subject is a unique combination of the two variables, the assumption that each subject is classified into a single cell is also satisfied. Because the four cells contain counts of subjects, the assumption that the data are counts or frequencies is satisfied. Finally, inspection of the cross tabulation table shows that all cells have information in them and that none contains a count of less than five. With no violations of the assumptions, we can proceed to interpret the chi-square test of association.

The Chi-square Test of Association

	VALUE	DF	ASYMP. SIG. (2 SIDED)
Pearson Chi-Square	9.154	1	0.002
N of Valid Cases	2136		

We expected a positive association between the presence of lung cancer and an affirmative answer to the question about smoking. We call such a question one-tailed, one-sided, or directional because a specific association is expected. To obtain the correct p-value (significance) for our directional test from the chi-square table, we halve the displayed value. Our correct p-value is 0.001, which, because it is less than the cut off value of 0.05, is considered statistically significant. There *is* an association between having ever smoked and lung cancer.

22. What type of conclusion error is associated with our decision that the result is statistically significant?

We have determined that there is a statistically significant association between smoking and lung cancer in our sample, a result that we would like to infer to the population of U.S. adults. If the association between smoking and lung cancer were only an artifact of our sample and not true for the population, we would have made a type I error (finding significance in the sample when it is not true in the population). If we had not found statistical significance in this situation, the relevant conclusion error would have been a type II error (not finding significance in the sample when it is present in the population).

23. What is the practical significance of our statistically significant chi-square result?

For practical significance, we go back to the cross-tabulation table (in question 21). Looking at the percentages of subjects with lung cancer who have or have not smoked, we see that three times the number of smokers (76.0%) as nonsmokers (24.0%) reported lung cancer. (Undoubtedly our results underestimated the true association because they did not include people who died from the disease and were not surveyed.) The counts are small, but the economic consequences for the health care system from such a finding are large.

24. What procedure should I use to test the hypothesis, "Current smokers have smaller body mass indices (BMIs) than nonsmokers"?

This hypothesis is a difference hypothesis. "Are there differences in BMI between current smokers and nonsmokers?" is an equivalent way of asking the question.

To use the figure on page 199, we must determine which of the two variables, smoking or BMI, is the dependent variable. If you think about cause and effect, it is easy to see that the hypothesis is framed in such a way that we would expect smoking to affect BMI, not the other way around. Consequently, BMI is the "effect" or dependent variable, and smoking is the "cause'" or independent variable. BMI is a ratio-level variable with a true zero. Smoking currently (SMKNOW from our example dataset) is a nominal-level variable, having only the groups or values "yes" and "no.".

We enter the figure on the topmost entry branch (Interval/ratio-level DV) and move along the difference hypothesis path. We have two groups or values for smoking (yes/no); thus we choose the "two groups in IV" path. Because each subject in our example dataset came from a different household, we may assume that subjects are unrelated. "Unrelated groups" finally leads us to the independent samples t-test, which is the procedure that we will use to test the hypothesis:

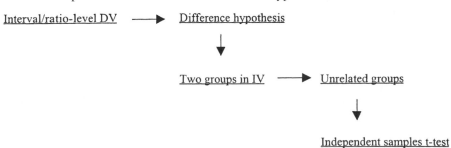

25. What results do I get when I use the independent samples t-test to investigate this hypothesis?

First we test the assumptions for the independent sample t-test: (1) the smokers and nonsmokers are different people and not related; (2) BMI is approximately normally distributed for both smokers and nonsmokers; and (3) smokers and nonsmokers have equal variances (variance is equal to the standard deviation squared) for BMI. We must assume that the research design (one adult per family) ensured that smokers and nonsmokers are not related. We can test approximate normality with the procedures described earlier.

Body Mass Index (BMI)

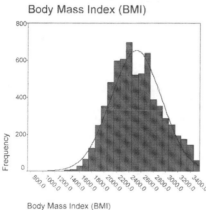

Histogram for BMI for smokers.

Body Mass Index (BMI)

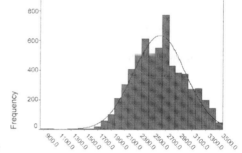

Histogram of BMI for nonsmokers.

These histograms obtained from the SPSS program look reasonably consistent with normality. The Fisher coefficients of skewness and kurtosis, however, are somewhat outside the limits for a normal distribution. Because the violations are not severe and the procedure is relatively immune to all but the most severe of problems, we will not worry about it. (Our alternative, if the violation were severe, is to use the comparable nonparametric procedure, the Mann-Whitney U test, which does not assume a normal distribution to produce accurate results.) The third assumption of equal spread in the smoker and nonsmoker groups is tested directly as a part of the t-test procedure, using the SPSS program.

Group Statistics

	SMKNOW (SMOKE CURRENTLY)	N	MEAN	STD. DEVIATION	STD. ERROR MEAN
BMI (body mass index)	1 Yes	6763	2520.15	412.533	5.016
	2 No	6189	2617.12	388.183	4.934

The two columns in the table on the next page under Levene's Test for Equality of Variances (again, the variance equals the standard deviation squared) give us the test of our third assumption. Because the significance (sig.) is less than 0.05, we conclude that the spread of the variable BMI is not the same for smokers and nonsmokers. We use this information to choose the uncorrected (equal variances assumed) *or* corrected (equal variances not assumed) row in the table. Because our variances are not equal in the groups, we interpret the corrected row of the t-test (equal variances not assumed). The t-test result is in the fourth column, labeled t. Because our hypothesis was phrased as a directional hypothesis (smokers have a smaller BMI than nonsmokers), we should divide the obtained p-value (sig. < 0.001) by 2 to obtain the correct value. However, half of less than 0.001 is still less than 0.001. We look at the means in the Group Statistics table to see that the answer to our hypothesis is that current smokers *do* have smaller BMIs than nonsmokers, on average.

Independent Samples Test

		LEVENE'S TEST FOR EQUALITY OF VARIANCE		T-TEST FOR EQUALITY OF MEANS						
		F	SIG.	t	DF	SIG. (2-TAILED)	MEAN DIF-FERENCE	STD. ERROR DIF FERENCE	95% CONFIDENCE INTERVAL OF THE DIFFERENCE LOWER	UPPER
BMI (body mass index)	Equal variances assumed	24.793	<0.001	–13.744	12950	<0.001	–96.97	7.055	–110.8	–83.14
	Equal variances not assumed			–13.781	12940	<0.001	–96.97	7.036	–110.8	–83.18

26. What do the columns labeled "95% Confidence Interval of the Difference" in the Independent Sample Test table mean?

Confidence intervals are a way of placing an interval around an obtained sample statistic (in this case, the difference between means), which locates the population parameter inferred with a certain level of confidence. Using the data in the Independent Sample Test table, we can say that 95% of the time the true difference between the means in the population will lie between the values –83 and –111. This 95% confidence interval on the mean difference is the same regardless of whether we use the corrected or uncorrected rows. It is also a repeat of the significance testing results; if the t-test were not significant, the 95% confidence interval would include the value zero.

27. True or false: Since we have statistical significance, the relevant conclusion error would be a type I error.

True. It is possible that we found statistical significance in our sample when none exists in the population.

28. Is our statistically significant finding practically significant?

To determine practical significance for the t-test, we look at the exact difference in BMI, shown in the Independent Samples text table as –96.97. This difference is less than 5% of the means (displayed in the Group Statistics table); thus, we would conclude that the practical effect of smoking on BMI is relatively small.

29. How do I test the hypothesis, "BMI differs based on perceived health status change"?

This hypothesis is a difference hypothesis; it contains the word "differ." To use the figure on page 199, we must determine which of the two variables, perceived health status change or BMI, is the dependent variable. Applying the same strategy as with the independent samples t-test, it is easy to see that the hypothesis is framed in such a way that we expect health status change to affect BMI, not the other way around (although undoubtedly there is some reciprocity to this interaction). For our purposes, however, BMI is the "effect," or dependent variable, and perceived health status change is the "cause," or independent variable. BMI is a ratio-level variable with a true zero. Perceived health status change is a nominal-level variable coded into three groups or values: 1 is Better, 2 is Worse, and 3 is Unchanged.

We enter the figure on the topmost entry branch (Interval/ratio-level DV) and move to the difference hypothesis path. With three groups or values for perceived health status change (better/worse/unchanged), we go next to the "More than two groups in IV" path. As each subject in our example dataset came from a different household, we may assume that subjects are unrelated. This path leads us finally to the analysis of variance (ANOVA) procedure, which we will use to test our hypothesis:

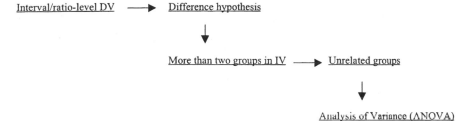

30. What do the ANOVA results look like when I test this hypothesis?

First we test the assumptions, which for ANOVA are identical to the independent samples t-test: (1) subjects in each group are different people and not related; (2) BMI is approximately normally distributed in all three groups; and (3) all three groups have equal variances (equal to the standard deviations squared) for BMI. We must assume that the research design (one adult per family) ensured that subjects rated themselves into only one group and that there were not many people in any given family. We can test normality with the procedures described earlier.

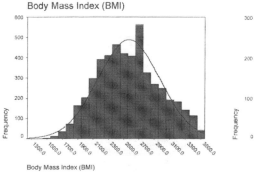

BMI, subjects in "Better" group.

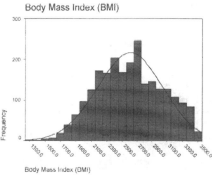

BMI, subjects in "Worse" group.

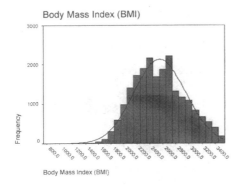

BMI, subjects in the "Unchanged" group.

The three figures depicted above show distributions that are consistent with approximate normality. The skewness and kurtosis indices were somewhat abnormal but the means, medians, and modes were close. This evidence, along with the knowledge that ANOVA is not particularly vulnerable unless the violation of normality is severe, allows us to proceed. (If the violation were severe enough, we could use the Kruskal-Wallis test, a nonparametric procedure that makes no distributional assumptions.) Again, the third assumption, that of equal spread in BMI in the three groups, is tested as part of the ANOVA procedure:

Descriptives

BMI (Body Mass Index)

	N	MEAN	STD. DEVIATION	STD. ERROR	95% CONFIDENCE INTERVAL FOR MEAN		MIN	MAX
					LOWER BOUND	UPPER BOUND		
1 Better	4958	2566.30	403.874	5.736	2555.06	2577.55	1291	3499
2 Worse	2356	2611.32	432.689	8.914	2593.84	2628.80	1297	3497
3 About the same	21313	2553.29	398.435	2.729	2547.94	2558.63	784	3499
Total	28627	2560.32	402.610	2.380	2555.65	2564.98	784	3499

Test of Homogeneity of Variances

BMI (Body Mass Index)

LEVENE STATISTIC	DF1	DF2	SIG.
21.020	2	28624	< 0.001

ANOVA

BMI (Body Mass Index)

	SUM OF SQUARES	DF	MEAN SQUARE	F	SIG.
Between groups	7359095	2	3679547.455	22.734	< 0.001
Within groups	4.6E + 09	28624	161848.723		
Total	4.6E + 09	28626			

Robust Tests of Equality of Means

BMI (Body Mass Index)

	STATISTIC*	DF1	DF2	SIG.
Welch	20.185	2	5252.426	< 0.001
Brown-Forsythe	21.193	2	7405.673	< 0.001

* Asymptotically F distributed.

In the second table (Test of Homogeneity of Variances), the significant result (sig. less than 0.05) tells us that the variances (equal to the squares of the standard deviations) are not equivalent for the three perceived health status groups. For teaching purposes, we will confirm our ANOVA result with the nonparametric Kruskal-Wallis test, which has the less restrictive assumption of similarly shaped (rather than normal) distributions.

The third table gives us the ANOVA results. The significance value of less than 0.001 tells us that BMI differences are associated with perceived health status change. The Kruskal-Wallis test (results not shown) confirms that this significant outcome is not due to the violations of the assumptions as do the two correction formulae shown in the fourth table (Robust Tests of Equality of Means).

The final step in the ANOVA is to determine which groups differ. This determination involves a procedure called a **multiple comparisons test**, which essentially is a series of t-tests with some protection built into the significance values so that we are not so likely to find significance inappropriately when we compare combinations of groups. Applying two commonly used multiple comparisons procedures (Tukey and Student-Neuman-Keuls—output not shown) to this analysis demonstrated that the significant differences in the ANOVA lay between the group reporting a change in health for the worse and the other two groups. Perceived health status *did* impact BMI; subjects who perceived their health to have changed for the worse had higher BMIs than subjects who perceived that their health status had either not changed or improved.

The 95% confidence intervals for the three group means are displayed in the first table (Descriptives). These confidence intervals indicate, with a certain level of certainty, the range in which the true population group means lie. Consistent with our ANOVA outcome, note that the lower bound of the 95% CI for the "change for the worse" group overlaps the upper bound of neither the "change for the better" nor the "no change" group. Conversely, there is considerable overlap in the 95% CIs between the "change for the better" and the "no change" groups.

31. Summarize the types of conclusion errors.

The table at the top of the next page is based on the results of statistical testing (p-values relative to alpha, α) and the "true" situation in the population. There are four outcomes, two of which represent no error and two of which represent conclusion errors. Careful attention to research design and analysis helps to ensure that your results fall into the "no error" categories.

32. How do I determine whether my statistically significant ANOVA result is practically significant?

Looking at the means displayed in the first table of question 30 shows us that the group reporting worse health has a larger BMI, on average, than either of the other two groups. The difference is approximately 50, less than 5% of the group means. As before, this result indicates that the impact of perceived health status change on BMI was small.

NULL STATISTICAL HYPOTHESIS (<u>POPULATION</u>)

		true	false
NULL	true		type-II
STATISTICAL	$(p > \alpha)$	no error	error
HYPOTHESIS			
DECISION	false	type-I	
(<u>SAMPLE</u>)	$(p \le \alpha)$	error (α)	no error

33. Statistics is a complicated subject. Where do I obtain assistance?

Experienced researchers and statisticians can provide statistical assistance to beginners. There may be a statistics department at your local university or college, or your hospital may employ statisticians to help staff with research projects. It is important to have a statistician involved at the beginning of your research study to assist in the planning of the statistical analyses. Otherwise you may have a difficult time when you are ready to conduct the analysis.

BIBLIOGRAPHY

1. Munro B: Statistical Methods for Health Care Research, 3rd ed. Philadelphia, Lippincott, 2001.
2. Pett M: Nonparametric Statistics for Health Care Research: Statistics for Small Samples and Unusual Distributions. Thousand Oaks, CA, Sage Publications, 1997.
3. Rowntree D: Statistics Without Tears: A Primer for Non-mathematicians. New York, Charles Scribner's Sons, 1981.
4. Vogt WP: Dictionary of Statistics and Methodology, 2nd ed. Newbury Park, CA, Sage Publications, 1996.

23. QUALITATIVE DATA ANALYSIS

Joanne Gladden, RN, PhD, and Katharine C. Cook, RN, PhD

1. Discuss the relationship between the philosophical framework of qualitative research and data analysis.

The philosophy underlying a research study directs the interpretation of results and, therefore, is inextricably linked with data analysis. For example, in phenomenology, whether a researcher uses **bracketing** depends on the specific philosophical framework. Bracketing refers to setting aside personal beliefs, expectations, and what is known about the phenomenon under study. In Heideggerian phenomenology, beliefs and assumptions are explicitly stated, rather than bracketed and are a part of the critical analysis of the text. The philosophy underlying the study helps the researcher and the consumer of research understand how reality is defined, the unique values that guide the study analysis, and the overall context of the analysis procedure. The terminology of the analytic procedure is related to the philosophical framework. This terminology (also called jargon) can be challenging to define and keep straight!

2. What steps are generally used in the analysis of qualitative data?

Data generation and analysis are interrelated steps in any qualitative study. Data are collected after careful attention to appropriate sampling methods. All data generation measures rely heavily on researcher involvement. Analysis of data involves examining words, descriptions, and processes. Data are analyzed using a nonstatistical approach that is consistent with the research philosophy, question, and design.

Data are generated using a wide range of methods that may include interviews, observation, audio-video taping, photography, and primary and secondary sources such as official documents, texts, reports, and journals. Multiple methods of data collection and analysis may be used simultaneously, such as rereading and coding of transcript while watching a videotape to enhance appreciation of nonverbal communication. Multiple methods often facilitate deeper understanding of the meaning of the data.

An important aspect of analysis is to let the meanings of the text evolve and not rush to judgment. It takes patience to let the relationships among categories, participants, actions, and events emerge. Many types of qualitative studies use transcribed interview text that is systematically analyzed through a process of coding.

3. What is a code?

After arranging data into a format that you can analyze, you are likely to feel overwhelmed at the daunting task ahead. Assuming that you have read and reread each interview in its entirety, you are ready to reduce the data into codes. Codes are generally 1-to-4-word descriptions that capture the broad meaning of paragraphs (chunks) of data. As you organize the data into these preliminary abstractions, you begin to see common elements among the participants' remarks. For example, in Cook's study of adult offspring making care decisions for cognitively impaired parents, three of the codes identified were *defining condition*; *comparing with others*; and *guessing needs*.[1]

211

Defining condition included remarks from informants such as:
- "There is no rhyme or reason to it."
- "Some things occur that just don't make any sense."
- "They just can't process everything that is going on around them."
- "Now in hindsight I think it was something that was coming years ago."
- "I thought we were just dealing with a nasty person."

Comparing with others included such statements as:
- "Actually my story is probably easier than many."
- "My neighbor . . . well you ought to talk with her about care giving."
- "I think I'm so lucky and yet here I am whining to you because I have it better than so many people do that you are going to interview, I'm sure."

Guessing needs included such statements as:
- "It is difficult to tell what she is responding to."
- "I can't get inside her head to figure out what is best for her."
- "I liked the casualness of it. Since my mother was a country person I thought she would like that."

Note that the researcher was careful to use every day language to word the codes. Professional and theoretical language should be avoided because it can confuse rather than enlighten the reader's understanding of the phenomenon.

4. What are common coding pitfalls for the novice researcher?

At first blush, the novice tends to become overwhelmed and attempts to take some control of the data while worrying that something important is going to be overlooked. This concern leads to an initial tendency to "over-code" the data by trying to find meaning in every word and sentence. Since coding is one of the first steps in reducing the data, it is advisable and more accurate to take large pieces of text and understand them by concise everyday language.

One of the most frustrating aspects of coding is determining what to do with irrelevant data, which quickly clutter data analysis. Reduce the initial transcripts into paragraphs that are relevant to the question at hand, and delete the extraneous references that occur in every story. It is important, however, to submit random edited transcripts for peer review to determine that you have not deleted information with the potential to enhance understanding of the phenomenon.

Another pitfall for beginning researchers is trying to be too narrow and specific during the initial coding. This tendency inevitably results in codes that need to be merged at a later point. This mistake is not fatal—just time-consuming. For example, in Cook's study, individual codes identified specific feelings (e.g., anger, frustration, acceptance, guilt) that were eventually merged into the code "feelings."[1] Even this code was eventually dropped from the completed study.

Again, beware of premature closure of the codes. Experienced researchers may have a good feel for repetitions that are most likely to occur in future data (saturation), but beginners need to avoid narrowing the options at an early stage. Trust your instincts. If you feel that you are treating the data superficially by deciding codes too early, you probably are missing important understanding of the data.

5. What is a theme? How are themes and codes related?

As the researcher begins to live more and more inside the data (dwelling in the data), an understanding of what life is like for those who experience a certain phenomenon emerges. This process takes a long time. It almost seems that the researcher must devote the time and energy with heart, head, and gut to experience vicariously the phenomenon experienced by the collective whole. Needless to say, at this stage endless patience with oneself and the data is needed. The researcher finally takes the leap from looking at discrete individual experiences of the phenomenon to understanding the commonalities of the experience for a given group of informants. At this magical moment themes begin to emerge from the data.

Themes are groups of codes that unify into more abstract common denominators and the researcher moves from analysis to synthesis of the data. As codes are read and reviewed in the context of the whole, patterns begin to emerge that further illustrate the experiences of the informants themselves. These patterns are identified and illustrated by clusters of codes, which are given thematic names. For example, in Cook's study (after many attempts), one theme that emerged was **Finding a voice**, which included the codes of *Defining condition, Safety concerns, Role-reversion,* and *Feelings.*[1]

As the identification of themes begins, the researcher writes and rewrites ideas of how the data fall together, sometimes literally sketching impressions and seeking feedback from colleagues. For the beginner, the codes at first seem to fit into some identified schemata with which the researcher is familiar. For example, Cook initially saw a pattern that seemed similar to the grieving process. Although this pattern of feeling did exist in the data, it overlaid something much deeper, which eventually emerged as a decision-making process. This deeper theme would have been missed if the researcher had stopped at themes that felt familiar and comfortable.

6. How can software help my data analysis? Where do I find such programs?

Much debate surrounds the use of computer software in qualitative analysis.[2,3] In an analysis of focus group discussions, Fielding and Lee[2] found that the advantages and disadvantages of computer-assisted qualitative analysis software (CAQDAS) are neither clear nor unambiguous but rather lie in the eye of the beholder. The issue of how computer software affects qualitative research also needs to be reexamined in light of the research environment and, in particular, the type of qualitative research method used. Tesch,[4] however, maintains that "strictly speaking, there is no such thing as qualitative research. There are only qualitative data"[4] (p. 55). So the question becomes, how do computer software programs change researchers' interactions with qualitative data?

Data are more easily managed with the use of software programs. Some researchers simply use folders created on the desktop to keep together chunks of data that are coded similarly. The use of word search in some proprietary programs, such as Microsoft Word, can also help in identifying repeated areas under discussion by the informants. Other researchers find the use of software programs that are specifically designed for qualitative research data analysis, such as NUDIST and Atlas.ti, quite helpful for various tasks;

- Managing large quantities of data
- Quickly coding data with an opportunity to see the whole chunk of data with the original transcript
- Schematically drawing representations of how codes might form themes

The software is also helpful in forming an exact audit trail since the software is usually able to generate a report of when each step in the analysis process was taken. Look carefully and try free software demonstration packages of particular programs that you are considering for your analysis. Software can be easily found on the Internet by going to sites such as Scolari.com and the CAQDAS World Wide Web Page <http://soc.surrey.ac.uk/caqdas/>. An excellent overview of several CADQAS programs can be found in table format at <http://www.Quarc.de/body-overview.html/>. Comparisons of several aspects of different programs, such as data entry, coding, retrieval of coded segments, visualization, quantitative elements, and team-work capabilities can be found and easily understood.

Once the software is selected and purchased, practice data analysis with a few transcripts before using the program to manage and analyze larger databases. This step helps you to realize the full potential of the software without getting over-whelmed and to work out peculiarities of how data are imported into the software package from original transcripts. Some programs do not use proprietary word-processing programs, and the data must be transformed to a public format before you can read it in the qualitative analysis program.

7. Define reflexivity.

Reflexivity is the ability to understand self to the degree that one can recognize biases and preconceptions about the phenomenon at hand while being part of the data and "exploiting self-awareness as a source of insight"[5] (p. 75). Although this sounds like a contradiction, the researcher must both "not use self" and "use self" as a mechanism in data collection and analysis.

8. How does reflexivity influence data analysis?

Early in the process, as the research question is articulated, the researcher needs to determine his or her unique view of the phenomenon at hand. This view is usually written down before data collection begins. As the researcher pro-gresses to field work, choices are made during and after interviews about which roads to pursue and what remarks need further clarification and understanding. This process occurs spontaneously and somewhat intuitively while the researcher listens to informants and more formally when field notes are recorded after each interview.

Journaling immediately after the encounter with the informant helps researchers to reflect on their own reactions to the interviewee and what they may mean to the interpretation of the data. For example, Cook interviewed a respondent who elicited feelings of helplessness that were hard to shake after the interview was completed. These feelings were duly noted in the field notes. Further examination revealed the this informant tended to interact with her whole environment in the same way that she interacted with the researcher: continuously trying to define what was going on (*defining condition*) but refusing all avenues to make adjustments to her situation or dealing with the situation differently internally as other interviewees readily did (*correcting course*).

As Aamodt points out, "Transformation of the data from one level of analysis to another requires a similar sense of awareness and an intuitive sense of the whole of the data, as well as the context in which the abstractions will probably be placed"[6] (p. 49). You, as the researcher, are an integral part of the data. Be aware that your presence at the interview influences the respondents' answers. Personality, personal baggage, age, gender, and socioeconomic status are among the many variables that can influence responses.

9. How can I best ensure that my interpretation is valid?

Throughout data collection and analysis, researchers typically record personal reflections, observations, questions, ideas, hunches, and feelings. These vital steps help you to judge and interpret data and, ultimately, to construct meanings.

Qualitative researchers generally agree that there is no genuinely objective, authentic information from which only one correct interpretation can be made. Interpretation is based on the researcher's careful self-reflection and reflection about text content and context. Although multiple valid interpretations may occur (especially in the case of research teams), the findings must remain trustworthy in relation to the data.

A mechanism called **member checking** and a standard called **credibility** help to preserve the integrity of participants' statements. The researcher goes back to the participants during data analysis to determine whether the participants recognize the experience as their own.

10. What happens if, in member checking, participants deny having made a certain statement?

If there is disagreement between a participant and researcher on what was said or how it was interpreted, the area of discrepancy needs further exploration. Sometimes participants feel embarrassed about what they said or feel that they exposed too much personal information. What was said originally may be denied. It is the researcher's role (not always easy) to interpret the disparity and make a judgment about how to put the new information into context.

11. What does the term *data immersion* mean?

This term is used interchangeably with phrases such as dwelling with the data. It represents the process of gaining deeper and broader understanding and familiarity with the data as they are collected. It usually involves carefully reading and rereading transcripts, listening to audiotapes, viewing videotapes, and reflecting on field notes and experiences with participants. The researcher becomes "immersed" in multiple dimensions of the data and in the process discovers groupings or classes of things, persons, and events and their characteristics. As might be expected, immersion in the data can be associated with the feeling of being overwhelmed. Systematically reducing the volume of data by grouping and classifying makes data analysis more manageable.

An important process within the phenomenon of immersion is gaining insight. There is no special, scheduled time when this phenomenon occurs. Place note pads and a pen in strategic locations so that you can script your "out-of-nowhere" flashes of keen insight, reflections, and puzzles. Although you probably do not want to place a note pad and pen in the shower or bed, you will find that times of relaxation and openness often stimulate amazing (sometimes inopportune) moments of new awareness. Write them down as soon as they occur.

12. How can I improve my qualitative analysis skills?

Finding a mentor experienced in using the specific research methodology that you intend to use is vital. The mentor can help you determine early in the process whether the data analysis method under consideration is appropriate based on your overall research purpose and design. The mentor may provide helpful feedback on all aspects of your research. Becoming an active team member in a group research project with more experienced researchers can also expose you to excellent mentoring in a supportive, collaborative environment.

Analysis is a component of critical thinking that can be learned and improved through a disciplined, systematic approach to the unique work of the research project. Experienced qualitative researchers anticipate multiple realities, surprises, ambiguity, and nonlinear ways of thinking. Intuition is valued. Like any skill development, analytical skills are refined through practice and continuing education. Exposure to diverse qualitative research articles helps build understanding of many methods of analysis in distinct contexts. Become actively involved in qualitative research conferences and workshops, present your research to colleagues, and seek and be open to constructive critique.

13. Will I lose touch with my data if I use computer software for analysis or have someone else transcribe it?

Although these are separate questions, they are related. Data analysis can never be completely turned over by the researcher to anything or anyone. Losing touch with the data can sometimes happen when the time between data collection and analysis is long and memory becomes dulled, notes are superficial, and important contextual information is difficult to recall.

The researcher, from the outset, must give clear directions to the typist and proof transcripts for accuracy and completeness. General guidelines for the usual procedure for transcribing include directions for indicating pauses in speech, spacing, margins, paragraphs, and numbering of lines and pages.[7] Even an excellent transcriptionist may not be able to hear or understand what is being said on a tape. The researcher—not the transcriptionist—is responsible for putting participant statements in context (e.g., consideration of feelings, emphasis, nonverbal communication, setting) so that data can be interpreted with insight and clarity. However, more than one qualitative researcher has made an interesting comment about transcriptionists: "Transcriptionists sometime know before I do that data saturation has occurred. They become aware of significant repetition of ideas and statements." Many times they are right!

Use of computer and other technologies in recording, processing, storing, and sorting data should not diminish the role of the researcher in analysis and critical evaluation of data. Newer software, however, offer possibilities for actual analysis and integration of the data.[8] Appropriate research software can free the researcher to be more efficient and attentive to data analysis because it reduces time spent on tedious functions that do not require personal involvement during specific phases. It can increase the feasibility of collecting and successfully managing larger quantities of data, if that is a goal. Weitzman and Miles and others provide a critique of currently available software.[9]

14. What is voice recognition software? Is it useful in qualitative data analysis?

Voice recognition software are programs that train the computer to understand your voice as you speak into a microphone. The computer will "type" words on the screen once it recognizes your voice. Like many technologies, this approach has advantages and disadvantages. If you are a slow typist or do not have the resources to hire a transcriptionist, you may want to try this software. Be aware, however, that you cannot use it during interviews unless the computer learns the voices of each of your respondents. Since this process involves access to a high-powered computer and a significant time commitment for all involved, you may simply want to tape the interview and repeat it in your own voice into the computer microphone once you return home. Speech recognition software is steadily improving. The three main programs are Naturally Speaking by Dragon Direct, Voice Direct, and Via Voice by IBM. Many computer journals rate these programs in terms of accuracy, system requirements, integration with other software programs, ease of use and installation, and cost.

15. How can multiple researchers manage data analysis?

Qualitative analysis using multiple researchers is a challenge, but, in the final analysis, the diversity adds to the depth, breadth, and richness of the analysis. Some of the most significant problems arise if researchers participating in qualitative analysis become stuck in a quantitative paradigm or in their own private worldviews.

Because no single reality exists and interpretation of the same data by multiple researchers can vary, it is important that the approach to analysis be clear to all involved. The principal investigator is responsible for delineating the plan for analysis based on the study purpose and its unique philosophical foundation.

Frequently, each researcher codes and interprets data independently. Then the team comes together to share insights and findings. Codes and interpretations of the data are discussed, and a consensus is usually reached on the findings and their meanings. In the process of resolving differences, the interpretations can be the more holistic, complex, and more meaningful. The process of "coming together" requires regular, open communication in which the views of others are respected. In reporting research findings, areas of variances in interpretation are identified and discussed.

16. What is the role of culture broker in data analysis?

In a multicultural society, nursing research increasingly involves communicating with persons of different cultures. Culture is defined broadly to extend beyond ethnic and racial characteristics. Persons who are deaf, blind, and homeless—to name a few—often have world views that are unique and important to understand. In ethnographic research, understanding cultural phenomena is the goal. Interpretation of language, customs, and events requires the inclusion of a "culture broker" on the research team or contracting with someone competent to serve in that role. A culture broker serves to mediate, negotiate, and/or bridge the gap between the health care culture and the participant's (individual, family, or community) culture and can be vital to generating insights into cultural phenomena that otherwise may be missed or misinterpreted by the researcher.

17. What factors should be considered in selecting a culture broker?

Including a person from a particular culture to serve as a culture broker does not necessarily create more accurate data generation and analysis. A Korean who is fluent in the general language may not be equipped to translate or interpret medical information important to a particular study. Differences in dialect can be particularly challenging. Whenever possible, researchers studying a particular cultural phenomenon should be an integral member of that culture or well versed in it. In selecting a culture broker as a team member or consultant, it is useful to know whether he or she has served in that role previously, the nature of his or her experience with the culture, and his or her understanding of the culture *and* language. Ensuring confidentiality, assessing the person's standing and acceptability within the culture, and skill level are important issues to be considered. Understanding only words or spoken language does not necessarily equate with understanding the culture. Achieving an understanding of context is critical to data analysis.

Finding a reliable list of culture-brokers is helpful but not always easy. Resources for finding translators and interpreters, even in large cities, can be disappointing and frustrating. If a reliable culture broker cannot be found, it is better to exclude certain subgroups from the research sample than to generate and publish misinformation and faulty, biased interpretations. In any grant submitted to federal or state sources, how sampling is done and how cultural differences are dealt with become critical criteria for funding.

18. How is the term *rigor* used in qualitative research?

In quantitative research, rigor is defined in terms of precise adherence to a quantitative design and statistical rules with the perceived achievement of objective, generalizeable findings.[8] Qualitative research attempts to organize and structure subjective data and to elicit meaning from them. There are fewer (some may say that there are none) systematic "rules" for analyzing and presenting qualitative data, and it is harder to make the validity of findings patently clear.

Scientific rigor in qualitative and quantitative research is different but no less valued or conscientiously established by the researcher. Rigor represents the striving for excellence and the use of discipline and adherence to detail and accuracy.[9] Criticism about rigor in qualitative research has generally come from people who have not understood the differences in the outcomes of the two approaches and seek more assurance that the researcher accurately captured the thematic patterns in the data. Problems with rigor occur in both types of studies, although they are somewhat different. It is important for qualitative researchers to be aware of issues of rigor and to pay close attention to ensuring and documenting how it was achieved.

19. What standards can I use to evaluate rigor in my research?

Burns and Grove[9] provide an excellent listing of standards that can help guide the evaluation of rigor. The research design and specific philosophical framework of the study determine which threats to these standards are most likely.

- Standard I relates to **descriptive vividness**, which includes essential descriptive information, clarity, factual accuracy, credibility of the description, and reactions of the researcher. Descriptive vividness implies that the context of the study is clear and adequate.
- Standard II relates to **methodologic congruence**, which includes rigor in documentation, procedural adherence, ethics, and auditability. The researcher should present the elements or steps of the study accurately and clearly. Type, quality, and quantity of informants and overall data need to be sufficient, trustworthy, and credible. Informed consent and protection of human subjects are part of this standard. Creating decision rules, recording nature of decisions, and providing evidence for conclusions so that other researchers can arrive at similar conclusions are dimensions of auditability.

- Standard III relates to **analytical preciseness**. In qualitative research, concrete data are gradually transformed across several levels of abstraction. Although the process is somewhat difficult because of the intuitive nature of some reasoning,[9] the researcher should make efforts to identify and record the decision-making processes through which the transformations are made. Does the schema (pattern) developed by the researcher fit the data? Member checking or asking participants to provide feedback on the researcher's interpretation is one way to help ensure that statements correspond with the findings. Analytical preciseness also reflects the logical connections among categories, themes, or common elements to form a whole picture.
- Standard IV, **theoretical connectedness**, requires that the theoretical schema developed from the study be clearly expressed, logically consistent, reflective of the data, and compatible with the knowledge base of nursing.[9] Data need to validate the basis for identifying concepts, propositions, and conceptual map.
- Standard V, **heuristic relevance**, means that the researcher describes the results of the study clearly so that the reader is able to recognize the phenomenon described in the study, its relevance and applicability to nursing practice situations, and implications for future research.

Other schema for evaluating rigor in qualitative research are discussed in Chapter 6.

REFERENCES

1. Cook KC: "It's a Hard Place Not to Be": Making Care Decisions for Cognitively Impaired Parents. Poster Presentation at The Southern Nursing Research Society 16th Annual Conference, February 7, 2002, San Antonio, Texas.
2. Fielding NG, Lee RM: Computer Analysis and Qualitative Research. Newbury Park, CA, Sage, 1998.
3. Kelle U: Computer-aided Qualitative Data Analysis: Theory, Methods and Practice. London, Sage, 1995.
4. Tesch R: Qualitative Analysis: Analysis Types and Software Tools. London, Falmer Press, 1990.
5. Lipson JG: The use of self in ethnographic research. In Morse JM (ed): Qualitative Nursing Research: A Contemporary Dialogue. Newbury Park, CA, Sage, 1991, pp 73–91.
6. Aamodt AM: Ethnography and epistemology: Generating nursing knowledge. In Morse JM (ed): Qualitative Nursing Research: A Contemporary Dialogue. Newbury Park, CA, Sage, 1991, pp 40–53.
7. Morse JM, Field PA: Qualitative Research Methods for Health Professionals, 2nd ed. Thousand Oaks, CA, Sage, 1995.
8. Polit DF, Beck CT, Hungler BP: Essentials of Nursing Research: Methods, Appraisal, and Utilization, 5th ed. Philadelphia, Lippincott, 2001.
9. Burns N, Grove SK: The Practice of Nursing Research: Conduct, Critique and Utilization. Philadelphia, W.B. Saunders, 2001.

24. INTERPRETING RESEARCH OUTCOMES

Katherine R. Jones, RN, PhD, FAAN

1. What is meant by interpreting research outcomes?

In the simplest terms, one interprets the outcomes of a research project by assigning meaning to the information reported. After the statistical analysis is done, the results must be turned into knowledge that is useful to others and to nursing science in general. This goal is accomplished through interpretation. The results of the data analysis are carefully examined, organized in a systematic manner, and given meaning.[1,2] Analysis of the study findings takes into consideration the overall research aims, specific hypotheses, existing scientific knowledge base, and any methodologic limitations.[1] Both the statistical and the clinical significance of study findings are assessed and reported.

2. What skills are required to interpret research findings successfully?

When the researcher moves from data collection and analysis to interpretation, a greater amount of abstract thinking is required. It is a time for reflection, logical reasoning, sensitivity, and intuition. Interpretation also provides the investigators the opportunity to be creative, as they assign meaning to the various findings of the study. The process of interpretation requires the investigator to do the following:[2]
- Evaluate the research process used
- Produce meaning from the results
- Forecast the usefulness of the findings to others

More specifically, the researcher must examine the evidence, form conclusions, explore the significance of the findings, generalize the findings, and consider the implications for further research and practice. Interpreting research findings is challenging because it demands creativity, critical thinking, intellectual insights, and courage. Courage, according to Talbot,[3] is demonstrated when investigators go beyond and even challenge established explanations for reality, making themselves vulnerable to doubts and disdain from both peers and the larger scientific community.

3. What steps are involved in examining research evidence?

The investigator looks at all evidence that either supports or fails to support the validity of the research results.[2] There are several different components of this process.

1. The research plan is reviewed to ensure that the methods were consistent with the conceptual framework, that potentially confounding variables were adequately controlled, and that the sample was appropriate for testing the study hypotheses. Instruments are also examined for their reliability and validity.

2. The data collection process is analyzed to evaluate the representativeness of the sample, identify any measurement issues, and explore contextual variations that may have influenced the study findings. Contextual issues relate to changes in the internal or external environment that may have interfered with the intervention or outcomes measured.

3. The data analysis approaches are examined to assess data entry errors, extent of missing data, whether statistical assumptions have been violated, and whether the appropriate statistical tests have been performed. Problems in any of these areas may cause difficulties or make it impossible to interpret the research results.

4. What are research findings? How should they be presented?

Research findings are the end-result of evaluating the evidence. The investigator synthesizes the results of the analysis related to each research question or hypothesis. A more general statement about what has been found as a result of the analysis is made. For example, an analysis of variance (ANOVA) may show statistically significant differences in staff knowledge scores about pain management across nursing homes in different geographic locations. The findings may be reported as follows: "Staff in rural nursing homes were more knowledgeable than staff in urban nursing homes on current pain management practices, especially pharmacologic approaches." Research findings can be presented in both narrative and graphic formats. Graphic formats such as tables or figures can present a great deal of information in a concise manner and can be used to support the narrative report. The investigator should make sure that information provided in the narrative and supporting tables is consistent.

5. What are research conclusions?

Conclusions are derived from a synthesis of the findings of a study. The researcher creates a meaningful message from the many pieces of information gained from the findings from this and previous related studies.[2] The researcher needs to maintain objectivity while generating the conclusions, trying to avoid bias and misinterpretation. It is preferable that the investigator be somewhat conservative in drawing conclusions and consider alternative explanations for the findings.[1] Conclusions may either support or fail to support (refute) the expectations of the researcher. It is important to remember that research never *proves* that an expected relationship between or among variables exists. However, multiple, well-controlled studies that report similar findings provide strong evidence for an expected relationship.

6. How should the interpretation of research outcomes be organized?

Talbot[3] has identified five steps for systematically interpreting study findings (see figure, top of next page):

7. How can the investigator organize the data in a coherent and consistent manner?

First, the investigator needs to examine the sample and population characteristics and identify any between-group differences. Then, the researcher should search for covariates (other variables that change in relation to the dependent variable). In addition, the investigator needs to evaluate the consistency of the intervention—was the intervention carried out in the same way across all settings and time periods? This concept is also referred to as the fidelity of the intervention.

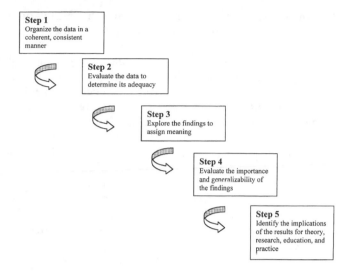

Step 1
Organize the data in a coherent, consistent manner

Step 2
Evaluate the data to determine its adequacy

Step 3
Explore the findings to assign meaning

Step 4
Evaluate the importance and generalizability of the findings

Step 5
Identify the implications of the results for theory, research, education, and practice

8. How do you know that your data are adequate for analysis and interpretation?
Ask yourself the following questions:
- Usable data: What is the extent of missing data, illegible responses, incomplete records or notes?
- Coding and data entry accuracy: Has data integrity been maintained? Was a double-entry method used?
- Psychometric testing of data collection instruments: Have reliability (test-retest, interrater, internal consistency) and validity (concurrent, discriminant, predictive) been established as appropriate?
- Do the instruments adequately measure the phenomenon of interest, and are they appropriate for the sample? Were better instruments available?

9. How do you assign meaning to the findings?
The researcher first needs to explore all statistically significant findings by comparing and contrasting the findings with existing or emerging theory. Searching for patterns in the findings by displaying the data on graphs may reveal important relationships.

10. How does the researcher know that the findings are important and can be generalized to other populations?
- Evaluate both the statistical and clinical significance.
- Ask yourself "So what?" and "Who Cares?"
- Assess power and error, including the possible occurrence of type I and type II errors. Type I errors occur when the null hypothesis (there is no difference) is rejected when it should have been accepted. Type II errors occur when the null hypothesis is accepted when it should have been rejected.
- Explore the cost and quality implications of the findings. How feasible is it to adopt the more effective intervention? Do the quality gains justify the incremental cost?
- Examine generalizibility and possible sampling bias. Is the sample representative of the target population? Are there crucial variables omitted from the study that might make a difference in the findings and recommendations?

11. How does the researcher go about identifying the implications of the results of a study for theory, research, education, and practice?

Ask the following questions:

- **Theory**. Is current theory supported or contradicted by the findings? Has scientific knowledge been expanded—in what ways? Were inconsistencies in the theoretical framework uncovered? Can new theoretical linkages be established?
- **Research**. How do the findings add to the existing knowledge base? Have measurement techniques been improved? Should the intervention be further developed for application in additional populations or settings?
- **Education**. Should changes be made in the substance or process of nursing or medical education? Are there implications for patient education?
- **Practice**. How should the results be translated into clinical practice? How should system policies or structures be altered as a result of the findings? Should the findings be incorporated into clinical practice guidelines? Should existing clinical practice guidelines or care protocols be updated to reflect the new knowledge?

12. What outcomes are possible when a researcher examines the results of a study?

According to Burns and Grove,[2] five outcomes are possible:

- The investigator may find significant results that are consistent with the predictions. The research findings support the expected links between the conceptual framework and research questions. However, as pointed out previously, such a finding does not prove causation—it simply supports the possible existence of such a relationship. The investigator should also consider alternative, plausible explanations.
- The investigator may find nonsignificant results; the study fails to show a difference or effect. In this case, the investigator needs to review the entire study for possible flaws in methodology or lack of power to detect statistical differences. Nonsignificant results may indicate the failure to detect relationships rather than the true absence of such relationships or suggest shortcomings in the conceptual or theoretical framework that guided the selection of study variables.[1]
- The investigator may find significant results that are opposite to the predictions. Such findings should be verified with additional studies as well as compared with findings of other studies. Data collection processes and analysis procedures should be reexamined.
- The investigator may find mixed results, which may reflect reliability or sensitivity issues and suggest the need to alter or modify the existing theory.
- The investigator may find unexpected results, which are useful in theory development or refinement.

13. How are the results of qualitative studies evaluated?

When the outcomes of qualitative studies are interpreted, a different set of questions needs to be asked. First, the trustworthiness of the study needs to be established. To be judged trustworthy, four objectives must be attained[3]:

- **Credibility** is similar to validity and means that the investigator has developed believable interpretations and conclusions based on the data analysis. Credibility can be established by comparing the data with data obtained from other sources (triangulation); having colleagues explore and clarify the investigator's interpretations to reveal potential biases; searching for disconfirming evidence; and returning to the study participants to validate and verify the investigator's conclusions and interpretations.

- **Transferability** refers to judgment by a noninvolved investigator that the findings are applicable to another setting or context.
- **Dependability** means that a noninvolved investigator can logically follow the processes and procedures used in the study.
- **Confirmability** means that the findings, conclusions, and recommendations are supported by the data and that there is internal agreement between the interpretations and the actual evidence.

A second set of questions relate to the quality of the study itself: the strength of its linkages with a theoretical framework, the authenticity of the study, its intellectual rigor, and its utility to the profession.

14. Why do journal editors require authors to identify the implications of their research findings?

Editors are interested in publishing studies that provide direction to clinicians, educators, managers, other researchers, and policymakers and administrators. The study findings may suggest the need to change system or organizational policies, institutional processes or structures, and/or clinical practices to improve patient outcomes. The findings may reflect content that needs to be updated or emphasized in nursing school curricula or staff development programs. Perhaps most importantly, the results identify areas requiring further study or logical next steps in this area of scholarly inquiry, thus facilitating the building and strengthening of nursing science.

15. How are future research projects identified?

Each study that is completed should culminate in recommendations for future research studies that build on the current study and related studies focused on the same research questions.[2] A good place for a new researcher to start is to replicate the current study or to extend the study to a new sample. For example, the transitional care model originally tested by Brooten[4] and her research team for very-low-birth-weight infants was extended to both maternity and geriatric patients in subsequent studies. The new study should incorporate the lessons learned in the original study to improve the methods and analytic techniques and pay particular attention to the limitations described in the original study. For example, the timing of the outcome measure may be altered to better capture the effect of the intervention. Or different procedures may be developed to better ensure the fidelity (integrity) of the intervention. Before replicating the study it may be wise to contact the original researchers, who are usually more than happy to discuss their projects.

Another way to identify future research studies is to find a gap between desired performance levels or outcomes and achieved levels. Benchmarking your institution's outcomes against those of comparable institutions is one way to identify such performance gaps. For example, a higher-than-average incidence of medication errors or patient falls may lead to a study to discover the processes most responsible for these outcomes or to a study of a particular intervention to reduce the incidence of adverse occurrences. Observations by unit staff that a particular problem seems to be occurring with increasing frequency, such as wound infections, may lead to a study to determine care delivery structures or processes associated with this problem. Nurse researchers who are beginning a program of research may want to visit the websites of federal agencies (National Institutes for Health [NIH], Agency for Healthcare Research and Quality [AHRQ], Health Resources and Services Administration [HRSA]) or foundations (Robert Wood Johnson [RWJ], Kellogg, Commonwealth) that support research projects in their areas of interest or to subscribe to a service that sends automatic alerts of program announcements and requests for proposals or applications in specific topic areas. Review of the current funding priorities is helpful, as is examining the list of studies currently funded by a particular agency. Many program announcements provide lists of research questions that have been identified by agency officials and advisory panels as having high importance to advance the state of the science in that area.

16. What are study limitations? Why should they be reported?

It is not possible to design the "perfect" study. Weaknesses in sampling, measurement, and analysis may occur. For example, it may not be feasible to include a large number of facilities in a sample because of budgetary constraints, which may limit the types of statistical analyses that can be performed. Or a study may include an overrepresentation of Caucasians so that the results cannot be generalized to the entire population. It is also possible that the timing of follow-up data collection may be inappropriate, and take place before or after the phenomenon of interest actually occurs. Other problems may relate to inconsistent application of the intervention due to inadequate training of the interveners, nonadherence by subjects, environmental changes, or other issues. Poor response rates, high dropout rates, and extensive missing data should also be reported in the limitations section. The strength of the conclusions may be substantially reduced if the limitations are considered serious. In addition, the researcher may "overdraw" conclusions, meaning that the conclusions go beyond what the data actually support.[2] Results should not be generalized beyond the study sample, particularly if the sample was not randomized. Study limitations should be reported so that other researchers may learn from and go beyond them in designing future research studies.

17. How do I know if the study findings are significant?

Most researchers think that their study findings are important. However, there are more objective means for assessing the significance of research results. The most common approach to determining the significance of study findings is from a statistical perspective. This quantitative analysis uses specific statistical tests to determine that the results are unlikely to be due to chance. If not likely to be due to chance, the results are deemed to be significant. However, findings that achieve statistical significance may not be clinically significant or of value to nurses or the community. Alternatively, a clinically significant change or difference may not achieve statistical significance but be important to patient care. It is therefore important to pay attention to the numerical values obtained in the analysis as well as the significance levels in assessing the implications of the findings. A third type of significance is the study's practical significance—that is, its importance to the profession's body of knowledge. Studies with the greatest practical significance are the benchmarks for the discipline. One can judge the practical significance of a study by examining the number of times it has been cited by other researchers. Studies that have served as such benchmarks include the study by Brooten et al.[4] of transitional care for low-birth-weight infants and the study by Aiken et al.[5] of magnet hospitals and mortality rates.

18. What resources are available to help me interpret research findings if I am new to research?

Classes on research utilization and evidence-based practice may be available through the institution's staff development program or from a nearby school of nursing. A nursing research journal club also may be helpful and can invite local experts to lead discussions focused on specific research reports. The Internet can be accessed to locate evidence-reports related to specific clinical interventions and treatments. A formal mentorship program may be established so that experienced investigators can guide novice researchers through the process of interpretation.

19. How do I translate research findings into practice?

One of the major challenges is to apply knowledge, derived from research, to routine clinical practice. To improve the quality of health care service delivery, existing research findings must be translated for health care organizations in such a way that they can be integrated into their routine structures and processes.[6] These quality improvement efforts themselves should be grounded in sound evidence. The "quality" of the evidence supporting research translation strategies can range from high (generated from randomized clinical trials [RCTs]) to low (generated by expert opinion or expert panels). Effective strategies for achieving clinical practice changes include reminder systems, face-to-face education outreach visits (academic detailing), involvement of peer-recognized local opinion leaders, patient-mediated interventions, and combinations of these interventions.[7] Researchers trying to persuade health care providers to change their clinical practice can use one of the following frameworks to guide their choice of intervention:[7]

- Epidemiologic: people make decisions in a rational manner.
- Educational: people have an intrinsic motivation to improve performance.
- Marketing: people respond to attractive, targeted messages.
- Behavioral: people respond to external influences such as feedback, reminder systems, and incentives.

No one method is superior. The selected approach must be appropriate for the specific setting and group. For example, to achieve incorporation of the latest pain management strategies into clinical practice, investigators may want to consider development of an intervention strategy that includes chart audits and feedback to staff about levels of pain being assessed and appropriateness of pain medications being used (a behavioral approach). They also may want to identify key clinicians (physicians, nurses, pharmacists) who are respected by their peers and willing to serve as change agents. However, before embarking on any initiative to improve clinical processes in a health care organization, it is important to understand the organization's readiness to change and its ability to use new knowledge. It takes time for an innovation to be diffused and adapted into practice.

20. How is organizational readiness to change and adopt new research-based practices assessed?

Organizational Readiness

CATEGORY	QUESTION
Ability or capacity to change	Are staff and other resources sufficient to support the change?
Compatibility of the proposed change with the value system of the organization and its staff	Is the change consistent with the organization's mission and culture?
Relevant information about the change being suggested	Is it credible? How strong is the evidence supporting the change?
Current circumstances that support or undermine the change	Is there a significant staffing shortage? Does the leadership support the change?
Timing of the change	Are other major initiatives also taking place that will compete for attention and resources?
The obligation required by the change	What level of commitment (time, money, personnel) is required to adopt the change?
Resistance and inhibiting factors	Does the change affect any contractual relationships, such as with unions or contractors?
The yield, reward or perceived payoff	Will there be measurable improvements in patient coutcomes or satisfaction? Will the workload become heavier with little or no observable change in patient outcomes?

From Borbas C: Translating research into practice [unpublished paper]. St. Paul, MN, Healthcare Education and Research Foundation, 2002.

21. What other sources of information about research evidence are available?

The emphasis in health care is now on evidence-based clinical and managerial practice. One aspect of this emphasis requires keeping abreast of current research findings. Several mechanisms are available to assist both clinicians and researchers. The Agency for Healthcare Research and Quality (AHRQ) website contains links to the National Guidelines Clearinghouse and evidence reports issued by AHRQ-funded evidence-based practice centers. In addition, the Cochrane Collaborative issues the results of meta-analyses of research findings for specific treatments and conditions. Membership on relevant list-serves sponsored by private sector and public agencies facilitates keeping up to date as well as provides the opportunity for dialogue with other professionals who face the same or similar challenges.

22. Can the results and recommendations of a published research study always be trusted?

Unfortunately, some investigators are not entirely truthful in the publication of research findings. This problem may occur when the investigator has a proprietary interest in a particular product or device or when the investigator receives financial support from a company whose drug, device, or product is evaluated or tested in the study. This support can come in the form of dollars to support the research, consulting fees, speaker's bureau fees, seats on boards of directors, and/or stock ownership. Many are concerned about the influence that such arrangements can have on the objective reporting of research findings, especially if the results are not favorable to the company's product. Many journal editors have taken steps to make sure that any financial arrangements between an investigator and a private company that stands to benefit from the findings of a study are fully disclosed. The consumer of research literature should examine the publisher's policies about disclosure of potential conflicts of interest and note whether such relationships are revealed in the published articles.

REFERENCES

1. Polit D, Hungler B: Nursing Research: Principles and Methods, 5th ed. Philadelphia, J.B. Lippincott, 1995.
2. Burns N, Grove SK: The Practice of Nursing Research: Conduct, Critique, and Utilization, 3rd ed. Philadelphia, W.B. Saunders, 1997.
3. Talbot LA: Principles and Practice of Nursing Research. St. Louis, Mosby, 1995.
4. Brooten D, Kumar S, Butts P, et al: A randomized clinical trial of early hospital discharge and home follow-up of very low birthweight infants. N Engl J Med 315:934–939, 1986.
5. Aiken LH, Smith HL, Lake ET: Lower medicare mortality among a set of hospitals known for good nursing care. Med Care 32:771–787, 1994.
6. Dickinson E: Clinical effectiveness for health care quality improvement. JCAHO J Qual Improve 18:37–46, 1998.
7. Berman S: Measuring and improving the quality of care in health plans. JCAHO J Qual Improve 25:434–439, 1999.
8. Strom KL: Quality improvement interventions: What works? J Healthcare Qual 23:4–14, 2001.
9. Borbas C: Translating research into practice [unpublished paper]. St. Paul, MN, Healthcare Education and Research Foundation, 2002.

V. Communicating the Findings

25. RESEARCH ETIQUETTE

Regina M. Fink, RN, PhD, FAAN, AOCN, and Kathleen S. Oman, RN, PhD

1. Why is it important to talk about research etiquette?

As more nurses become involved in research, there has been an increase in the dissemination of research findings. Nurses who decide to write for publication must adhere to ethical principles in writing and publishing, paying close attention to proper etiquette procedures.[1] Understanding the strategies that have been developed to prevent ethical violations enhances the integrity of the publication and assures readers that the information is accurate and trustworthy.

2. What specific criteria are used for determining authorship of a publication once the research study has been completed?

A group of editors, also known as the Vancouver Group,[2] developed guidelines for authorship, entitled *Uniform Requirements for Manuscripts Submitted to Biomedical Journals*, stating that an author must make substantial contributions in the following three areas:
- Formulation of the research question, input into the design and analysis
- Development of a draft or revision of a manuscript
- Approval of the final manuscript prior to publication ensuring accuracy

All authors of a publication should be able to understand and critically discuss all aspects of the research study. Huth[3] suggests that legitimate authors must be able to take responsibility for the content in the paper and should be able to defend the paper under public or professional scrutiny. All authors should be able to verify their participation in the research process by providing documentation of attendance at research meetings, assistance with data management, and participation in writing drafts of manuscripts.

3. In this age of large research groups with the potential for multiple authors, should the Vancouver Group's requirements still apply?

The Vancouver recommendations still apply. However, some researchers suggest that authors publicly define their contributions to the project so that the reader can critically evaluate the merit of their authorship.[4,5] Many journal editors require authors to define their roles and contributions to the study at the time of manuscript submission.

4. What is the difference between an author and a contributor?

Traditionally, a contributor provides technical or intellectual support, but his or her contributions have not met the criteria for authorship as outlined above.[6] Examples of contributors include data collectors, statistical consultants, persons enrolling subjects, and data managers. A contributor may qualify as an author when he or she has collected or analyzed all of the data or provided some other significant contribution to the research study.

5. How are contributors acknowledged in a publication?

It is customary to list contributors in an acknowledgment at the end of the paper. Written permission from contributors mentioned in acknowledgements should be obtained before publication. This step is critical for the following reasons:

- Acknowledgement may imply endorsement of the project.
- Contributors may not want to be associated with the study.
- Acknowledgement of a prestigious contributor may not be warranted.
- Verification of an article's accuracy and content must be ensured.

6. If numerous investigators are involved in a research study, how do you decide who is the first author?

The first author is usually the person who has the strongest commitment and investment in the research project (the person who does the most work). The decision of authorship should be made early in the manuscript-writing process by all involved.

7. What are the responsibilities of the first author?

The first author usually organizes the preparation of the manuscript, which includes making writing assignments, editing the final draft into a cohesive manuscript, acquiring permissions, coordinating references, and communicating with the publication's editor.

8. What is the role of coauthors? How are they ordered in the manuscript?

Coauthors need to participate actively by writing a portion of the manuscript. The level of commitment and contribution determines the order of authorship. Coauthors are not alphabetically ordered, nor are seniority and credentials a deciding factor. The coauthors should collectively decide on the order of authorship before the first draft of the manuscript. The final decision should be communicated to the group in writing so that there is no misunderstanding.

9. Is the principal investigator always the first author?

No. The principal investigator is responsible for the development and implementation of the research study but may be peripherally involved in the actual writing of the manuscript. This point should always be negotiated before manuscript preparation.

10. When should you define roles and responsibilities of the research team?

As in the case of defining authorship, roles and responsibilities should be delineated early in the research process, mutually agreed on by all involved, and documented.

11. What is the relationship of the statistician to the research team?

It depends on the statistician's wants or desires. Some statisticians like to be listed as a contributing or co-primary author and should have that distinction if they meet the suggested criteria for authorship as listed in question 2. Others are happy to be listed in an acknowledgment for their contribution to the research study.

12. What do you do if the research team disagrees on authorship order?

It may be necessary to involve an objective mediator who understands the ins and outs of publication to help the group reach consensus. Making authorship decisions early in the research/manuscript writing process can help prevent misunderstandings about roles and clarify individual responsibilities. A written contract may be necessary to delineate the roles and responsibilities of all authors and contributors.

13. What is a research collaborators' contract?

It is a written contract (Appendix A) that formalizes an agreement among researchers about their roles, rights, and responsibilities as members of a research team. Developed by three members of the University of Colorado Health Science Center School of Nursing faculty,[7] it has been successfully used in hospitals both regionally and nationally. It has been effective both in influencing the progress of research being conducted and in ensuring appropriate recognition of all members of the research team.

14. How is the research collaborators' worksheet used?

Early in the research effort, researchers use the definition of research elements on the worksheet to assign the percentage that each collaborator has contributed to the project. At regular intervals the agreed on worksheet is reviewed and revised as necessary to ensure that researchers are fulfilling their responsibilities and adhering to the proposed timeline. Ultimately, the worksheet is used to determine authorship and other recognition in the dissemination of findings.

15. Why is something like the research collaborators' worksheet needed?

The worksheet may be helpful in clarifying and specifying roles, responsibilities, and accountability of all members of the research team. As with any team effort, clarity of roles is essential if the project is to be completed. In addition to defining responsibilities, the worksheet can protect the rights of individual researchers. For instance, if a clinical nurse identifies the research problem and invites a nurse researcher/faculty member to consult or to become a member of the research team, the contract can ensure that the contributions of the clinical nurse are recognized and maintained.

16. What should be done when a coinvestigator who assists with the start of a research study relocates or someone joins the project at a later time?

At times health care professionals may make employment changes during the course of a research study. When this occurs, it is important to discuss the individual's desire to remain connected to the project. If it is not feasible for the contributor to participate in the project, a consensus needs to be reached on what, if any, acknowledgment will be given for his or her contribution. Similar discussions need to take place when health care professionals join a project already in progress.

17. What should you do when you have assisted with a research study and receive no acknowledgment of your help in the manuscript?

This problem should never happen if an open discussion about roles and responsibilities has taken place at the beginning of a research project. If a contributor has been mistakenly omitted from an acknowledgment at the end of a journal article, it is possible for the journal to publish an erratum with the correct information in a subsequent issue. Therefore, it is important to bring this error to the attention of the first author.

18. If a colleague critiques your manuscript in preparation for publication, should he or she be listed as an author?

Critique does not mean authorship. If a colleague critiques a manuscript for you at your request, this is usually considered a kind professional gesture and does not require acknowledgment.

19. How are acknowledgments noted in a manuscript?

Typically acknowledgments are included as a separate paragraph at the conclusion of the manuscript and before the references. Acknowledgments should specifically address each individual's contribution to the research project, which may include the following:
• Data collection
• Statistical analysis
• Technical consultation (e.g., writing the proposal, instrument testing, pilot study)
• Intellectual inspiration
• Emotional or financial support
• Manuscript preparation

20. Can more than one article be written about the results of a particular research study?

Duplicate or fragmented publication of the same information or research, otherwise known as salami publishing, is considered irresponsible authorship[8] (see Chapter 27). Multiple articles containing the same content in different journals build up an author's biography, inflate the amount of research work done on the topic, and impede the publication of new material by wasting space in multiple journals. Sometimes journal editors are not even aware of concurrent or prior publication of similar material. Authors have an ethical responsibility to notify editors of both journals. The International Committee of Medical Journal Editors[2] suggests that the following conditions should be met:
• Both editors should be knowledgeable about the duplicate publication.
• The primary journal publishes the article first; the second paper is published with a different audience in mind.
• The second version of the article accurately reflects the primary article.
• A footnote tells readers of the secondary paper of the existence of a primary publication.

21. How do you negotiate the roles when an experienced faculty researcher works with an inexperienced or novice nurse who had the idea for the research study?

It is vital that nurses new to research have a mentor available for instruction, supervision, and guidance throughout the research process to ensure high standards and rigor in research. At times, it is difficult for experienced nurses and nursing faculty to have time for this mentorship process. Development of a research team can allow sharing of workload and use of multiple resources in the research process. Although there is pressure to publish among nurse researchers and nurse faculty as evidence of scholarly productivity, it is important that those who do the work receive appropriate credit and acknowledgment.

22. What is plagiarism? How do you avoid it?

Plagiarism is defined as presenting another's work as one's own.[9] Plagiarism can be avoided by referencing the author and publication information when someone else's work or ideas are presented. Sometimes it is not easy to determine what is another's work or intellectual property (ideas). One may not remember that an idea originated from another source, and it is hard to separate what may be the influence of thought from the plagiarism of ideas. Another practical matter concerns defining when an idea or information becomes general knowledge. Winkler and McCuen[10] state that a piece of information that appears in five or more sources may be considered general knowledge.

Self-plagiarism is possible when an author copies his or her own work, published in another publication, without permission.[/] Self-plagiarism can be avoided by obtaining written permission to use copyrighted material. A copyright is a property right. Copyright laws that protect an author's work from being used without permission protect published materials. Written permission is needed to reproduce material that has a copyright and is obtained from the publisher.

APPENDIX A

Research Collaborators' Worksheet   ©Stoner, Pepper, Keefe, 1987

StudyTitle _____   _____
COMIRB #_____ **Date**_____ **Initial**_____ **Review** _____ **Final**___

<u>Collaborators</u>
1._____ _____
2._____ _____
3._____ _____
4._____ _____

Elements of Research	**Collaborators' Contributions (%)**			
1. Research Idea	1.	2.	3.	4.
2. Review/Critique of Literature	1.	2.	3.	4.
3. Methodology/Design	1.	2.	3.	4.
4. Procedures/Instruments	1.	2.	3.	4.
5. Proposal Writing/COMIRB/HRRC	1.	2.	3.	4.
6. Pilot Study	1.	2.	3.	4.

7. Clinical Access/Subject Recruitment	1.	2.	3.	4.
8. Data Collection	1.	2.	3.	4.
9. Data Analysis	1.	2.	3.	4.
10. Manuscript/Poster Preparation	1.	2.	3.	4.

Options for Dissemination

Presentation/Poster	Percentage (%)	Publication
1. Co-presenters (alternate alphabetical order)	50/50	Co-authors (research/clinical journal)
2. Primary and Secondary		Primary and Secondary
3. Acknowledgement	85/15	Footnote

Definition of Research Elements

1. **Research Idea**—Specify an innovation or intervention; recognize patterns in a phenomenon; identify clinical problem or issue; delimit the problem; assess feasibility of study of the problem.

2. **Review and Critique of Literature**—Locate, read, organize, critique and synthesize previous literature; identify theoretical/conceptual model for study; specify the implications of prior research for the study design.

3. **Methodology/Design**—Refine the question; designate major variables; develop predictions about relationships of variables; formulate hypotheses; select the type of design; specify techniques for control of extraneous variables; formulate the sampling plan including sample size.

4. **Procedures/Instruments**—Operationalize variables; locate potential tools or techniques for data collection; select instrument to fit question and design; obtain author permission to use instruments; assess established reliability and validity and/or specify techniques to assess psychometric properties; prescribe research protocol including inclusion/exclusion criteria, order of data collection, and other technical details.

5. **Proposal Writing/COMIRB/HRRC Application**—Formulate the text, critique drafts; revisions; establish budget, timeline and consent form; compile supporting material and appendices; complete appropriate COMIRB and HRRC forms and submit paperwork for study approval.

6. **Pilot Study**—Collect data; analyze and write results; revise proposal as indicated; train research assistants and data collectors.

7. **Clinical Access/Subject Recruitment**—Secure entry into system and obtain institutional approvals; locate appropriate population; publicize study; orient managers and staff; secure necessary space and equipment; arrange for modification of routines; obtain informed consent; advise other health care professionals; serve as contact or liaison for staff, family and subjects.

8. **Data Collection**—Gather and record data.

9. **Data Analysis**—Organize; summarize; code; clean; enter data; select and calculate statistics; interpret results; make inferences; explain results.

10. **Manuscript/Poster Preparation**—Formulate texts, figures, charts; plan visual displays (PowerPoint, slides, poster), construct displays.

Use of Worksheet/Contract

Place initial of responsible person above each task in list of definitions. Assign percentage responsibility for each element. Average the responsibility over all elements. Assign credit according to average responsibility for the study. At any level of authorship, as opposed to footnote acknowledgement, the author should be able to defend the study and explain his/her contribution within the context of the entire study.

REFERENCES

1. King CR: Ethical issues in writing and publishing. Clin J Oncol Nurs 5(Suppl 3):19–23, 2001.
2. International Committee of Medical Journal Editors: Uniform requirements for manuscripts submitted to biomedical journals. JAMA 277:927–934, 1997.
3. Huth EJ: Preparing to write. In How to Write and Publish Papers in the Medical Sciences, 2nd ed. Baltimore, Williams & Wilkins, 1990, pp 43–54.
4. Rennie D, Yank V, Emanuel L: When authorship fails: A proposal to make contributors accountable JAMA 278:579–585, 1997.
5. Smith R: Authorship: Time for a paradigm shift. Br Med J 314:1009, 1997.
6. Duncan A: Authorship, dissemination of research findings, and related matters. Appl Nurs Res 12:101–106, 1999.
7. Stoner M, Keefe M, Pepper G University of Colorado Health Sciences Center School of Nursing, 1987.
8. Blancett SS: The ethics of writing and publishing. JONA 1:31–36, 1991.
9. Clark AJ: Responsible dissemination of scholarly work. J Neurosci Nurs 25:113–117, 1993.
10. Winkler AC, McCuen JR: Writing the Research Paper: A Handbook, 3rd ed. Philadelphia, Harcourt, Brace, Jovanovich, 1985.

BIBLIOGRAPHY

Wilcox L: Authorship: The coin of the realm, the source of complaints. JAMA 280:216–221, 1998.

26. WRITING A RESEARCH ABSTRACT

Regina M. Fink, RN, PhD, FAAN, AOCN, Kathleen S. Oman, RN, PhD, and Mary E. Krugman, RN, PhD

1. What is a research abstract?

A research abstract is a brief report that communicates essential elements of a research project.[1] The abstract often precedes a published article and provides a summary of the research project, alerting the reader to the relevancy of the study. Sometimes a research abstract may be written in response to a call for abstracts for a research conference. A research abstract highlights the research report and helps to provide a framework for reading the body of the text.[2] Writing a research abstract is the first step in communicating research.

2. How long are research abstracts?

The length and content of the abstract depends on the group to whom you are presenting your study. Research symposium planning committees publish a call for abstracts in flyers, newsletters, journals, and professional mailings approximately 6–9 months before a research conference. The instructions for abstracts specify the format, length, line spacing, font, and margins. Abstracts are usually 1 page ($8\frac{1}{2} \times 11$) in length, 100–250 words, using 10 or 12 Times New Roman font, single-spaced.

3. How should I structure an abstract?

Many calls request structured abstracts in which the elements of the research project are included as headings in the abstract. The following headings are frequently used:

- Title
- Author and affiliation
- Introduction/background
- Purpose of the study
- Methods/data analysis
- Results/outcomes
- Clinical implications

4. What content is typically included in each element of an abstract?

- **Title**: Titles for abstracts should reflect the study and promote an interest in reading the abstract.
- **Introduction/background**: Begin with a background sentence stating the scope or nature of the problem addressed in your research. This is the rationale supporting the need for the study. The importance of the study should be emphasized, and a theoretical or conceptual framework should be included if applicable.
- **Purpose of the study**: Clearly state the objectives of your study, including the study purpose, specific aims, research question, or hypothesis.
- **Methods/data analysis**: Describe how your study was implemented. State the general design of the study, describe the study setting, and include the procedures for sample selection (inclusion and exclusion criteria). Briefly outline the study procedure and describe the interventions. Instruments or tools used

in the research study should be described using reliability and validity information. Define your variables and measurements used. Discuss which data analytic procedures were used, including statistical tests.

- **Results/outcomes**: Present the specific data that addresses your research question or study purpose. Include statistical results and significance.
- **Clinical implications**: State reasoned conclusions with implications for clinical practice, education, and research. These conclusions are based on the significance of your data and findings.

5. Do you have any helpful hints for writing an abstract?
- Abstracts should be clear, logical, and grammatically correct.
- Make each sentence brief but maximally informative.
- Define abbreviations and unique terms.
- Use verbs and active voice rather than nouns and passive voice.
- Describe results and clinical implications in the present tense.
- Adhere to the suggested guidelines in the call for abstracts.

6. Describe the usual procedure for abstract submission.
Abstracts are submitted with a cover letter that includes the abstract title, authors, affiliation, correspondent, and whether you prefer to present by poster or podium. All authors' names and titles are usually removed from the submitted abstract to allow a blinded review. Abstracts can be submitted on a diskette with hard copy attached. Some professional organizations have their call for abstracts on their website with electronic abstract submission. It may be helpful to have a peer researcher or colleague review an abstract before submission.

7. Who reviews abstracts after they have been submitted?
A group of health care professionals with research and clinical experience review all abstracts on submission. Abstract review forms with specific criteria are used in the critique process. Scores are tabulated, and abstracts meeting criteria are chosen for either poster or podium presentation. An abstract review form used to critique abstracts at the University of Colorado Hospital Multidisciplinary Clinical Research Symposium is found in Appendix A.

8. What is the notification process after submission of an abstract?
The standard procedure is that the submitter is notified by a written correspondence. If the abstract is accepted, the letter may outline further steps for meeting program or publication deadlines and requirements. Typically, forms are included for audiovisual or other program needs.

APPENDIX A

Abstract Critique Form

Title of Abstract_____

Reviewer _____

1. Background:
• Is the topic significant/important/relevant to patient care and outcomes?
Missing   0   (Low) 1   2   3   4   5 (High)

• Is the conceptual framework/rationale sound and logical?
Missing   0   (Low) 1   2   3   4   5 (High)

2. Purpose:
• Is the purpose clearly stated?
Missing   0   (Low) 1   2   3   4   5 (High)

3. Methods:
• Are the methods and/or practices described in the abstract appropriate?
Missing   0   (Low) 1   2   3   4   5 (High)

4. Results/Outcomes:
• Are the results/outcomes sound and justified?
Missing   0   (Low) 1   2   3   4   5 (High)

5. Clinical Implications:
• Is the impact on clinical practice clearly described?
Missing   0   (Low) 1   2   3   4   5 (High)

6. Presentation:
• Is the abstract well written?
Missing   0   (Low) 1   2   3   4   5 (High)

• Are the ideas clearly communicated?
Missing   0   (Low) 1   2   3   4   5 (High)

7. Overall Merit:
• Is this an innovative, cutting edge topic?
Missing   0   (Low) 1   2   3   4   5 (High)

TOTAL POINTS   _____
Podium   _____   **Evidence based research project**   _____
Poster   _____   **Conduct of research**   _____
            _____   **Performance improvement project** _____
Completed Research   _____   **Other, please specify**   _____
Research in Progress   _____

Adapted from Oncology Nursing Society Abstract Guidelines, 1999.

REFERENCES

1. Burns N, Grove S: The Practice of Nursing Research: Conduct, Critique, and Utilization, 3rd ed. Philadelphia, W.B. Saunders, 1997.
2. Downs FS: How to cozy up to a research report. Appl Nurs Res 12(4):215–216, 1999.
3. Oncology Nursing Society Abstract Submission Guidelines, 1999.

BIBLIOGRAPHY

1. Beyea S, Nicoll L: Writing and submitting an abstract. AORN J 67:273–274, 1998.
2. Blix A, Rogers B: Writing abstracts. AAOHN J 45:513–514, 1997.
3. Cole F, Koziol-McLain J: Writing a research abstract. J Emerg Nurs 23:487–490, 1997.
4. Kachoyeanos M: The process of writing an abstract. MCN 23:50, 1998.

27. WRITING FOR PUBLICATION

Rose Mary Carroll-Johnson, MN, RN

1. What are the ingredients of a successful publishing experience?

A publishing experience is usually successful if the manuscript is a high-quality product and there is an optimal match between the manuscript and the journal.

2. What constitutes a high-quality paper?

First and foremost, the science behind the research must be sound. If the research was poorly executed there may be little that can be done to salvage the report. Clear and concise writing alone cannot hide the sins of a poorly designed or conducted study. Conversely, if the study report is poorly written, the paper may be rejected or publication can be delayed by the need to revise (and usually re-review) a manuscript that is incomplete or confusing. Although poor writing can be fixed, a sloppy presentation often raises red flags in the minds of the editor or the reviewers about the clarity of the author's thinking and ability to attend to detail.

3. How do you decide where to submit the paper?

When choosing a journal, consider the following points:
- Your paper needs to be consistent with the type and scope of articles usually published in the journal.
- The journal's readership (who and how many) should be consistent with the audience that you want to reach.
- Your paper needs to be appropriate in content and level for the journal's audience.
- The frequency and size of the publication should be considered because they affect time to publication after acceptance.
- If you need or desire help, what editorial support (e.g., editor's help, copyediting) is available?

4. What author characteristics contribute to successful publication?

There are no "make-or-break" attributes, but successful authors seem to have (or soon develop) desire, persistence, perspective, and a productive work ethic based on setting schedules and meeting deadlines.

5. What are the ground rules of biomedical publication?

Most biomedical publications follow Ingelfinger's rule. Ingelfinger was editor of the *New England Journal of Medicine* when the policy was established that no paper would be considered for publication if its substance has been submitted or reported elsewhere.[1] Simply stated, you may submit your paper to only one journal at a time. Most journals do not consider appearance of an abstract in a proceedings as publication per se. The published abstract does not, under most circumstances, preclude publication of the full text.

6. What is salami publishing?

Also known as redundant publication, it is the practice of inappropriately dividing the results of a single study into more than one paper or reworking results reported in one paper into a slightly different but essentially similar manuscript. Academic pressure to publish or perish sometimes drives this practice. It is undesirable because it can overemphasize the research results, clog up the literature, and overburden reviewers.[2]

7. How do I avoid duplicate publication?

You need to develop the ability to be objective about your papers. Some authors are prolific writers on basically one topic. They are experts and share their knowledge widely, shaping the content to the audience. Other writers report on an ongoing and lengthy program of research that appropriately involves sequential reports. Drawing the line between a legitimate publication and one that merely rehashes previously published work may not always be clear. Probably the best way to avoid the pitfall is to explain any concern to the editor of the journal to which you submit your paper. Include a copy of any paper that you have published and that may be too similar to the paper submitted for peer review and ask the editor for his or her opinion.

8. Why does the publication process take so long?

Time to publication is influenced by a number of variable and fixed factors. The time required to review a manuscript can vary from a few weeks to few months, depending on the journal's systems, the number of manuscripts that it receives, and the number of reviewers in place. After the review, the author may need to revise the paper, and the paper may need to be re-reviewed and, possibly revised yet again before acceptance. Once the manuscript is accepted, scheduling for publication may depend on available space, frequency of the publication, backlog of articles accepted before yours, and timeliness or interest level of your article. Some journals have a substantial backlog of manuscripts. Unless the editor has a specific reason for moving your paper forward in the queue, you may need to wait months for publication. Obviously, journals that publish larger issues more frequently can accommodate a larger number of papers. As a general rule, however, all print publications have limits as to the number of pages per issue. Finally, authors need to be aware that the physical production of an issue of a print journal usually takes from 3 to 4 months. This time is fixed and not amenable to change.

9. How can I shorten the time involved?

Papers that are considered particularly timely (i.e., a new or current topic or one with startling results) or papers that contain content that is likely to be out of date very quickly (e.g., genetics-related topics) are often "fast-tracked" by the editor. Occasionally an editor is looking for papers on a particular topic for a special issue. If your paper comes along at the right time, it may be published quickly. However, the reverse is also possible. An editor may want to delay publication of your paper for a special issue. If you are not happy with the time to publication for your accepted paper, discuss it with the editor. Often your perspective on the importance or timeliness of the paper will be seriously considered, but do not be surprised if an editor is not as convinced as you of the value of your paper to nursing science and practice. In reality, few papers need to be published as quickly as possible. Online publication formats are becoming increasingly more available and often can result in faster publication.

10. What is online-only publication?

There is a small but growing number of online journals to choose from these days. Online journals do not exist in print. Their articles are accessed only via the Internet. The procedures used by these journals vary, but most of the time articles are peer-reviewed and, once accepted, published (i.e., posted on the Internet) as quickly as the editorial work can be completed. These articles are indexed in the standard databases (e.g., MEDLINE, CINAHL) but are usually accessible only to subscribers.

Some print publications are beginning to publish a portion of their articles "online only." These articles are subject to regular journal acceptance procedures but never appear in full in the print issues. They become available only online. The ability to avoid the 3- to 4-month production schedule usually means that a journal can publish these articles relatively quickly.

11. What should I consider in regard to online-only publishing?

If you need publication credits for tenure or employment purposes, check with your administration to ensure that online-only publication is acceptable. Other questions you may want to ask the editor include the following:

- Will access to the article be limited?
- How will information about the availability of your article be disseminated?
- Can access to the article be monitored?
- What mechanisms are available to access the article if someone is not internet-capable?
- How will the article be archived?

12. What is the best way to approach the task of turning a long dissertation or thesis into a publishable article?

Trying to figure out how to come up with a 12-page synopsis of the 150- to 200-page dissertation or thesis has stopped more than one newly minted PhD from writing for publication. The paper that you write for publication is not just a scaled back version of your dissertation. Its purpose is completely different. Research reports and dissertations have a basic organizing framework in common, but the similarities end there. The paper written for publication needs to address a defined and specific topic; thus, more than one publishable paper can legitimately emerge from your doctoral work (see question 6). Start with one or two main research questions and build your report from there. Stay focused on the topic of the paper. Consider the balance of the paper, given your page allotment. Each section is important, but the space devoted to presentation must be balanced according to importance. In other words, do not devote eight pages to introductory material and leave yourself only one or two pages for the discussion.

13. What do I leave out of an article based on a dissertation?

Articles written for publication have a diverse audience. That, coupled with the fact that you are working with a limited number of pages, means that your writing must be clear, pertinent, and succinct. Avoid research-speak. Convey your hypotheses/research questions in paragraph form rather than lists of formal, repetitive statements. Avoid the use of long explanations of statistical methods and manipulations, long quotations, and details about the content of tools. Do not add supplements, appendixes, or bibliographies. If tool development was part of your work, consider writing a separate paper about that process rather than trying to incorporate all details into your research report. Above all, avoid redundancy and repetition throughout the paper.

14. What is the best reporting format for my research?

A quick review of published research demonstrates that most research is reported using a basic organizing framework. Pilot studies, preliminary research, or quantitative studies with small samples may be well suited to some sort of brief-report format. Check the individual journal guidelines to see if such a format is offered.

15. What is a good length for a research report?

Full research reports most commonly consist of 15–20 double-spaced pages, exclusive of references, tables, and figures. In general, it is difficult to offer a complete report in less than 12 pages. Manuscripts that exceed 20 pages consume too much space in a journal whose page length is limited. In addition, long papers tend to lose the reader at some point. Reports of qualitative research may be allowed somewhat more latitude, particularly if there is a great deal of good quotational material. Nevertheless, the author needs to strive for as lean a presentation as possible. If you reach an impasse in conforming to the journal's preferred page length, you may want to contact the editor for advice or permission to submit something longer. Page limits are usually not a major concern if the article will be published online-only.

16. What are the parts of a classical research report?

- Introduction/background
- Theoretical/conceptual framework
- Literature review
- Purpose
- Methods
- Results/findings
- Discussion
- Conclusion/summary

17. What should the introductory material encompass?

You need to substantiate briefly the need for interest in your topic and provide some background information. The literature review needs to address current knowledge and statistics. Some critique of the studies highlighted should be offered. Be sure that you explain and substantiate why there is a need for your particular research study. The need for a detailed description of your theoretical/conceptual framework depends on the type and depth of your research. The framework may be implied or familiar to your audience and thus requires little explanation in the research report itself. Qualitative research, by definition, has few if any preconceived ideas. Presenting an elaborate framework before doing the research is not appropriate. Your framework is the justification for your methods and provides the underpinning for the discussion of your findings. You must provide enough information so that the reader can logically follow you through the remainder of the paper.

18. What is included in the methods section?

The methods section is fundamental to assessing the scientific value of the research. It needs to be complete enough so that readers have a clear idea of how the research was conducted (i.e., it could conceivably be replicated based on the information provided) and can ascertain that your methods have a high likelihood of leading to reliable findings. At a minimum you must detail the following:

- Study design (with a rationale for your choice if appropriate)
- Sample selection criteria and procedures (sample demographics may be detailed in this section or in the results/findings section depending on journal preference or custom)
- Instruments/tools, including reliability and validity assessments (either calculated by you or offered in supporting literature)
- Procedures (a step-by-step description of how you conducted the research including institutional review board approval and consent processes)
- Data analysis procedures

Labels for these categories of information are different for reports of qualitative research, but similar concepts must be addressed.

19. What is the most effective way to present results?

Results are best presented succinctly and supported by tables and figures. The organization of this section should be logical, based on categories of data collected or perhaps the research questions posed. If not presented in the methods section, begin with a description of the sample. In general, key findings can be highlighted in the text and details provided in supporting tables and figures. The goal is not to duplicate information displayed in tables and figures with lengthy discussions in the text. A number of resources are available to assist authors in appropriate construction of tables. The best way to display statistics in the text is usually covered by the journal's choice of reference style and can be determined by consulting the style manual. Finally, avoid the tendency to explain or interpret results, which is more properly done in the discussion section.

20. What are the hallmarks of the discussion section?

The discussion section may be the most important section of your report[3] and thus the most difficult to prepare. Here you make the case for the importance and meaning of your findings and their implications for nursing practice and research. A well-written discussion avoids making some of the most common mistakes that editors and reviewers address:

- Avoid simply reiterating your findings or presenting new findings. The discussion section can highlight the salient findings, but an explanation for your results must be the primary focus.
- An explanation of your findings should properly begin with the framework that you chose for the study and the existing knowledge about the topic. Too often the discussion section avoids mention of these key elements, leaving readers to wonder about the connections. Negative findings, findings contrary to findings of similar studies, or particularly unexpected findings also must be explained or discussed.
- When writing the discussion section, researchers walk a fine line between overstating their findings and completely avoiding the implications of the work. Reviewers often complain that the discussion goes way beyond the scope of the data gathered. Editors often have to force researchers to articulate the potential contribution that their findings make to research and practice. All results of well-conducted research make some contribution to knowledge, and no legitimate research ends with all questions answered. It is important to address these issues in your paper and not leave it to the imagination of the reader.

- Somewhere in this final section of the paper the limitations of the research must be addressed.
- Write a brief, to-the-point conclusion or summary. Do not just stop writing, leaving the reader hanging.

21. How should acknowledgments be handled?

Once your paper is accepted for publication, you may want to forward to the editor an acknowledgment of persons who were key to the research or report (e.g., subjects, research assistants, statisticians, key faculty members, typists). Please take the time to ensure that anyone who is acknowledged by name is told and agrees to the acknowledgment before publication. Acknowledgments are not a dedication but a recognition of substantive participation in the work that falls short of requirements of coauthorship. Those acknowledged by name need to be aware that their name will appear (see Chapter 25).

22. Is there room for innovation in the report format?

Although some editors have tried to devise new formats for reporting research, the traditional structure remains the best and most preferred. You can try submitting a research report using a nontraditional format, but it is most likely that reviewers or the editor will insist that the paper be reformatted. Reformatting requires additional work and, more importantly, additional time.

23. Is there a rule of thumb for the number of tables and figures?

Too few or too many tables/figures can handicap an article. The goal is to facilitate presentation of information and not to complicate or overwhelm it. In general, a standard research report contains 2–5 tables. Figures are less frequently included but can present certain types of information quite effectively and, with the computer software available today, are fairly easy to produce.

24. What guidelines apply to development of tables and figures?

A well-presented table or figure addresses one category of data or one notion. Just as the text of a dissertation or thesis needed to be adapted for publication, so too will the tabular material. Keep the material in the table relevant to the article and free of extraneous information.

Choosing whether to present your information in tabular form or as a figure depends, in part, on the nature of the information. If numbers are important, tabular presentation is preferred. If the author wants to convey a trend or overall impression of the data, some sort of figural presentation may be more appropriate. Three sources of assistance in designing tables include the style manual used by the journal, a good reference book on research or presentation of statistics, and a copy of the journal itself. If you devise a particularly long or detailed table, examine it carefully to see whether it can or should be broken up into smaller, more easily appreciated parts. By the same token, a handful of smaller tables with small amounts of similar types of content or categories may be better combined into one comprehensive table.

Refer to each table or figure by number in the text. Put each table or figure on a separate page, and place it at the end of the manuscript. The addition of color to tables and figures is easy and often appealing to the eye, but the ability to reproduce color exceeds the financial capability of many journals. Avoid the use of color unless it is absolutely necessary. If you prepare a color figure, have a plan to convert the categories of information into some sort of visual discriminators (e.g., lines, dots, hash marks) if color cannot be used.

25. When do you need to request permission to use material from another source?

Tables or figures previously published may be included in your paper if you receive permission from the copyright holder, usually the publisher (see questions 39 and 40). Even if you alter the original material by deleting content or adding your own nuances, you must request permission to adapt the material. These principles apply even if you were the original author of the material. Once material has been published and the copyright has been signed over to the publisher, even the author of the material needs to request permission to use it in another publication.

Tabular material that is based on textual information from another source should simply credit the source or sources. Permission is not required to use the information. Textual quotations must be referenced specifically, including the page number of the quote. You must request permission to quote material that exceeds 50 words.[4]

26. How do you request permission to use material from another source?

The request must be made formally and in writing, either by mail or, if allowed, by e-mail. Letters can be brief and to the point. Some publishers have request forms that you can fill out and forward to the permissions editor. The request should be accompanied by complete information about what you want to use, where specifically the material is located (i.e., the journal or book/book chapter, authors, page numbers, volume and issue or edition), how you plan to use the material, and in what publication it will appear. If you plan to adapt the information, include a copy of the planned adaptations.

Allow enough time to process the request. If you have not received a response in 3–4 weeks, however, you should follow up with a phone call or another letter.

27. Whom do you ask for permission?

Permission to reprint or adapt material must be requested from whoever holds the copyright—usually the publisher. Some copyright holders request that you seek permission directly from the author in addition. Unless specifically directed to do so, you need not ask the author. If the author is not the copyright holder, his or her permission is insufficient legal basis to use the information in your article.[5]

28. What if there is a charge to use material from another source?

Unfortunately, it is becoming more common for publishers to charge authors who want permission to reprint tables and figures. These costs can range from a few dollars to a few hundred dollars. As the author, you are responsible for these costs. Before paying you may want to consider the following:

- Check with the publisher of the journal to which you are submitting your paper. It is possible that the publisher has access to other versions of the material without needing to charge you.
- Look for other versions of the material in different publications, and try to find permission to reprint from someone who will not charge you.
- Consider taking the time to create the material yourself.
- Decide not to include the material at all.

29. What guidelines govern the use of references?

The difference between too little and too much referencing can be a fine line. The extensive referencing in a dissertation or perhaps in a grant proposal is not appropriate in a journal report. In general, cited references need to be:

- Current (generally less than 5 years old. If you have waited some time before submitting a report for review, an updated literature review is advised.)
- Pertinent (directly related to the material that you are discussing)
- Comprehensive (demonstrating that you have explored the literature well and recently)
- Accurate (Do whatever you need to do to ensure both citational and contextual accuracy.)
- Primary (Cite review articles sparingly; go to the original source, particularly for quotations and statistics.)

30. What resources are available to assist writers in the preparation of reference lists?

Some word-processing programs have end-note functions that allow writers to collect references as they go along, assigning numbers automatically. Reference information still needs to be entered, however, and the format checked for accuracy. Depending on the reference style used by the journal, other, more elaborate software support is available. If you anticipate writing a great many articles for publication, investing in a more expensive software program that will assist you in formatting your references according to a wide range of styles may make the most sense. Spend a little time shopping around for a product that meets your needs. Some possibilities include:

Lower-cost, narrower-capability programs
- APA-Style Helper available through <www.apastyle.org>
- Format Ease (Guilford Publications at <info@guilford.com>)
- Reference Point Software available through <info@referencePointSoftward.com>
- Scribe Reference Formatting (an online subscription-type service at <www.scribesa.com>)

Higher-end, wide-range capability programs
- EndNote at <www.endnote.com>
- ProCite at <www.procite.com> (searches PubMed and Internet libraries)

Information sources
- <NIHlibrary@NIH.gov>
- <www.ISIresearchsoft.com>

31. What is considered good etiquette for submitting a paper for peer review?

Read and adhere to the manuscript preparation guidelines (number of copies, reference style, length). Prepare the disk, if requested, according to specifications. *Always* accompany the manuscript with a typed cover letter that includes complete contact information (address, telephone numbers, e-mail address). Address the letter to the editor, using his or her correct name and credentials.[5]

32. What dos and don'ts apply to preparing manuscript copies for peer review?

Most journals employ a double-blind peer review process (i.e., reviewers are not told the identity of the author and vice versa). Many peer reviewers review for a variety

of journals and have a good deal of reading to do. Although styles vary, most reviewers and editors appreciate having some room to make notes for themselves or the author directly on the pages. Specifics in the author guidelines are designed to support these realities. Avoid common mistakes by following these rules:
- Remove your name from a running head/foot.
- Use a high-quality printer or copy machine.
- Paginate the manuscript, ensuring there are no blank pages and that all pages are present in the copy.
- Use a readable typeface and size (Times Roman or Courier, 10- or 12-point size).
- Provide acknowledgments after the manuscript has been accepted for publication.
- Avoid extensive self-referencing if possible.
- Supply the requisite number of copies.

33. What is a reasonable length of time for peer review?

Peer review done by hard copy through the mail takes 3–4 weeks at a minimum. Reviewer delays, problems mailing to large institutions, and editorial time to assess and compile the reviews add more weeks to the process. As electronic review becomes more commonplace, the amount of time involved across the board (from submission through acceptance) will be considerably shortened. Unfortunately, shortening review time is not likely to have a direct effect on shortening time to publication (see question 8).

34. How should you respond to the peer review?

Many authors agree that the peer review process is sometimes the most difficult part of writing for publication. Negative feedback is difficult for even the most experienced author to receive. Evidence indicates, however, that peer review results in stronger papers. In general, the quicker you sit down to respond to the peer review the more likely you are to fix the paper. As you undertake the review, follow these guidelines.
- Do not ignore the reviewers' comments. If you do not agree with the criticism, make your case to the editor. If you believe the reviewer "just doesn't get it," take another look at how you have presented your information and ensure that you make your points clearly.
- It is not uncommon to receive feedback that covers the spectrum of responses from positive to negative. Consider everyone's point of view. The truth usually lies somewhere between two highly divergent points of view.
- Look for common themes in the reviews. Reviewers often address the same issues, using different descriptors or assigning different importance, but the problem to be addressed may appear consistently in all reviews.[6]
- Prepare a careful synopsis of the major changes made and include it in a cover letter when returning the manuscript for final acceptance or second reviews. You are under no obligation to do what the reviewers suggest, but you should be prepared to explain your choices to the editor and possibly to the reviewers if a second review is required.[7]

35. What is the role of the editor at this point?

Each editor may approach the editorial role somewhat differently, but the editor is the final arbitrator and decision maker. If the direction that you should take on an issue is unclear, ask the editor for advice. If the editor has addressed specific problems in the manuscript, pay careful attention. Remember that publication is a collaborative process. The editor and reviewers have an obligation to readers to ensure as best they can that a paper meets the journal's standards, but they also have a responsibility to the authors to be helpful, supportive, courteous, and professional.

36. What can you expect once the paper is accepted for publication?

Once a manuscript is accepted for publication the editor should be able to give you a planned publication date. The date must be considered tentative. The editor must remain flexible to accommodate unforeseen journal problems or the need to readjust publication plans. Some weeks in advance of the publication date the manuscript is edited by the editor or associate editor and copyedited by trained individuals. The paper is returned to you, either as computerized copy or "typeset," and presented as a "layout" or actual journal page. As the author, you need to scrutinize this version of your paper word for word, including every table and figure, to ensure the following:

- No errors were introduced during the editing process.
- No content was inadvertently dropped.
- You answer all questions posed by the editor and copyeditor.
- The headings and subheadings have been interpreted and displayed appropriately.
- Tabular information has been displayed correctly and in correct alignment.
- You supply all requested details about references.

This is not the time to request addition of large blocks of text or substantive revisions to the manuscript. Avoid arguing over small details that have been changed to ensure that the manuscript conforms to journal style. Restrict your feedback to the content of the paper, factual errors, or misinterpretation of your text.

It is likely that the turnaround time at this point will be short. If, in the course of waiting for publication, your contact information changes, keep the editor up to date. Problems with contacting you at time of publication can result in postponement. Adhere to the deadlines that you are given, and respond quickly and completely. If your schedule does not allow a great deal of flexibility, ask the editor for advance warning so that you can be prepared to devote necessary time to reviewing the final version of the manuscript.

37. What is financial disclosure? Why is it important?

Financial disclosure refers to the process of identifying sources of funding for your research (e.g., scholarships, grant funding) or your affiliations with or involvement in any organization or entity with a direct financial interest in the subject matter or materials discussed in the manuscript.[8] The types of affiliation/involvement include (but are not limited to) employment, consultancy, ownership interest (stock), honoraria, gifts and travel expenses, paid expert testimony, board or advisory committee membership, and other financial or material interest. Financial disclosure seldom precludes publication in and of itself, provided the manuscript meets journal standards. However, an accurate appraisal of the objectivity of the author during collection and interpretation of data is not possible unless the editor, reviewers, and ultimately the readers have all of the information.

38. When should you provide financial disclosure?

Financial disclosure is appropriate when the manuscript is submitted for peer review. It should be reiterated at the time of submission of the final version of the manuscript. In the event that you forget to disclose a financial association or neglect to do so out of ignorance of the policy, you should disclose even after the article has been published.

39. What is copyright?

Copyright is the exclusive legal right to publication of a written work. It exists automatically, but a copyright can be registered with the Library of Congress for a small fee. This registering process affords a stronger legal position. In most cases, a publisher requires the author or authors to sign over copyright to the publisher or professional association that owns the journal.[4] The article then becomes the property of the publisher who registers the copyright, processes permissions to reprint copies of all or part of the article, and assumes legal responsibility for the article. Transferring copyright to the publisher means that even the author needs to request permission to use his or her own material in future publications. This arrangement may seem problematic, but in fact it seldom results in problems and certainly is considered the industry norm.

Copyright assignment forms can be as simple as a brief typewritten statement that the author signs or as involved as a multipage legal document. Regardless, the assignment should be read carefully and a copy signed by every author of the paper.

40. When should I retain copyright of my article?

In general, you want to consider signing over the copyright of your article to the publisher or association, but occasionally you may elect to retain copyright to some of your material. You may decide to retain copyright to original material such as a tool, survey, or artwork separate from the body of the manuscript. In such cases, you need to give the publisher written permission to reprint the material in the publication and to register the copyright, process all requests to use the material, and defend the material in the unlikely event of some sort of litigation. Discuss such concerns with the editor or the publisher.

41. Should I order reprints?

Before publication you are likely to be asked if you wish to purchase reprints of your article. Reprints must be purchased in large lots and are often quite expensive. Access to libraries, document delivery services, and online access to many publications have decreased the need for authors to supply copies of their articles in response to large numbers of requests from outside parties or nonsubscribers. Most authors do not assume the expense of purchasing reprints. If requests come to you, alternatives include providing information about how the article may be accessed on the Internet or how to obtain a copy via a service such as the Copyright Clearinghouse or interlibrary loan programs. If you find yourself in the situation of needing a number of copies (e.g., for a presentation), you need to request permission from the publisher to make such copies.

42. What if my paper is rejected?

Manuscripts are rejected for various reasons that may not have too much to do with the quality of the paper. Perhaps the paper was not a good fit with the journal. Other reasons may have to do with the fact that the content has recently been covered in the journal or the editor has recently accepted a similar paper, although these types of rejection do not usually apply to research reports.

Rejected papers should be submitted to another journal. However, carefully read the reviewers' comments and the editor's letter and take sometime to correct the manuscript's deficiencies before sending it elsewhere. Expect another round of peer review. In addition, ensure that the manuscript is re-prepared according to the author guidelines of the new journal.

Occasionally, a research report is rejected based on what is perceived to be a "fatal flaw" in the research process. If you truly do not foresee being able to publish successfully, consider whether a part of the manuscript can be salvaged for publication. Perhaps the literature review can be embellished and submitted as an integrative review. Persistence and imagination are important to the process of writing for publication; both need to be developed.

REFERENCES

1. Ingelfinger F: Definition of "sole contribution." N Engl J Med 281:676–677, 1969.
2. Kassier J, Angell M: Redundant publication: A reminder. N Engl J Med 333:449–459, 1995.
3. Woodward FP: How to Teach Scientific Communication. Reston, VA, Council of Science Editors, 1999.
4. Sigler B: Signing on the dotted line. Clin J Oncol Nurs 5(Suppl 3):17–18, 2001.
5. Carroll-Johnson RM: Submitting a manuscript for peer review. Clin J Oncol Nurs 5(Suppl 3):12–16, 2001.
6. Johnson SH: Dealing with conflicting reviewers' comments. Nurs Au Ed 6(4):1–3, 1996.
7. Cupples S: Responding to reviewers' comments. Nurs Au Ed 11(1):1–4, 2001.
8. King C: Ethical issues in writing and publishing. Clin J Oncol Nurs 5(Suppl 3):19–23, 2001.

28. ORAL PRESENTATION

Mary Beth Flynn, RN, MS, CNS, CCRN

1. How do you disseminate the results of your research study?

Many professional organizations have research symposia or conferences that solicit a call for abstracts for both poster and oral presentations. Nursing journals, hospital websites, professional nursing organizations, and most schools of nursing have information about upcoming research symposiums seeking abstract submissions. Look for organizations that match your research focus. Contact the organization for abstract submission guidelines. Read the abstract submission form carefully. Your ability to comply with the abstract submission requirements is the first step in the review process.

2. Can I present research in progress as an oral presentation?

Typically research that has not been completed is presented in poster format.[1] If you are submitting for a podium presentation, it is expected that your research will be completed by the time of the presentation. Oral presentations are more formal and usually draw a larger audience; thus completed research is presented.

3. What title should I use for my abstract?

The title of your abstract needs to be interesting and should invite the reader to learn more from your oral presentation. Think about the mission of the organization to which you are submitting. Review the title of the conference. Can you identify a theme in the conference title? (For example, quality outcomes, evidence-based practice, or caring.) Will you be speaking to nurse administrators? Nurse practitioners? Staff nurses? Academic nurses? Or a mixed audience? Succinctly convey the "soul" of your research. Avoid long titles if at all possible, and if you identify a theme, try to tie your title to the conference theme.

4. Once your abstract is accepted, what next?

First, celebrate! Next, begin your preparation early; do not procrastinate. Determine what you want the audience to take away from your presentation. Consider how much time you have to present. Oral presentation time frames vary but usually range from 15 to 30 minutes. Typically the last 5 minutes are allotted for questions. Start organizing your thoughts so that you will be able to stay within the suggested time frame. It is highly embarrassing if you run out of time and the audience is no longer listening.

5. Anticipating the audience: to whom will you present?

Most people in the audience are much like you. They do not critique every word or slide. However, audience members are interested in your research and want to leave more informed than when they sat down. Ask some of the following questions to help define your audience, which in turn will help you prepare your presentation:
- How many people attend this conference?
- Will I present as a part of a break-out session?
- What are the nursing roles of the audience members?
- What level of knowledge may the audience have about my research topic?

• What level of knowledge may the audience have about the research process?
• Is the language or jargon related to my research common to all nurses?[2]

Before the final conference brochure arrives, you may not know what colleagues are also presenting, nor whether similar topics will be presented. Review the brochure closely, examining the topics to get a better feeling for the type of audience that the organization is trying to attract. A final option is to contact the organization and ask what type of audience mix you should anticipate.

6. Organizing your thoughts: how do you formulate your research into a presentation?

In preparing your presentation, stay focused on what information you want the audience to understand at the close of your talk. Usually the content of the presentation follows the format of the written abstract. Review the classic literature that is part of your research, and conduct a brief literature review to ensure that no new material has been published before your presentation date. The table below describes the elements most often included in an oral presentation[1]:

Elements Included in an Oral Presentation

ELEMENT	DESCRIPTION
Title with authors and institution	
Acknowledgments	Support from colleagues, consultants; any grant or financial support.
Introduction	Background to the development of the research question.
Purpose of the study and specific aims	The answer to these questions are most likely what you would like the audience to remember at the close of your presentation. Tie the remaining sections of your presentation back to this questions/answer.
Theoretical or conceptual framework	Keep this section brief.
Review of the literature	Include a review of classic and the most relevant literature. The purpose of this section is to support the importance of your research question. Keep this section brief, but provide enough information that the listener has a good understanding of what research may/may not have discovered relative to your area of study.
Methods, study design, and data analysis	Typically this information includes specific information about the instrument(s) used and should be briefly reviewed.
Results/outcomes	This section should tie back to the purpose of the study and is where you want to spend the majority of your time.
Clinical implications	Why was your research important? Tell the audience the impact your research can/will have on nursing practice and patient outcomes. Again, tie the purpose, results and clinical implications together for the listener.

7. Should I write out my lecture?

Everyone's presentation style is different, but the act of writing your lecture offers the opportunity to reexamine and condense your research. It also forces you to become increasingly familiar with the content format that you plan to use when you are at the podium. Your comfort with the material and progression of your presentation will give you confidence at the podium. While writing the presentation, do not include words with which you are not comfortable. If you struggle with the words on paper, you will surely struggle during your oral presentation. Once the presentation is written, you can more easily progress to audiovisual development.

8. Should I practice the presentation before giving it?

Absolutely. Practice is essential to a smooth, professional, and rewarding presentation experience. Frequently it is suggested that you give the presentation to a friend who knows nothing about your research topic. If your friend can understand the message that you had intended, you have mastered the content! Ask your friend to critique elements of the delivery of your presentation, including body language, grammar, pauses, and "umms." Time yourself as you practice. If you end on time while practicing, you will finish on time during your podium presentation. If you are over the time limit, edit your content.

9. How do I avoid reading my notes?

Develop audiovisual materials that provide cues or key elements of information. Avoid bringing a written lecture to the podium. Instead, create note cards or brief note pages to which you may refer while you are speaking. Many computer-generated presentation programs provide a note-page option that works well for creating lecture note cards. Keep the number of cards and pages to a minimum. You do not want to be shuffling through papers for information as you present. Number your notes so that you can easily re-organize the pages if they become disorganized.

Practice your presentation without using your cards. This step helps you identify which note card you most likely will need during the presentation. Frequently, it is the statistical analysis section or limitations section of your presentation. Color-code this note page with a highlighter to assist you during the presentation. Avoid yellow highlighter because it can be difficult to read when the lights are dimmed. Pink or light blue show up nicely in a dim room.

10. How do I engage the audience?

- Use eye contact and smile. If at all possible, stand away from the podium. This strategy allows you to feel more engaged with the audience. Scan the audience slowly and methodically as you talk. Focus on an individual for 2–3 seconds, smile, and continue talking to other members of the audience. Seek the faces of those who are smiling back and nodding their heads. Use humor, either verbal or visual, to lighten your presentation and reengage the audience. Do not worry if people get up to leave the presentation; people leave for multiple reasons.
- Arrive at your room early, and engage in casual conversation with participants at the front of the room as they enter and assume their seat. As you become more comfortable with public speaking, you will be able to draw elements of the participant's conversations into your presentation.

- Another presentation skill is the ability to pull elements from previous presenters and/or keynote speakers into your presentation. This skill demonstrates the ability to focus and complement the work of colleagues as you present your work.

11. What if someone else presents results on the same type of research?

If you can attend the other presentation, do so. Attempt to identify how your results may be similar or different and the reason for any differences. If you present after the research with similar content, try to address the similarities and differences during your oral presentation. Avoid the temptation to think that your research presentation will not be interesting. If you have similar conclusions, the two presentations help to validate the results of both researchers.

12. What if the audience asks questions?

Anticipate questions and prepare answers. Questions at the end of your oral presentation are a compliment. Listen carefully to the question, and repeat it to ensure that you understand the participant. If you do not know the answer, admit it. Depending on the size of the audience, you may ask if anyone in the audience has an answer. You may also offer to speak to the participant later to exchange addresses so that you can research the answer. Consider putting your e-mail address on your title slide, and carry ample business cards for participants who may want to contact you in the future.

13. How do I develop visual aids?

- Review the abstract acceptance form. You may be limited to slides, overheads, or computer-assisted presentation aides (PowerPoint). Slides or computer presentations are most frequently used. Overheads or flip charts are typically used when audience participation is desired during the oral presentation. If you are using a computer presentation, find out whether you must bring your own laptop, whether one will be provided, and computer compatibility (IBM or Apple). Most conferences offer only IBM computer support.
- A few words to the wise in developing your slide presentation, whether it consists of hard copies or is computer-generated. If the slide background is a dark color, use yellow or white lettering for text. If the slide background is white or a light color, use black lettering. Typically, computer programs provide templates that have been tested for colors that project best in dark rooms. Avoid the use of red, pink, purple, or green for text; they are difficult to read in the dark.
- Animation can be humorous and definitely gets the attention of your audience. However, too much animation is distracting and can cause the listener to focus on the animation rather than your message. Use animation on your slides tastefully and in moderation. Animation for a summary slide is appropriate and adds closure to your presentation.
- Avoid using graphs that do not project well or will be difficult to read. You and the listener are frustrated when all participants cannot view the audiovisual. If a graphic will be poorly projected, put the information into text.
- A good rule of thumb for slides is one slide every 60 seconds. Some slides may be briefer, whereas others may require more time. But if your presentation is 15 minutes, do not have more than 20 slides.

• Slides are tools to help cue you during your presentation. General rules include no more than 7–8 lines of information and no more than 8 words within each sentence. Chose a simple font design such as Arial or Times New Roman. Avoid the use of all capitals; use upper- and lower-case typing. A font size less than 24 points will be difficult to read in the back of the room. Add pictures when they augment the text or speak for the text.

14. How do I time my presentation with my visual aids?

Practice speaking with your slides as the primary cues and your notes at your side. Many computer programs have a notes feature. Optimize this feature for use with slides that convey challenging information. Ensure that the font is large enough (usually 14 or 16 points) to be read from a distance and in the dark.

15. How do I deal with stage fright?

Preparation and practice before the presentation help you gain confidence. But even the most seasoned presenters can be nervous. If possible, arrive at the conference the day before you present. Examine the room, podium (relative to projection screen), arrangement of participant seating, and audiovisual (AV) equipment. Have a relaxing evening, review your presentation, visualize the room as you practice, and go to bed early. You want to be rested on the day of the presentation. Arrive at your presentation room ahead of schedule, and become comfortable with the AV equipment and microphone. After you have been introduced, take a deep breath, stand tall as you walk to the podium, and smile. Smiling lets your audience know that you are excited to be with them.

16. What happens if I realize that I am running out of time?

Always keep a timepiece that you can easily see near your notes. Glance at it casually as you speak. If you are running behind, gently increase the speed in which you present the slide information, summarizing the slide instead of discussing every line. Avoid the temptation to speak faster or to skip slides. The purpose, results, and clinical implications are the primary information that you want the audience to remember. If you are behind, summarize other elements of your presentation to allow ample time for results and clinical implications. If you do not have time for questions, invite participants to speak with you at the close of the session. If you have included your e-mail address on a cover slide, encourage participants to e-mail you so that you may address their specific questions.

17. When should I use the laser pointer?

Use a pointer when you want to emphasize a statistic or statement. Avoid the temptation to read the slide using the laser pointer. If you are feeling nervous, use two hands to hold the pointer; this technique steadies the light beam and gives you time to take a deep breath and calm your nerves. Try to avoid the urge to create large, rapid circles with the laser pointer.

18. What type of handout should I prepare?

Review the abstract acceptance paperwork carefully. The deadline for participant handouts will be clearly outlined. Typically the participant handout is due several weeks to months before your actual presentation date. You must ensure that your handout matches the actual presentation that you plan to deliver. Some conferences allow only the abstract to be the participant handout. If additional handouts are permitted, keep the handout brief yet informative. A print-out copy of your slide presentation, 3 slides to a page, provides an adequate handout and resource for participants.

19. Should I list selected references?

Typically, a page of references is included in the handout. References may be included in your presentation by multiple methods. You can type a reference at the bottom of a specific slide, or create a final slide with selected references and include it in your handout but not as a part of your presentation.

20. Any tips on how to anticipate the unexpected?

Anything that is vital to your presentation should be available on your person. If you are using slides or a computer-generated presentation, bring your slides and/or computer disk with you. Carry your lecture notes with you along with a few of the key supporting articles for your review. Avoid packing any essential information or materials in your luggage.

21. How should I dress?

Choose an outfit that you "feel good" in. You want to look professional, yet you need to be comfortable and not distracted by clothing. Give careful consideration to comfortable shoes.

22. What if I feel disappointed when the presentation is over?

First, you did it! Celebrate your achievement. Usually the audience provides immediate and positive feedback in the form of questions and applause. However, not all presentations conclude with the audience seeking more information, and you may feel that your presentation was unsuccessful. Focus on the positive aspects of your presentation and critique elements that you will change for your next presentation. It is important to be objective about your presentation as well as celebrate your accomplishment.

BIBLIOGRAPHY

1. Fink R: Communicating research through podium presentation. In Fink R (ed): Professional Resources Practice Outcomes Research Manual. University of Colorado Hospital, Denver, CO, 2000.
2. Martin V: Making presentations. Nurs Times 96(20):43, 2000.
3. Adams Z: Presenting in style. Nurs Times 94(43):66–67, 1998.
4. Clark VB: The ABCs of highly effective presentations: A customer-centered approach. J Nurses Staff Develop 15(1):23–26, 1999.
5. Law LH: Preparing your presentation. Pract Midwife 4(2):40–42, 2001.
6. McConnell E: Giving an outstanding presentation. Am J Nurs 12:62–64, 1997.
7. Miracle VA, King KC: Presenting research: Effective paper presentations and impressive poster presentations. Appl Nurs Res 7(3):147–157, 1994.

29. POSTER PRESENTATION

Barbara Krumbach, MS, RN, CNS, CCRN

1. What is a poster?

A poster is a visual presentation of a project or research findings to communicate ideas to a selective audience. An effective poster requires thoughtful planning and development so that it can convey the idea of the project with or without the presence of the presenter to answer questions about the content.

2. Why would I want to consider doing a poster?

A poster is used to communicate research work, either completed or in progress. Posters are also used to present new ideas, policies, and procedures; to enhance staff and patient education; or to teach a new skill. Poster presentations are often an integral part of conferences and may be simple or complex. The overall goal is to get your message across to the audience for which it is intended. According to Bushy,[1] "a good poster cannot rescue a bad idea, but a poor one can easily sink the best idea as well as the viewer's impression of the author."

3. If I want to do a poster presentation, how do I get started?

Start by asking yourself, "What is the purpose of my poster? What do I want to convey, to whom and where?" Many conferences put out a call for abstracts, which may include posters as well as podium presentations. Conference planners give guidelines for the abstract submission. The goal of the abstract is to summarize the study, describe the purpose and methodology used, review data strategies and analysis, discuss project outcomes, and summarize implications for use in practice. The description is usually written in 250 words or less. The abstract is the starting point for the poster.

4. After I write the abstract and it is accepted for presentation, what do I do next?

The two major factors that you should consider are (1) the guidelines from the conference or organization accepting the poster and (2) your resources. Poster guidelines instruct you on when and where you will be presenting the poster, the audience for whom the conference is intended, size requirements, and display restrictions. You need this information before developing your poster.

Resource considerations include the amount of time you have to complete the poster, your budget, and who is available to assist you. Determining a timeline and a budget contributes to your success. Including others to critique your poster helps ensure that the content is easy to read and understand. Consider them part of your poster team, since what may seem clear to you may not appear so to the intended audience.

5. What resources are available to assist in creating a poster?

Look for educational support services in your institution. They can give you suggestions about material to use and identify the type and cost of available services. Check out art and supply stores for materials. Use computer programs such as PowerPoint, Excel, or Corel Draw to write the text, obtain images, and develop charts. Seek the expertise of clinical nurse specialists/educators, managers/directors, members of a research council, or peers who have experience developing a poster. Consider all of them part of your team.

6. What should be kept in mind in developing the content?

The hardest part of writing content for the poster is to keep it simple. There is a tendency to put everything about your project into the poster. People viewing the poster have limited time. When selecting the content, use the **KISS** principle: **keep it** simple and short. Display only the major ideas. You can add to the information when discussing the study at your poster session. The information should be eye-catching to attract the attention of the viewer and readable in 5 minutes or less.

7. What parts of the research project should be included?

You want to include the title, introduction/background, highlights, research question or hypothesis, research methodology, data analysis, findings/results, conclusions, and implications for practice. Use the abstract as a guide. Elicit feedback from your peers for clarity.

8. How is a poster displayed?

The poster project may be displayed on a tripod, a table, a special premade display board, or a larger display board supplied by the sponsoring conference/institution. You need to know what options are available before creating your poster.

9. What materials are used to make the poster?

Guidelines and space dictate how the information is displayed. Various materials are available for use in creating your poster. When choosing the type of materials, consider your budget and the guidelines obtained from the conference. If you are traveling, you will want to choose something that is easy to carry. A professional graphics department can display information on special paper. Although this may be expensive and takes time to produce, the poster can be rolled up for easy transport and attached to a display board with tack pins at the conference. Another method is to mount the material on several smaller boards. The boards can be fixed onto a larger display board with Velcro or pins. The following materials are commonly used to construct posters:

MATERIALS	COMMENTS
Poster board	Less sturdy Can be placed on a tripod Can be used to mount individual pieces of material
Matte board	Sturdy material Can be used to mount paper Can be cut into individual pieces and mounted on pre-cut board, a display board or a portable display.
Foam core	Very sturdy Comes as one piece or-pre-made to fold in sections Can be used to mount paper or matte board
Cardstock construction paper	Can be used to mount paper When mounting the content onto boards be sure there are no wrinkles and that it is mounted straight.

Always carry scissors, sprays or glue, Velcro or two sided tape to mount smaller units, a ruler, and some type of tacks or pins.

10. How should the material be arranged?

The arrangement should be carefully planned. Divide the display area into quadrants, and organize the content into a logical sequence. Place the introduction, abstract, and background in the left upper quadrant and the conclusions/implications for practice in the lower right quadrant. Place the rest of the materials in between so that they can be best read from left to right or top to bottom. Margins should always be aligned. Avoid handwritten or typewritten material; computer-generated text is the easiest to read. The following are key points to consider when constructing your poster:

Title
- Mount and center at the top of the poster.
- Needs to catch the eye of the viewer.
- Keep short (10–12 words and no more than 2 lines).
- Use bold print and readable font (Roman).
- Make letters 1–3 inches high.
- Black lettering on white background is easiest to read, but other dark colors may be used.
- Use upper- and lower-case letters.
- Should be visible from 20–25 feet.

Authors
- Place authors, credentials, institution/affiliate beneath title.
- Consider keeping credentials to a minimum if there are too many authors.
- Use bold print and upper- and lower-case letters.

Text
- Keep it simple.
- Use bullet points when possible.
- Use plain lettering; avoid italics.
- Place captions with each section.
- Double-space the material, if possible.
- Keep letters at $\frac{1}{2}$–1 inch high.
- Check for readability at 3–5 feet.

Graphics
- Balance with text.
- Use captions with charts.

Color
- Can enhance your poster.
- Do not overuse.
- Keep to 3–4 colors with two major ones.
- Use to enhance photos, contrast data in charts, bullet points, or use as background for text.
- Keep plenty of background or whitespace.

11. How do I know if I am conveying the information that I want to convey?

It is wise to have peers critique the mock-up of your poster as you prepare it, assessing the clarity, content, spelling, grammar, arrangement, use of color and graphics, and overall presentation. Revise the poster until you are satisfied that someone can read your poster in less than 5 minutes and is able to understand the information you want to convey.

12. How do I transport the poster?

It depends on how far you are going and the size of the poster. You definitely want to prevent it from being damaged. Large posters can be rolled up and placed in carrying tubes. Posters constructed in smaller pieces can be carried in a briefcase or a box. Protect the poster from being bent and from coming in contact with any type of fluid (e.g., moisture, drinking fluid). If flying to a conference, you should carry on the poster, if possible, so that you know it will arrive with you. You may also send it ahead by UPS to the facility, in care of the conference contact, or by special arrangement to the hotel where you will stay.

13. What should be considered when the poster is presented?

If you are attending a conference, start by reviewing the sponsor's instructions about when to set up and remove the poster and the times to be at your poster to answer questions. Arrive early so that you can familiarize yourself with the area and do not feel rushed in the set-up. It is wise to come prepared with extra supplies in case a touch-up is needed or the display area has changed. Dress comfortably, yet professionally. You may be standing for long periods. Be prepared to greet the participants with a smile. Allow them time to view your poster. Remember that the poster should speak for itself. Ask viewers if you can answer questions or if they want additional information. Thank them for stopping by. It is generally recommended to bring extra materials (i.e., copies of your abstract, the instruments you used, business cards, and pen and paper) so that participants can write their name, address, and the additional information that they want. Take time to view other posters; this is a great opportunity to network with your colleagues, add to your knowledge base, and learn from them. You have been successful in presenting your material. Be proud, compliment yourself, and enjoy it!

REFERENCES

1. Bushy A: A rating to evaluate research posters. Nurse Educ 16:11–15, 1991.

BIBLIOGRAPHY

1. Beyea SC, et al: Developing and presenting a poster presentation. AORN J 67:468–469, 1998.
2. Biancuzzo M: Developing a poster about a clinical innovation. Part I: Ideas and abstract. Clin Nurse Spec 8:153–155, 1994.
3. Biancuzzo M: Developing a poster about a clinical innovation. Part II: Creating the poster. Clin Nurse Spec 8:203–207, 1994.
4. Biancuzzo M: Developing a poster about a clinical innovation. Part III: Presentation and evaluation. Clin Nurse Spec 8:262–264, 1994.
5. Horn P, et al: A systematic evaluation of a poster presentation. J Contin Educ Nurs 24:232–233, 1991.
6. McCann SA, et al: The poster exhibit: Guidelines for planning, development, and presentation. Dermatol Nurs 11:373–379, 1999.
7. Moore L, et al: Insights on the poster preparation and presentation process. Appl Nurs Res 14:100–104, 2001.
8. Morin K: Poster presentations: Getting your point across. Matern Child Nurs 21:303–310, 1996.
9. Windle P: Celebrating successes through poster presentation. J Perianesthes Nurs 16:337–339, 2001.

INDEX

Entries in **boldface type** indicate complete chapters.